GENETIC
EPIDEMIOLOGY

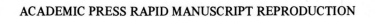
ACADEMIC PRESS RAPID MANUSCRIPT REPRODUCTION

GENETIC
EPIDEMIOLOGY

Edited by

NEWTON E. MORTON AND CHIN SIK CHUNG

University of Hawaii
Honolulu, Hawaii

ACADEMIC PRESS   New York   San Francisco   London   1978

A Subsidiary of Harcourt Brace Jovanovich, Publishers

ACADEMIC PRESS, INC.
111 Fifth Avenue, New York, New York 10003

United Kingdom Edition published by
ACADEMIC PRESS, INC. (LONDON) LTD.
24/28 Oval Road, London NW1 7DX

Library of Congress Cataloging in Publication Data

Main entry under title:

Genetic epidemiology.

Based on a symposium on various aspects of
human genetics held at the University of Hawaii,
October 17-18, 1977.
1. Medical genetics—Congresses. 2. Human genetics—
Congresses. I. Morton, Newton E.
II. Chung, Chin Sik, Date
RB155.G384   616'.042   78-18296
ISBN 0-12-508050-6

Contents

v

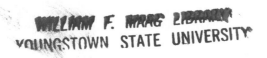

COMMON DISEASES

CONCLUSION

Participants

V. E. ANDERSON, University of Minnesota, Minneapolis, MN
G. C. ASHTON, University of Hawaii, Honolulu, HI
B. M. BENNETT, University of Hawaii, Honolulu, HI
C. L. CARTER, University of Hawaii, Honolulu, HI
L. L. CAVALLI-SFORZA, Stanford University, Stanford, CA
R. CHAKRABORTY, University of Texas at Houston, TX
B. CHAPPELL, University of Hawaii, Honolulu, HI
J. CHEN, University of Hawaii, Honolulu, HI
M. CHERN, University of Minnesota, Minneapolis, MN
C. S. CHUNG, University of Hawaii, Honolulu, HI
C. R. CLONINGER, The Jewish Hospital of St. Louis, MO
C. C. COCKERHAM, North Carolina State, Raleigh, NC
R. ELDRIDGE, National Institutes of Health, Bethesda, MD
R. C. ELSTON, University of North Carolina, Chapel Hill, NC
I. EMANUEL, University of Washington, CDMRC, Seattle, WA
G. R. FRASER, Department of Health and Welfare, Ottawa, Ontario,
    Canada
A. S. GOLDBERGER, University of Wisconsin, Madison, WI
B. D. HALL, University of California-San Francisco, CA
J. HANKIN, University of Hawaii, Honolulu, HI
E. B. HOOK, New York State Birth Defects Institute, Albany, NY
Z. D. HRUBEC, National Research Council, Washington, DC
Y. E. HSIA, University of Hawaii, Honolulu, HI
J. A. HUNT, University of Hawaii, Honolulu, HI
J. F. JACKSON, University of Mississippi, Jackson, MS
P. A. JACOBS, University of Hawaii, Honolulu, HI
R. C. JOHNSON, University of Hawaii, Honolulu, HI
K. W. KANG, Indiana University Medical Center, Indianapolis, IN
B. J. B. KEATS, University of Hawaii, Honolulu, HI
K. K. KIDD, Yale University School of Medicine, New Haven, CT
H. N. KIRKMAN, University of North Carolina, Chapel Hill, NC
A. G. KNUDSON, The Institute for Cancer Research, Philadelphia, PA
D. KOLAKOWSKI, University of Connecticut, CT
L. KOLONEL, University of Hawaii, Honolulu, HI
J. M. LALOUEL, University of Hawaii, Honolulu, HI
K. LANGE, University of California, Los Angeles, CA

C. C. LI, University of Pittsburgh, Pittsburgh, PA
B. MacMAHON, Harvard University, Boston, MA
R. C. MARVIT, University of Hawaii, Honolulu, HI
S. MATTHYSSE, Mailman Research Center, Belmont, MA
D. McLAUGHLIN, State of Hawaii Department of Health, Honolulu, HI
A. MEADOWS, The Institute for Cancer Research, Philadelphia, PA
P. MOLL, University of Michigan, Ann Arbor, MI
N. E. MORTON, University of Hawaii, Honolulu, HI
A. G. MOTULSKY, University of Washington, Seattle, WA
J. J. MULVIHILL, National Cancer Institute, Bethesda, MD
N. C. MYRIANTHOPOULOS, National Institute of Neurological and
    Communicative Disorders and Stroke, Bethesda, MD
W. E. NANCE, Medical College of Virginia, Richmond, VA
J. OTT, University of Washington, Seattle, WA
C. B. PARK, University of Hawaii, Honolulu, HI
D. R. PETERSON, University of Washington, Seattle, WA
M. PIETRUSEWSKY, University of Hawaii, Honolulu, HI
D. C. RAO, University of Hawaii, Honolulu, HI
T. E. REED, University of Toronto, Ontario, Canada
G. C. RHOADS, University of Hawaii, Honolulu, HI
T. REICH, Washington University, St. Louis, MO
D. REMONDINI, National Institutes of Health, Bethesda, MD
J. I. ROTTER, Harbor General Hospital Campus, Torrance, CA
B. SANDERS, University of Hawaii, Honolulu, HI
R. M. SIERVOGEL, The Fels Research Institute, Yellow Springs, OH
C. F. SING, The University of Michigan, Ann Arbor, MI
M. SKOLNICK, Latter-Day Saints Hospital, Salt Lake City, UT
M. A. SPENCE, University of California, Los Angeles, CA
Z. STEIN, Columbia University, New York, NY
M. SUSSER, Columbia University, New York, NY
P. VAN DE VERG, University of Hawaii, Honolulu, HI
D. K. WAGENER, University of Pittsburgh, Pittsburgh, PA
R. WARD, University of Washington, CDMRC, Seattle, WA
C. WHITE, Yale University, New Haven, CT
W. WILLIAMS, University of Hawaii, Honolulu, HI
P. WORKMAN, University of New Mexico, Albuquerque, NM
S. WRIGHT, University of Wisconsin, Madison, WI
H. ZOCHLINSKI, University of Hawaii, Honolulu, HI

Preface

Genetic epidemiology is concerned with etiology, distribution, and control of disease in relatives and with inherited causes of disease in populations. *Inherited* is used here in a broad sense to include both biological and cultural inheritance. The set of *relatives* may be as close as twins or as extended as an ethnic group. *Cultural* subsumes any environmental factor distributed nonrandomly among families, whether social, behavioral, nutritional, or other. Behavior genetics and anthropological genetics, to the extent that they deal with traits of biomedical significance, are part of genetic epidemiology, which is differentiated from evolutionary genetics by preoccupation with contemporary health-related problems, and from biometrical genetics by absence of controlled matings or selection programs and by inclusion of major loci, chromosomal aberrations, and cultural inheritance.

Inbreeding and outcrossing effects, group comparisons, and population surveillance are aspects of genetic epidemiology, but the central problem is to unravel the causes of family resemblance. An inference must satisfy both epidemiological and genetic criteria of validity, with no bias for or against genetic hypotheses. It must reflect the contemporary state of molecular genetics, without assurance that genes characterizable in molecular terms by current techniques play a major role in any particular disease. Therefore statistical approaches should not be rejected on philosophical grounds: The best analysis at a given state of the art is informative and potentially useful.

Genetic epidemiology is a challenge not only to the ingenuity of its practitioners, but to the rigidity of social theory. We remember our predecessors in Nazi Germany who succumbed to racism, and the martyrs of the Soviet Union who lost liberty and life to mindless environmentalism. We cannot forget that today in the United States a group called Science for the People enjoys much ignorant support for its attacks on human and experimental biology. Their influence extends to professional journals, congresses, and grant review groups.

At a time when antiscientism makes such headway, we who represent the rationalist tradition in those societies where it is nominally tolerated and fitfully encouraged have a precious opportunity to participate in the development of a new science at the interface between genetics and epidemiology. Although little represented in peer review groups and editorial boards, genetic epidemiology already accounts for about one-fourth of papers published in human genetics journals and presented at related congresses. We are divided by differences in language and methodology, but united in the conviction that any hypothesis may be entertained providing it can be tested, and that no untested hypothesis should be accepted.

At this initial stage it is difficult to steer a middle course between methodological preoccupation and neglect. Some readers will consider that we have not given enough attention to methodological variants, while others will regret that problems common to genetics and epidemiology are sometimes obscured by technical details. We hope that references will be helpful to the ravenous, and discussions to the fastidious.

Union of genetics and epidemiology is impeded by conservatism of research support and graduate training. If genetics were to neglect diseases of complex inheritance, or if epidemiology were to ignore familial aggregation of disease, genetic epidemiology would develop not through collaboration of two disciplines, but unilaterally from one. Science and health would be the losers. This workshop will have served its purpose if, by furthering the synthesis of genetics and epidemiology, it contributes to understanding and eventual control of the major diseases and causes of death.

We are grateful to the National Science Foundation, the National Institutes of Health, and the University of Hawaii for support of the conference.

NEWTON E. MORTON
CHIN SIK CHUNG

INTRODUCTION

Two founders present the epidemiologic and genetic background. Brian MacMahon discusses environmental and genetic aspects of family resemblance as a special case of space-time clustering. Sewall Wright gives the early history of path analysis, which Haldane considered "may replace our old notions of causation" (Perspect. Biol. Med. 7:353, 1964). The confluence of these two streams is the beginning of genetic epidemiology.

GENETIC EPIDEMIOLOGY

EPIDEMIOLOGIC APPROACHES TO FAMILY RESEMBLANCE

Brian MacMahon

Walcott Professor of Epidemiology
Harvard School of Public Health
Boston, Massachusetts

I understand this conference to be an attempt to describe
the middle ground between human genetics and epidemiology.
Before looking for a middle ground, it seems appropriate to
define the points between which it may be expected to lie. I
prefer to define both epidemiology and human genetics in terms
of their substance - the knowledge which their practitioners
endeavor to assemble - rather than of their methods. The
common ground of this substance is knowledge of the effects of
the environment, broadly defined, on mankind. The primary
characteristic distinguishing genetics and epidemiology is the
time at which the relevant species-environment interaction
took place. When investigating the origins of a characteristic
of an individual human the geneticist seeks determinants which
are now largely intrinsic to the species - the results of all
the diverse environments that have existed since its origin
(or origins) - and for results of those interactions that have
been transmitted to the individual by a specific mechanism.
The epidemiologist, on the other hand, searches for events
that have occurred and circumstances that have existed during
the lifetime of the individual or individuals whose characteristics are of interest. Having made the point that genes have
environmental origins, I will, in the remainder of this paper
use the word environment to refer only to those environments
that have existed during the life of the individual of

interest. This dual terminology is unfortunate but necessitated by the fact that I know of no term that describes the
sum of the environments experienced by a species during its
existence.

There can be no question that there is a large middle
ground between these two disciplines. It has been the scientific hunting ground of many giants of human biology, past and
present. Whether it is usefully considered a separate field
or discipline I do not know; I certainly can see no clear
separation between it and either epidemiology or genetics.
Indeed, the methods employed by practitioners of subspecialties of the two fields (e.g. population genetics and statistical epidemiology or clinical genetics and clinical
epidemiology) are often much more similar than are those of
the subspecialties within either field.

I thought I might attempt to outline some components of
this middle ground by taking a central theme of genetic work
and asking how it relates to epidemiologic investigation.
Family resemblance is that theme. Family resemblance is to
the geneticist what time-place clustering is to the
epidemiologist - it is not the whole story, but if it is not
present there is a strong temptation to look for work elsewhere. Parenthetically, the vagueness of disciplinary borders
becomes immediately apparent in thinking of family resemblance
and time-place clustering, for family resemblance is no more
than time-place clustering with measurement units somewhat
different from those to which the epidemiologist is accustomed.

I propose to indicate some ways in which family resemblance has been, or could be, used to identify environmental
causes of human characteristics, particularly human diseases.
I should emphasize that I am concerned with ways to utilize
the patterns of family resemblance themselves, not the
epidemiologic study of traits or diseases that show family
resemblance. For example, it has been common in diseases
which evidence recurrence in sibships to study the patterns of
risk by birth order and parental age. Not a great deal has
come of such studies to date, in spite of the compilation of
a great deal of information, but nevertheless these are
logical variables to study and the practical import of the
information that has been assembled on them may one day become
apparent. However, associations with birth order or maternal
age are not intrinsically related to the fact of sibship recurrence, and it makes as much sense to study them in diseases
that do not recur in sibships as in those that do. I therefore do not plan to discuss variables of this nature.

I will consider the major patterns of family resemblance
individually.

I.   RECURRENCE IN SIBLINGS

     Every disease of which I can conceive - and for that
matter every human trait - either has been shown to occur more
frequently in the siblings of affected individuals than in the
population at large or can, on theoretical grounds, be
expected to show this feature if sufficient and appropriate
data were collected. Both shared environment and common genes
contribute to this sibship clustering. If the probability of
recurrence in sibships corresponds to that expected of a trait
determined by a single, fully penetrant, major gene, the
inference is strong that the sibship clustering is in fact
genetically determined, since the likelihood that an environmental cause would fit such a prediction precisely is small.
However, to show that the pattern does not fit any such
prediction is insufficient evidence on which to conclude that
the sibling resemblance is environmentally determined - the
geneticist has a large armamentarium of penetrance, expressiv-
ity, polygenes and other Acts of God to counter that play.
What features of sibship clustering might, then, an epidemiologist examine for evidence that the clustering is due to
shared environment rather than shared genes?
     Thoreau wrote: "Time is the stream in which I go a-
fishing". In this statement he went to the heart of a substantial component of epidemiologic methodology. A question
that an epidemiologist will ask early in his investigation of
a disease showing sibling clustering is whether there is
clustering of risk with respect to time within affected
sibships. Several approaches to this question have been
suggested:
     1. One can simply compute the time interval between
onset or diagnosis of disease in affected siblings. In
congenital defects the appropriate interval would be the
interval between births of affected individuals. In the acute
infectious diseases of childhood, useful information has been
obtained by computing secondary attack rates in siblings,
limiting observations to some interval - usually corresponding
to the known range of incubation periods of the disease in
question - following the introduction of the first case into
the sibship. However, evaluation of lower recurrence rates
than are commonly seen in such diseases requires some basis
for comparison. One possible approach is to compare the
interval between affected sibs with the interval between all
possible pairs of siblings in the same sibships, excluding the
affected pair. I know of only one instance where this
technique has been used - a study of Hodgkin's disease in
siblings by Grufferman et al. (1).
     2. All siblings of affected individuals - in singly as

well as multiply affected sibships - can be characterized with respect to interval between their birth and that of the affected proband, and recurrence rates estimated according to that interval. In a study of neural tube defects, Yen and I saw suggestive, though not statistically significant, evidence of higher recurrence rates among sibs born close in time to the propositus (2). I am not aware that such a pattern has been sought in the other large bodies of data existent on these defects, or for that matter on other congenital malformations for which recurrence in sibships has been demonstrated.

3. Differences in secular time of onset of disease may be compared with differences in age at onset within sibships. If risk within a sibship were distributed uniformly with respect to time, then on average the cases within a sibship would be expected to have a similar age at onset - given that the disease is age-related, as all diseases are. A temporal clustering of risk within a sibship will tend to lengthen the difference between siblings in age at onset of disease, since not all siblings will be at their peak risk with respect to age during the temporal high risk period. This method has been applied to Hodgkin's disease and multiple sclerosis - both chronic diseases with a 7 to 8 fold increase in risk to siblings of affected individuals. Shapira et al. noted that there was little difference between members of affected sib-pairs in year of onset (1.4 years) but a larger difference (4.7 years) in age at onset (3). A similar phenomenon has been reported in two studies of familial Hodgkin's disease (4,5). Superficially, it would seem that a lower mean difference in time of onset than in age of onset of sibship cases would be suggestive of temporal clustering, and therefore of environmental determination. However, the examination is often confounded by methodologic problems, including truncation of the observation period. These problems have been discussed by Mantel and Blot (6,7). The problems discussed by Mantel and Blot relate to the constraints on the method imposed by specific study designs or data sets and not to the utility of the method in concept.

4. An analysis may be undertaken of the contiguity of affected siblings, irrespective of time lapsed between births. For example, there is some evidence that the pregnancies immediately before or after the birth of a child with neural tube defect are more likely to miscarry than are others in the same sibship (8). If birth order of all siblings of a series of affected individuals is known, then recurrence rates can be computed by ranked distance from the proband. If, as is sometimes the case, birth order is known only for the sibships with multiple cases, the method of all possible pairs may again be invoked (1).

All the above are methods for identifying temporal

clustering in sibships. If such is found it is evidence that the sibship recurrence originates in environmental rather than genetic similarities. None of these methods has been exploited to anything like the extent that it deserves and none has achieved an appropriate status as a routine component of the evaluation of observed clustering in sibships.

There are other characteristics of sibship recurrence that intrigue the epidemiologist. In a disease that shows no overall predominance of one or the other sex, a genetic analysis of sibship recurrence - or for that matter an epidemiologic one - will frequently treat male and female siblings without discrimination. In the study of Hodgkin's disease already referred to, it was noted that siblings of the same sex as the affected proband had a risk of Hodgkin's disease double that of siblings of the opposite sex (1). The observation needs confirmation, but if confirmed would be rather strongly suggestive that an environment shared more closely by siblings of the same sex than by sex-discordant siblings was responsible for the pattern of sibship recurrence.

Although difficult to ascertain and study in adequate numbers, half-siblings would seem to have special value for research in the area with which we are concerned in these two days. They sample the gene pool of only one parent of a proband; some share his family environment, others do not. In a study of 98 half-siblings of 41 alcoholic probands, Schuckit found the likelihood of alcoholism to be related to the commonality of an alcoholic parent, regardless of whether the half-sib shared the familial environment of the proband (9). Criteria and ascertainment in the field of alcoholism are, to say the least, difficult and the numbers in this study are too small for definitive conclusions. However, the study illustrates a method which should receive broader application.

II. OCCURRENCE IN TWINS

The geneticists here will be amused by the recency of the epidemiologist's discovery of twins. Of course, we have known they exist; we have even had some curiosity as to how they come about; but as a vehicle for the study of disease etiology we have been content to leave them to the geneticist, more or less.

However, some intriguing individual patterns of twin association that lie outside the mainstream of genetic interest have caught the epidemiologist's attention. After clarification of some confusion over the expected prevalence of twins in a series of individuals with a given trait - a clarification

consequent to the realization that a successful twin gestation
produces two, not one, twin individuals, an interest in twinning per se as a risk factor for disease remains. So far,
little has developed, but it would seem wise to pursue this
line, particularly in the context of prenatally-determined
interference with fetal growth and postnatal psycho-social
influences.

The extremely low concordance rate for neural tube defects
among twins - seemingly lower than that among non-twin
siblings - presents a problem whether one is thinking in
environmental or genetic terms (2). Recent data from New York
State suggest that this low concordance rate may not prevail
in that area (10), but these data are so much at variance with
extensive data from other areas that one is reluctant to
generalize from them before confirmation in other studies.
Similarly, apparent lack of difference between concordance
rates for monozygous and dizgous twins is a feature that
prompts epidemiologic attention.

Apart from these individual curiosities, an important
potential for the use of twins in epidemiologic research has
been illustrated in recent studies of coronary artery and
respiratory disease among twins in Swedish, Danish and American
twin registries. In these studies, investigation has focussed
not on twins who are concordant but on monozygous twins who
are discordant with respect to some suspected environmental
cause of disease - in this case, cigarette smoking. Of
particular importance have been the observations of lack of
difference in cardiovascular symptomatology or mortality
between monozygous twins who are discordant for cigarette-
smoking practice, leading to the inference that the association
of cardiovascular disease with smoking among non-twins may be
the consequence of indirect genetic determinants rather than a
direct causal relationship (11-14). The respiratory
symptomatology was found to be different between monozygous
twins discordant for smoking (11,13). This would appear to
be a powerful methodology for investigating the effects of
environmental agents that occur with some frequency in the
population. The limitation of such studies to relatively
frequent exposures is necessitated by the requirement to have
reasonable numbers both of discordant and of concordant
monozygous twins. The difficulty of assemblying reasonable
numbers of such twins is also likely to limit its application
to the most common of human diseases and traits. In addition,
Friedman has noted the importance of correct classification
of twins with regard to exposure (15). Relatively low rates
of misclassification of individual twins can lead to high
rates of misclassification of twin sets. One must be cautious
in drawing negative conclusions from apparently discordant
twin sets since a high proportion of such sets may in fact be
concordant.

III. ILLNESS IN PARENT AND CHILD

Some of the features described in the context of sib-sib
resemblance may also be examined when a disease is found to
affect parent and child. For example, many of the reported
cases of Hodgkin's disease in parent and child involve cases
with onset within relatively short periods of time (4). This
feature is even more striking in parent-child combinations than
in sib-sib pairs, since in the former the result is frequently
a pair of cases with a 20 to 25 year difference in age at
onset. On the other hand, the numbers of reported parent-child
sets is quite small, and there is considerable room for
ascertainment bias, since a set in which the disease occurs
in both members within a short time is presumably more likely
to come to attention than one in which 20 to 25 years separates
the onset of disease in the two members.

Unusual sex combinations are also of interest. Some years
ago, McKeown and I noted that the pattern of parent-child
combinations in pyloric stenosis indicated that the risk to
the child of an affected mother was four times that of the
child of an affected father (16). This seemed to us at the
time inconsistent with a genetic origin of the increased risk
experienced by the children of affected parents. Subsequently,
an ingenious model of polygenic inheritance was proposed in
which an affected mother, because she is female and therefore
intrinsically less susceptible, must carry a heavier burden
of the predisposing genes to manifest the disease and therefore
transmits a heavier load to her offspring (17). The model,
despite its ingenuity, still seems contrived, and a less
attractive explanation than the existence of an environmental
risk factor closely associated with the mother.

A major opportunity for studying environmental causes of
parent-child clustering is provided by adopted children raised
by non-related parents. Like half-siblings, such children are
relatively few in number and their study involves many social,
ethical and legal difficulties. The difficulties can be
overcome. Goodwin et al. compared the frequency of alcoholic
and other psychiatric problems in a group of 55 men who had
been separated from their biological parents early in life,
and at least one of whose parents was alcoholic, with that in
a matched group of adoptees without a history of alcoholism
in the parents (18). Substantially more of the children of
alcoholic parents had alcohol problems, as measured by such
objective criteria as morning drinking, delirium tremens and

arrests, hospitalization and treatment for drinking problems.
Other forms of psychopathology, such as depression and
character disorder, did not differ between the two groups.
Interestingly, the alcohol consumption levels did not appear
to be increased in the proband group - only the frequency with
which that consumption led to trouble. As with the study of
alcoholism in half siblings already referred to, the results
of this study may not be entirely to the epidemiologist's
liking - since it points to genetic determination of the
disease under study. The investigation illustrates, however,
a technique that should receive more attention from practitioners of both disciplines.

IV.   OTHER FAMILY PATTERNS

     The use of family patterns other than those described
above for epidemiologic inferences has been episodic and
largely anecdotal. The fact that the tendency to carcinoma
of the breast is inherited as much through the paternal as
through the maternal line has suggested that if a vertically
transmissible factor is involved it is not likely to be
transmitted via the milk, as it is in mice (19). Instances
of temporal clustering of cases of Hodgkin's disease in
relatives other than sib-sib or parent-child have been
reported.
     Apart from an early study of mortality in spouses reported
by Ciocco (20), studies of conjugal disease have also largely
been anecdotal. However, a study by Segall showed a substantial increase in mortality from stomach cancer among spouses
of probands who died of the same disease, particularly when
the first to die was the husband (21). Further data on
conjugal mortality and morbidity would be extremely valuable
both in testing existing hypotheses and in formulating new
ones. Apart from disease due to manifest infections, however,
conjugal disease is generally sufficiently rare to necessitate
the collaboration of multiple large data sources to provide
adequate numbers.
     In this presentation I have considered only one of the
geneticist's primary areas of interest - family resemblance.
My main objective has been to describe how relevant to the
epidemiologist's goal is one pattern of disease occurrence
commonly considered the prerogative of the geneticist. I
believe the same objective could have been accomplished by
consideration of other areas of endeavor in human genetics -
tribal or ethnic resemblance, consanguinity, linkage, and so on.
I hope that some day I might be invited back to Honolulu to

document that belief.

V.   REFERENCES

1.   Grufferman, S., Cole, P., Smith, P.G., Lukes, R.J.,
     New Engl. J. Med. 296, 248-250 (1977).
2.   Yen, S., MacMahon, B., Lancet ii, 623-626 (1968).
3.   Schapira, K., Poskanzer, D.C., Miller, H., Brain 86, 315-
     332 (1963).
4.   MacMahon, B., Cancer Res. 26, 1189-1200 (1966).
5.   Vianna, N.J., Davies, J.N.P., Polan, A. et al., Lancet
     ii, 854-857 (1974).
6.   Mantel, N., Blot, W.J., J. Natl. Cancer Inst. 56, 413-
     414 (1976).
7.   Mantel, N., Blot, W.J., J. Natl. Cancer Inst. 58, 10-11
     (1977).
8.   Clarke, C., Hobson, D., McKendricks, O.M. et al., Brit.
     Med. J. ii, 743-746 (1975).
9.   Schuckit, M.A., Goodwin, D.W., Winokur, G., Am. J. Psychi-
     atry 128, 122-126 (1972).
10. Janerich, D.T., Piper, J., J. Med. Genet. in press.
11. Cederlof, R., Friberg, L., Jonsson, E. et al., Arch.
     Environ. Health 13, 726-737 (1966).
12. Hauge, M., Harvald, B., Reid, D.D., Acta Genet. Med.
     Gemellol. 19, 335-336 (1970).
13. Cederlof, R., Friberg, L., Hrubec, Z., Arch. Environ.
     Health 18, (1969).
14. Friberg, L. Cederlof, R., Lorich, U. et al., Arch.
     Environ. Health 27, 294-304 (1973).
15. Friedman, G.D., Amer. J. Epidemiol. 105, 291-295 (1977).
16. McKeown, T., MacMahon, B., Arch. Dis. Childh. 30, 497-500
     (1955).
17. Carter, C.O., In Second International Conference on
     Congenital Malformations, pp. 306-316. International
     Medical Congress, Ltd., New York, 1963.
18. Goodwin, D.W., Schulsinger, F., Hermansen, L. et al.,
     Arch. Gen. Psychiatry 28, 238-243 (1973).
19. Fraumeni, J.F. Jr., Miller, R.W., Lancet 2, 1196-1197
     (1971).
20. Ciocco, A., Human Biol. 12, 508-531 (1940).
21. Segall, A.J., Personal communication.

THE APPLICATION OF PATH ANALYSIS TO ETIOLOGY

Sewall Wright

University of Wisconsin
Madison, Wisconsin

This paper begins with the origin of path analysis in
an attempt at etiological interpretation of a matrix of correlations among bone measurements from a rabbit population
(Wright, 1918), a study of heritability of variations of the
piebald pattern of guinea pigs (Wright, 1920) and a first
general account (Wright, 1921). This is followed by derivation of the basic formula. Four very different applications
of this formula are discussed: (1) to the calculation of the
correlation between linear functions (mathematical rather
than etiological), (2) to statistical estimation (in which it
becomes identical with multiple regression), (3) to representation of a correlation matrix in a pattern on the surface of
a hypersphere (in which it becomes identical with factor analysis), (4) to the etiological interpretation of a correlation
matrix (the original purpose).

The first is the one that has been used the most (in
deriving the theoretical genetic consequences of patterns of
inbreeding, assortative mating and population structures in
general). This is not discussed here as not etiological.
The second needs no discussion. The relation of path analysis
to factor analysis has required more discussion. Several very
diverse illustrations are given of the fourth application,
that to etiological interpretation.

ANALYSIS OF MEASUREMENTS OF RABBIT BONES

I developed path analysis while a graduate student in Zoology at Harvard, 1912-15, specializing in genetics under the supervision of Prof. W. E. Castle. Knowledge of statistical methods among biologists was very limited in America at that time, consisting largely of a few descriptive statistics: mean, standard deviation, correlation coefficient and their probable errors. Castle was among those who had made considerable use of these, especially in his studies of artificial selection. He had gotten into a controversy on the nature of the genetic difference between large and small breeds of rabbits. In connection with this and to give us training, he set his graduate students, Harold Fish and myself, to the task of calculating all of the correlations among five bone measurements in a population of rabbits, obtained by a previous student, E. C. MacDowell. These were the length (OM) and breadth (ZP) of the skull and the lengths of humerus (H), femur (F) and tibia (T). He published the results (Castle, 1914), noting that the high correlations (.658 to .857) supported his thesis that genetic differences in size had to do largely with general size rather than with sizes of separate parts.

I became interested in the nature of the residual factors. At that time, Raymond Pearl was promoting Pearson's coefficient of partial correlation as a somewhat magical device for disentangling causal relations. The formula,

$$r_{XY \cdot A} = (r_{XY} - r_{XA} r_{YA}) / \sqrt{(1 - r^2_{XA})(1 - r^2_{YA})}$$ gives an

estimate of the correlation between two variables, X and Y, expected with any given value of another, A. By repetition, estimates can be made for constancy of more than one variable. I calculated all of the possible partial correlations. Table 1 shows the ten total correlations and the ten with constancy of the three measurements other than the pair in question. Only three of the latter were greater than 0.23. These suggested the existence of factors for size of the skull as a whole, sizes of the hind legs as wholes and sizes of homologous bones of fore and hind legs.

A method of evaluating the relative importance of these and of the factors determining general size and of ones affecting the measurements separately was needed. I was familiar with the formula for the squared standard deviation of a sum

$$\sigma^2_{(A + B)} = \sigma^2_A + \sigma^2_B + 2\sigma_A \sigma_B r_{AB}$$

TABLE 1

Correlations among five bone measurements, made by
E. C. MacDowell from a population of 370 to 380 rabbits,
and their probable errors, and the partial correlations
for each pair with all of the other three constant. The
measurements were the skull length, OM (occipital to
maxilla), skull breadth, ZP (zygomatic arch, posterior),
and lengths of humerus, H, femur, F, and tibia, T.
(Wright, 1918)

Measures (AB)	r_{XY} PE	$r_{XY \cdot ABC}$
OM - ZP	.750 ± .015	.448
- H	.743 ± .016	.172
- F	.760 ± .015	.224
- T	.701 ± .018	.022
ZP - H	.675 ± .019	.119
- F	.674 ± .019	.004
- T	.658 ± .020	.136
H - F	.857 ± .009	.463
- T	.791 ± .013	.161
F - T	.858 ± .009	.517

It appeared that the ratio of the squared standard deviation of
a given factor effect to the total gave the most appropriate
measure of the degree of determination by that factor. There
would be correlational terms, possibly negative, from correlated factors but these would not occur in the case of independent factors. I found that the correlation between any
pair of the factors was given by a simple formula. Letting
a, b, c, etc. be the degrees of determination of variable x
by a number of factors and a', b', c', etc. those of variable
Y by these factors

$$r_{XY} = \pm \sqrt{aa'} \pm \sqrt{bb'} \pm \sqrt{cc'} \quad \cdots$$

Where a given cause produces effects in the same direction,
the sign of the term is +; where the effects are in opposite
directions, the sign is -.

I arrived at the estimates of degrees of determination given in Table 2 by a rather crude method of averaging the estimates from different ratios of correlations, and got around to writing it up for publication a couple of years later, after settling into a position in the Animal Husbandry Division of the U.S. Bureau of Animal Industry that I had accepted after graduation.

TABLE 2

Estimations of degrees of determination of
five bone measurements from a population of rabbits
by postulated factors. (Wright, 1918)

Variable	General size	Skull	Legs	Hind Legs	Proximal leg bones	Special	Total
OM	.746	.077				.177	1.000
ZP	.620	.065				.315	1.000
H	.739		.083		.030	.148	1.000
F	.755		.085	.064	.030	.066	1.000
T	.680		.076	.058		.186	1.000

I became convinced by this study that the pattern of causal relations among variables cannot be extracted automatically from the array of correlation coefficients by means of partial correlations or any other set program, although such procedures might yield useful suggestions. Tentative patterns must come from consideration of everything that bears on the matter, including spatial and temporal relations and experiments as well as the correlations. If it is reasonable to suppose that variable A is causally related to both variables X and Y and $r_{XY \cdot A} = 0$, it is strongly suggested that A is the only common factor, and similarly if it is reasonable to suppose that A is an intermediary in the chain $X \to A \to Y$. It is, however, quite possible that X, A, and Y are connected by a complex of common factors such that $r_{XY \cdot A}$ may be zero or nearly so without any simple explanation. Useful interpretation depends on bringing together all available evidence and is likely to remain tentative even if this is done.

HERITABILITY OF WHITE SPOTTING IN GUINEA PIGS

The term path coefficent was first used in a paper published in 1920 on "The relative importance of heredity and
environment in determining the piebald pattern of guinea
pigs." I had come to realize that the square root of the coefficient of determination used in 1918, is a more convenient parameter than the latter. It was defined here as
follows:

> "The path coefficient, measuring the importance of
> a given path of influence from cause to effect,
> is defined as the ratio of the variability of the
> effect to be found when all causes are constant
> except the one in question, the variability of
> which is kept unchanged, to the total variability.
> Variability is measured by the standard deviation."

This implies that if the standard deviation of the
effect actually is reduced by constancy of the other factors
because of correlation, the total standard deviation must be
scaled down proportionately, in order to obtain the path coefficient.

In this case there was no question about the nature of
the primary etiologic factors, heredity and environment.
Secondarily, heredity could be divided in principle into an
additive component, dominance deviations, and deviations due
to interactions among loci. In the case of the piebald
pattern the results of crosses among inbred strains with
widely different mean grades gave no clear indication of any
sort of nonadditive effect and only additive heredity was
assumed in this paper. No genotype-environment correlation
was to be expected in the laboratory strains. The environmental factor was most conveniently divided into that common
to littermates, and that peculiar to individuals. The former
would seem to include practically all tangible aspects but
analysis showed that the latter was overwhelmingly the more
important. This was, indeed, obvious from the first because
of the variability from one extreme to the other in strains
tracing to a single mating, after many generations of brother-
sister mating had eliminated practically all genetic variability. The only tangible environmental factor found was the age
of the mother.

Figure 1 shows the path diagram that was used in the
analysis of the random-bred stock. The phenotypes of two
offspring O and O' and the sire and dam are each represented as determined by heredity (H), common environment of

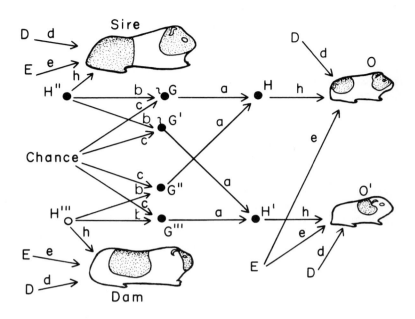

Figure 1. Path diagram illustrating the causal relations
           between litter mates (O, O') and between each
           of them and their parents. H, H', H'' and H'''
           represent the genetic constitutions of the four
           individuals, G, G', G'', and G''' that of four
           germ cells. E represents such environmental
           factors as are common to littermates. D repre-
           sents other factors, largely ontogenetic
           irregularity. The small letters stand for the
           various path coefficients. "Chance" should not
           be treated as a common factor of the G's (Wright,
           1920, fig. 5).

littermates (E) and accidents of development (D). The values
of the coefficients for the paths from parental genotype to
gamete and from gamete to offspring genotype are easily derived under the assumption of diploid autosomal heredity,

$b = \sqrt{1/2}$, $a = \sqrt{1/2}$. I had been able to demonstrate that
any correlation in such a diagram is equal to the sum of
contributions from all connecting paths in which the arrows
trace back from one to the other variable or to a common
factor and that these contributions are equal to the product

of the coefficients, one perhaps a correlation coefficient, along the path. Thus r_{OP} = habh $\leftarrow$ $(1/2)h^2$, and $r_{OO'}$ = $2 h^2 a^2 b^2 + e^2 = (1/2)h^2 + e^2$. The values of the two unknown path coefficients, h and e, could thus be calculated at once from the two equations, and d from the equation, $h^2 + e^2 + d^2 = 1$.

With more extensive data (3881 OP entries, 2080 OO' entries from the random-bred stock) it became apparent that heritability is about twice as great in males as in females (and variability also greater), making it necessary to make separate analyses for the sexes (Wright, 1977, Chapter 4). I will not go into more detail on the analysis here but merely give the most recent apportionment of degrees of determination in terms of percentage and of actual variance on the transformed scale that was necessary because of damping near each extreme (Table 3).

TABLE 3

Estimated degrees of determination and variance
components with respect to piebald spotting
in guinea pigs of a random-bred stock, B
(by sex) and inbred strain no. 35. Somewhat less than half of the variance common
to litter mates is due to age of the dam.
(Wright, 1977, Chapter 4)

	Random-bred (B)				Inbred (35)	
	♂(%)	♀(%)	Av.(%)	σ^2	%	σ^2
Genetic						
Additive	50	25	38	0.219	0	0
Dominance	4	2	3	0.014	0	0
Sex	–	–	2	0.011	3	0.010
Nongenetic						
Common to litter mates	9	9	9	0.049	10	0.036
Accidental	37	64	48	0.280	87	0.294
Total	100	100	100	0.573	100	0.340

An interesting check is provided by comparison of the analysis of the random-bred stock, B, and of inbred stock, 35 (numbers nearly the same) which traced to a single mating in the 12th generation of sib mating. The nongenetic components are essentially the same.

FIRST GENERAL PRESENTATION OF A PATH ANALYSIS

The first general presentation of the method was in 1921. The purpose of the method was stated as follows. A sentence often overlooked is here italicized.

"The present paper is an attempt to present a
method of measuring the direct influence along
each separate path in such a system and thus
of finding the degree to which variation of a
given effect is determined by each particular
cause. *The method depends on the combination
of knowledge of the degrees of correlation
among the variables in a system, with such
knowledge as may be possessed of the causal
relations.* In such cases in which the causal
relations are uncertain, the method can be
used to find the logical consequences of any
particular hypothesis in regard to them."

Several new examples of the method were presented.

I learned of Pearson's method of multiple regression in time for inclusion as a related method but not in time to recognize that the demonstration of the basic equation of path analysis could be derived much more simply by considering a path coefficient as a standardized partial regression coefficient (but often with respect to a hypothetical variable) than as the ratio of the standard deviation of the dependent variable, expected from the direct effect of the given factor, to its total standard deviation.

THE GENERAL FORMULA OF PATH ANALYSIS

Assume that V_O (Figure 2) is <u>completely</u> determined as a linear function of a number of variables (known and unknown) with coefficients c_{oi} for each V_i including an unknown independent residual factor, V_u, if necessary.

$$V_o = c_o + c_{o1} V_1 + c_{o2} V_2 + \cdots + c_{om} V_m + c_{ou} V_u$$

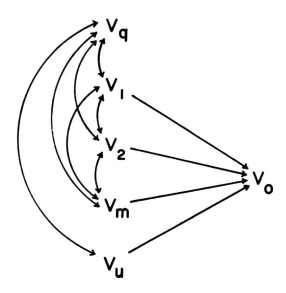

Figure 2. Path diagram for derivation of r_{oq}. (Wright, 1968, fig. 13.1)

Express this in terms of standardized deviations from the means such as $X_i = (V_i - \bar{V}_i)/\sigma_i$ and let $c_{oi} = p_{oi}\sigma_o/\sigma_i$ in order to absorb the σ's.

$$X_o = p_{o1}X_1 + p_{o2}X_2 + \cdots + p_{om}X_m + p_{ou}X_u$$

Let V_q be any linearly related variable. Since $r_{iq} = (1/n)\overset{n}{\Sigma}X_iX_q$, the correlation r_{oq} is as follows:

$$r_{oq} = p_{o1}\,r_{1q} + p_{o2}\,r_{2q} + \cdots + p_{om}\,r_{mq} + p_{ou}\,r_{uq} =$$
$$\Sigma\,p_{oi}\,r_{iq}$$

This is the basic equation of path analysis. The p's are the path coefficients.

The correlation of a variable with itself gives the useful identity equation $r_{oo} = \Sigma\,p_{oi}\,r_{oi} = 1$, still assuming complete determination of V_o. If any of the variables other than V_o are themselves represented as completely determined by others as linear functions, the basic equation may be applied to the terms r_{iq} themselves.

On representation of a system in an arrow diagram, the
correlation between any two variables is equal (in the absence of circular paths) to the sum of contributions from all
paths by which one may trace from one to the other without
going forward along an arrow and then back, and without going
through any variable twice in the same path.

THE CORRELATION BETWEEN LINEAR FUNCTIONS

Path analysis has come to be used for very different
purposes, not necessarily etiological. The most direct is in
the calculation of correlation coefficients from path coefficients as standardized multiple regression coefficients.
This application was involved, though not mentioned, in a
mathematical note (Wright, 1917) preceding publication of the
etiological interpretation of rabbit bone correlations, with
which I began. I had been brought into the Animal Husbandry
Division to analyze data from 24 inbred lines of guinea pigs
(23 maintained by sib-mating, 1 by parent-offspring mating),
started 9 years before. It was important to understand the
relations among all of the recorded characters. Thus I
wished to know the correlation between birth weight and year
weight of animals born in litters of a given size, litter
size being much the most important factor affecting birth
weight. This could be obtained easily for the entire array
in litters of 3 (560 animals) and for the array of 24 strain
means, weighted by the numbers of entries. But what I most
wanted was that within strains. I started calculating this
from the data of each strain before it occurred to me that
there should be some way to deduce it from the other two.
Since beginning the analysis of the rabbit bone correlations,
I had acquired the habit of making diagrams to clarify statistical problems. I made a path diagram in which birth weight,
B, and year weight, Y, were represented as determined by their
strain means ($\bar{B}$, $\bar{Y}$) and the necessarily independent deviations from these means (δB, δY), and each pair was connected
by double-headed arrows to represent the correlations (Figure
3).

The single-headed arrows do not represent causal
relations here, and their directions are merely arbitrary
choices of a point of view. The correlations represented by
double-headed arrows are the results of causation by common
factors but are accepted here merely as empirical facts.
The answer to my problem was immediately apparent. The
correlation between birth weight and year weight of the
guinea pigs was obviously the sum of contributions from two
connecting paths.

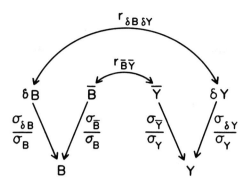

Figure 3. Path diagram for derivation of $r_{\delta B \delta Y}$.
(Wright, 1973, fig. 8)

$$r_{BY} = p_{B\bar{B}} \; r_{\bar{B}\bar{Y}} \; p_{Y\bar{Y}} + p_{B\delta B} \; r_{\delta B \delta Y} \; p_{Y\delta Y}$$

Substitution of the values of the path coefficients, each the ratio of the standard deviation of component to that of the total, gave:

$$r_{BY} \; \sigma_B \; \sigma_Y = r_{\bar{B}\bar{Y}} \; \sigma_{\bar{B}} \; \sigma_{\bar{Y}} + r_{\delta B \delta Y} \; \sigma_{\delta B} \; \sigma_{\delta Y}$$

The desired correlation $r_{\delta B \delta Y}$ could obviously be calculated from the other terms, making use of the well-known formula for the analysis of the squared standard deviation of a sum, referred to earlier. Table 4, taken from the 1917 paper, shows the work of calculation. Probable errors are shown instead of standard errors. The results deduced for an average strain are compared with the average of separate determinations that had been made from the 8 larger strains.

The analogy between the analysis into components of Pearson's product moment $(r_{BY}\sigma_B\sigma_Y) = (1/n) \; \Sigma(B - \bar{B})(Y - \bar{Y})$, and that of the squared standard deviation, may have led Fisher to rename the former the "covariance" several years after introducing (in 1918) the convenient term "variance" for the latter.

This property of the covariance could be demonstrated so easily by conventional algebra, after I had recognized it

TABLE 4

Calculation of the average correlation between birth weight and year weight within strains from that in the total array and that of strain means (Table 1, Wright, 1917)

	σ^2_B	σ^2_Y	σ_B	σ_Y	$\sigma_B \sigma_Y$	$r_{BY}\sigma_B\sigma_Y$	r_{BY}
Total (560 pigs)	130.53	14,852	11.425	121.87	1,392.4	522.15	+0.375 ± 0.024
24 family means	20.50	4,837	4.528	69.55	314.9	198.39	+0.630 ± 0.083
Average family (deduced)	110.03	10,015	10.49	100.08	1,498.8	323.76	+0.308 ± 0.026
Average 8 families with 297 pigs	108.78	8,915	10.43	94.42			+0.256 ± 0.036

from the path analysis, that I assumed that it must have been
known to Pearson though I had not seen any reference to it.
Thus I merely stated in my 1917 paper that "the very simple
formula discussed below has been useful to the writer and does
not seem to be well known."

I have found this direct use of path analysis for calculation of the correlations between linear functions useful in
many other cases. Much the most important use of the method
has, indeed, been of this sort, the calculation of fixation
indices, F, from diagrams representing breeding systems, including regular ones like that representing double-first
cousin mating (Figure 4), and irregular ones like the pedigrees of the foundation Shorthorn bulls, Favourite and Comet
(Figure 5). Calculations have been made for the Shorthorn
breed as a whole (Figure 6). Another application was to the
expected grade of a synthetic randombred stock derived equally
from n unselected closely inbred strains. It was shown that
this should have 1/nth less superiority over its inbred
ancestry than the average of all of the first crosses among
the latter (Wright, 1922). Formulas have been made of fixation indices from local inbreeding in continuous populations
and for that under assortative mating and so on. This index
is the theoretical correlation between uniting gametes,
easily shown to measure the change in heterozygosis from that
in a random breeding population. Since it is not concerned
with etiology, I will not discuss it further here (cf. Wright,
1921b, 68, 69, 77).

MATING OF DOUBLE FIRST COUSINS

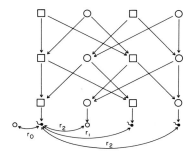

Figure 4.   Path diagram for derivation of the inbreeding
            coefficient under mating of double first cousins.
            (Wright, 1973, fig. 11)

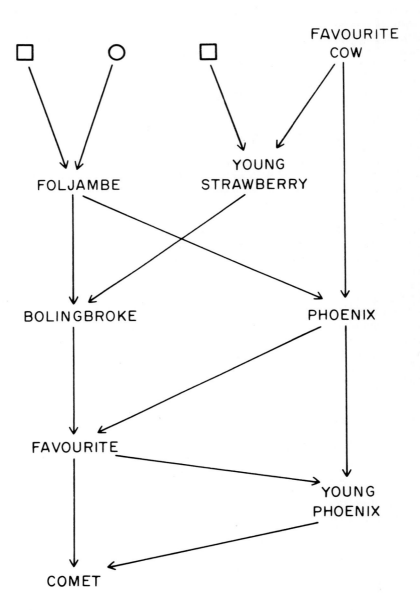

Figure 5.   Pedigree of the foundation Shorthorn bulls,
            Favourite (252) and Comet (115), used as a
            path diagram for calculation of their inbreeding
            coefficients. (Wright, 1977, fig. 16.1)

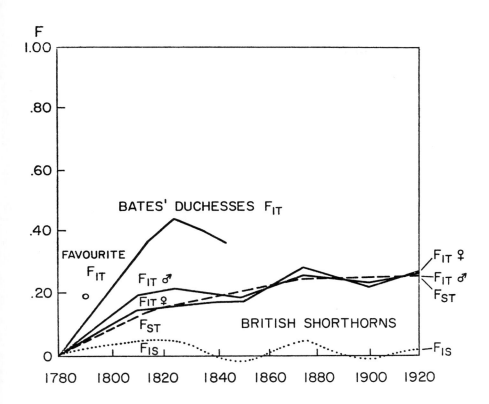

Figure 6. Inbreeding coefficients of British Shorthorn cattle from 1780 to 1920. Inbreeding of bulls and cows relative to the foundation stock, F_{IT}, of the breed as a whole and that of the Bates' Duchesses are in solid lines. Those for the hypothetical offspring of randomly mated animals, F_{ST}, are in a broken line. Those for individuals relative to the contemporary breed, F_{IS}, are in a dotted line. The inbreeding coefficient of the foundation bull, Favourite, is indicated by a circle. (Wright, 1977, fig. 16.2)

MULTIPLE REGRESSION

   In the second class of application (Figure 7), an
observed variable is treated as a linear function of a number
of other such variables for the purpose of estimation. Application of the basic equation to the simple diagram leads
at once to the normal equations of multiple regression (or
to those of the method of least squares for standardized
variables). Such estimation equations, tracing to Gauss more
than a century and a half ago, are also not concerned with
etiology and will not be discussed further here.

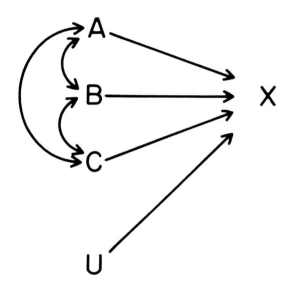

Figure 7. Path diagram corresponding to multiple regression.
           (Wright, 1973, fig. 4)

FACTOR ANALYSIS

   The third application of path analysis is as closely
related to another established method, "factor analysis," as
it is to multiple regression. The term factor analysis implies a method of dealing with etiology and this was clearly
the purpose of Spearman (1904) when he suggested that the
usually high correlations among mental tests implied the
existence of a single common factor: general intelligence,
supplemented in each case by a special factor. Others such
as Thurstone (1931) have postulated multiple mental factors.

The aim has been an algorithm for automatically extracting etiologic factors from correlation matrices. Unfortunately there is little likelihood that the pattern utilized by any automatic method will correspond to the complex irregular network of causal relations in the real world. Etiological analysis must use whatever evidence is available at the expense of becoming dependent on more or less subjective judgements.

What actually emerges from factor analysis in its most objective form is the location of the observed variables at points on the surface of a hypersphere of unit radius, a concept that traces at least to Pearson in 1900. The so-called factors are merely a set of (usually) orthogonal axes, chosen from the infinite array of possible axes by some convention. The factor loadings (corresponding to path coefficients) are merely the projections on these axes or in other words the coordinates of the points representing the observed variables. Strongly correlated variables come out closely clustered, independent ones 90° apart, and that with correlation -1, 180° away.

According to the convention proposed by Hotelling (1936), the first axis is to be that on which the sum of the squared projections is maximized, the second that on which squared orthogonal residuals are maximized and so on until no residuals are left, which, he showed, requires the same number of orthogonal axes as the number of variables. He devised an interation method for arriving at the factor loadings for the axes in succession. All factor loadings for the first axis are likely to be positive if there really is an important general factor common to all observed variables. Those for the other axes, however, necessarily show a balancing of positive and negative values under the method used.

The corresponding path diagram is one in which arrows are directed toward each of the n observed variables A, B, C ··· from each of just n hypothetical "factors" U, V, W ····. Thus an equation can be written for each of the n $(n + 1)/2$ correlation coefficients including the self correlations $r_{AA} = 1$, etc. of the type $r_{AB} = P_{AU} P_{BU} + P_{AV} P_{BV} \cdots$. Hotelling's method is one for solving the set of simultaneous quadratic equations.

Most factor analysts remove the self-correlations before calculating the $n(n - 1)/2$ remaining correlations and solving by Hotelling's interation process (or some less tedious approximation). The number of common factors for practical elimination of the residuals is usually considerably reduced

but n axes are added for special factors, one for each observed variable. The recognition of the likelihood that there
are special factors is a step toward a pattern representing
etiology. The factor loadings on the first axis may be
interpreted as measuring roughly the influence of the general
factor but they are complicated by contributions of other
factors. The factor loadings on the other axes are again
necessarily balanced in sign and are unlikely to measure
effects of any real factors.

     Table 5 shows the correlations among 6 bone measurements
from a flock of White Leghorn fowls (Dunn, 1928) recalculated
to apply to the 276 birds in which all measurements were
available (Wright, 1968).

TABLE 5

Correlations among 6 bone measurements of
276 White Leghorn hens. L = length of skull;
B = breadth of skull; H = humerus length; U = ulna
length; F = femur length; T = tibia length.
Data of Dunn (1928)

	L	B	H	U	F	T
L	1.000	0.584	0.615	0.601	0.570	0.600
B		1.000	0.576	0.530	0.526	0.555
H			1.000	0.940	0.875	0.878
U				1.000	0.877	0.886
F					1.000	0.924
T						1.000

     Table 6 gives the 6 factor solution by Hotelling's
method including the 6 self-correlations. Table 7 gives that
for 3 common factors and 6 special factors, found by Hotelling's method after exclusion of the self correlations.
Figure 8 shows the locations of the 6 variables relative to
the 1st and 2nd axes and to the 2nd and 3rd. They show the
clustering of the two measurements of head, of a wing and of
a leg. There would be less clustering on the surface of the
9-dimensional hypersphere because of the orthogonal separation of the loadings of the special factors.

TABLE 6

Factor analysis of correlations of Table 5 with
inclusion of self-correlations, by Hotelling's method
(Wright, 1954).

	P_{X1}	P_{X2}	P_{X3}	P_{X4}	P_{X5}	P_{X6}	
L	0.743	+0.454	+0.492	−0.021	+0.007	−0.001	
B	0.698	+0.589	−0.409	−0.001	+0.002	−0.014	
H	0.948	−0.158	−0.026	+0.218	+0.047	+0.162	
U	0.940	−0.213	+0.007	+0.203	−0.042	−0.165	
F	0.929	−0.235	−0.038	−0.214	+0.184	−0.032	
T	0.941	−0.191	−0.030	−0.195	−0.195	+0.045	
Σp^2	4.568	0.714	0.412	0.173	0.076	0.057	6.000
%	76.1	11.9	6.9	2.9	1.3	0.9	100.0

TABLE 7

Factor analysis of correlations in Table 5 with
exclusion of self correlations, except in determination
of factor loadings for special factors (Wright, 1954).

	P_{X1}	P_{X2}	P_{X3}	Special	
L	+0.685	+0.361	+0.007	+0.632	
B	+0.639	+0.409	−0.030	+0.651	
H	+0.951	−0.083	+0.162	+0.250	
U	+0.946	−0.152	+0.168	+0.232	
F	+0.930	−0.180	−0.166	+0.274	
T	+0.942	−0.124	−0.154	+0.271	
Σp^2	4.429	0.375	0.107	1.088	5.999
%	73.8	6.3	1.8	18.1	100.0

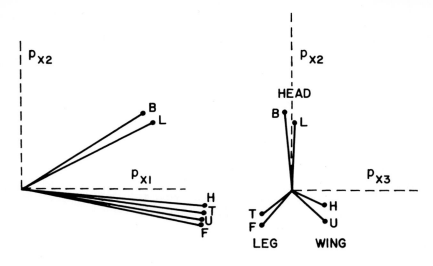

Figure 8.   Vectorial representation of relations among six
            measurements in a population of White Leghorn
            fowls.   The two most important axes are shown
            to the left, the second and third to the right.
            (Wright, 1954, fig. 2.1)

ETIOLOGIC INTERPRETATION

        This brings us to the fourth class of applications:
etiologic interpretation.   It is usually easy to suggest a
plausible interpretation of any single correlation coefficient.   It is much more difficult to arrive at an interpretation of an array of correlations, that is demonstrably
consistent throughout.   The etiologic application of path
analysis is intended to replace the usual verbal interpretation of an array of correlations.   As already noted, it must
take account of all available evidence: spatial relations and
homology in interpreting morphological correlations; temporal
relations where these are known; results of experiments
designed to throw light on causal relations; and perhaps
suggestions from partial correlations and from factor analysis.
It necessarily involves much subjective judgement.   An
algorithm for grinding out an etiologic interpretation completely objectively is, in general, an impossibility.

CORRELATIONS AMONG BONE MEASUREMENTS OF FOWLS

In the case of an array of morphological measurements, the action of factors affecting general size is usually the first class of factors that should be considered. This is not done in pure form by applying Hotelling's interaction method even by excluding the self correlations. One may, however, find which of the correlations deviate significantly from the values derived from the primary set of factor loadings and thus which probably involve one or more additional factors. These may then be excluded, together with the self correlations followed by application of Hotelling's method to those left. If there are still no significant deviations, the factor loadings may be considered to be the desired path coefficients for general size. In the case of the White Leghorn bones, 12 of the 15 correlations depended solely on general size by this criterion, leaving three that were significantly in excess of the amount due to general size. These three, r_{LB}, r_{HU}, and r_{FT}, were, not surprisingly, the correlations between different measurements of the same organ, head, wing and leg, respectively.

It remains to interpret the excess contributions to these three correlations. Since there is no overlap in this case, this can be done separately. There seems to be nothing substantially better than merely taking the square roots of the excess contributions as the path coefficients relative to factors for sizes of head, wing and leg respectively. (Figure 9.)

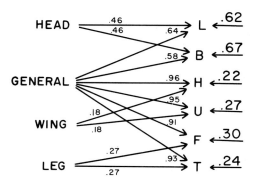

Figure 9. Path analysis of the correlations between bone measurements of Table 5 on the hypothesis that as many as possible are due solely to general size. (Wright, 1973, fig. 6)

TABLE 8

Path analysis of correlations in Table 5 on hypothesis
that as many as possible (12) trace to only one
common factor. Self correlations and r_{LB}, r_{HU} and
r_{FT} excluded in calculation for the general factor
(Wright, 1954)

	General	Head	Wing	Leg	Special	
L	+0.636	+0.461			+0.619	
B	+0.583	+0.461			+0.669	
H	+0.958		+0.182		+0.222	
U	+0.947		+0.182		+0.265	
F	+0.914			+0.269	+0.304	
T	+0.932			+0.269	+0.243	
	4.263	0.426	+0.066	+0.144	1.101	6.000
	71.1	7.1	1.1	2.4	18.3	100.0

Note that the path coefficients for each organ have come
out with the same sign, indicating that they relate to the
size of the organ in question, instead of to its form (contrary to the factor loadings from factor analysis, other than
the first). Form-determining factors certainly exist, as
Sinnott (1935) demonstrated in the case of Mendelian genes
that distinguish between disk, sphere and elongate squashes,
with no effects on volume. If there are factors for dolicho-
cephaly vs brachycephaly in hens (as probably in the human
species), they must be overwhelmed by other factors that make
for large or small heads relative to body size and similarly
for factors that effect the apportionment of length of wing
or leg.

HERITABILITY OF HUMAN IQ

I have evaluated the degrees of determination of variability by heredity and environment, and by components of
these, for several other characters than white spotting in
strains of guinea pigs (Wright, 1977, Chapter 4), but these
merely repeat the general pattern of etiologic interpretation
and need not be discussed here.

An analysis that I made in 1931 of data of Dr. Barbara Burks (1928) on the heritability of human IQ is of more interest here. She investigated the IQ's of 214 adopted children and the mental ages of their foster parents in comparison with similar data from a carefully chosen control array of 105 children reared by their own parents. All were White and non-Jewish, living in California. They covered the range of socio-economic classes but with much less representation at the lower levels than that in the general population. The standard deviations of the children's IQ's, were, however, typical (foster and control both 15.1) even though the means were well above the norm (foster 107.4; control 115.4).

I made this single excursion into human genetics in order to clear up a confusion from treatment of a path analysis as identical with multiple regression and thus merely an estimation equation, instead of one designed for etiologic interpretation. I suggested an etiological path diagram.

There was much indeterminacy because the number of independent equations available for solution was less than the number of unknown path coefficients, under the simplest etiologic pattern that seemed at all adequate. Even so it was necessary to assume that the genetic factors affecting the IQ's of children played much less of a role in determining parental mental ages, in order to avoid impossible results (negative coefficients of determination and hence imaginary path coefficients). The demands of consistency implied surprising narrow limits.

There was another wholly different sort of indeterminacy, one that makes it logically impossible for anyone to arrive at definitive estimates of heritability from human data unless data from monozygotic twins are included. Otherwise there is no adequate means of distinguishing the roles of nonadditive heredity (dominance and interaction effects of genes) from those of unmeasured environment and of genotype-environment interaction.

My maximal estimate in 1931 of heritability of child's IQ from Burks' data came out 80%. This was associated with 8% from graded home environment and 12% from genotype-environment correlation (a wholly different thing from genotype-environment interaction). This maximal estimate was under the unlikely assumption of no other environmental effects, no dominance or gene interaction, and no genotype-environment interaction.

My minimal estimate of heritability was about 50% based on the assumption, also unlikely, that the pertinent heredity was wholly additive.

Heredity for IQ is certainly not wholly additive in view of the well documented inbreeding depression, but neither is it tenable to suppose that the graded home environment is all of the child's environment that affects his or her IQ.

I have recently restudied the same data. While I have somewhat modified my interpretive path diagram, the maximal and minimal estimates of heritability remain about the same.

A new path diagram is shown in Figure 10. The immediate factors back of child's IQ (O) are heredity (H), genotype-environment interaction (J), graded home environment (E), and residual environment (U). Back of heredity are its additive component (G), dominance deviations (D), and gene interaction (I). Allowance is made for correlation between genotype and environment (r_{GE}). Parental mental age (P) is represented here (but not in 1931) as determined by parent's IQ as a child (O'), itself determined exactly as is child's IQ; and by a factor X which may be partly genetic but if so of a different sort from H. Child's environment is represented as determined by O' and X of the parents and a residual factor V. This can be transformed optionally into determination by the P's, X's and V. This differs from determination by the P's, parental home environments as children, E' and V on the 1931 diagram. The O's and P's are duplicated in the present diagram for convenience in taking account of strong phenotypic assortative mating (about .70 in the controls, corrected for attenuation as are all of the statistics). These duplications are made in such a way that the correlations between dupli-cants are perfect ($\Sigma p_{O'i} r_{O'i} = 1$, and $\Sigma p_{Pi} r_{Pi} = 1$), and spurious correlations are avoided by the convention that no compound path may pass through a given bracket (associated with O' or P) more than once.

As indicated earlier, definitive estimates in human data require the inclusion of monozygotic twins (identical in nonadditive as well as additive heredity). These introduce certain difficulties such as possible effects of prenatal competition and postnatal close association but the results of several studies involving such twins indicate strongly that heritability in White populations, comparable to that studied by Burks', is closer to the maximal than to the minimal estimates from her data and thus roughly in the neighborhood of 70%.

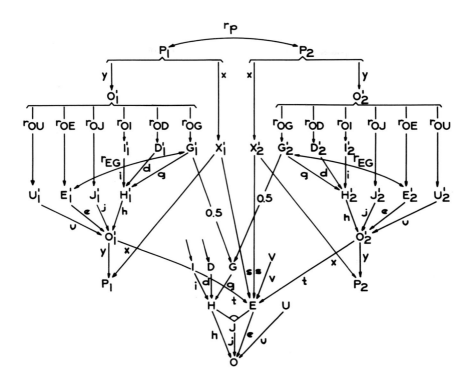

Figure 10. Path diagram of the factors, genetic and non-genetic, that affect child's IQ and parent's mental age in the White California population studied by Burks. (Wright, 1978, fig. 9.7)

The high average socio-economic level of the population that she studied does not seem to have curtailed the range of variability, with the implication that the estimates from her data applied roughly to the general White population of California. It is possible, however, that differences in the lower part of the range of socio-economic classes may have an inordinate environmental effect on IQ so that heritability may have been somewhat lower in the general White Californian population.

PERINATAL CHARACTERS OF THE GUINEA PIG

It was important in my investigation of the effects of
inbreeding and cross-breeding on guinea pigs to understand
the etiologic relations among such characters as size and
frequency of litters, mortality at birth and from birth to weaning
(33 days) and birthweight and gains to weaning (Wright,
1960c). There are important genetic differences among inbred
strains in all of these respects as shown by annual averages
but these cannot be demonstrated with confidence among individuals of a randombred strain. There are, however, important etiological relations among these characters, partially
illustrated in a path diagram (Figure 11). They can be illustrated only partially because of nonlinearity.

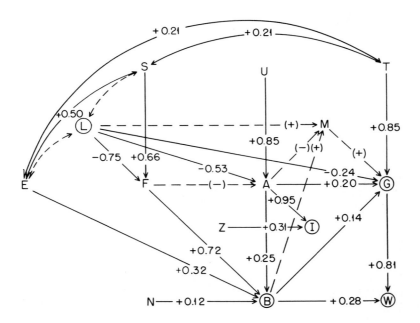

Figure 11.   Path diagram of the factors affecting birth
weight (B), gain to 33 days (G) and their
sum, weight at 33 days (W), in a population
of guinea pigs. (Wright, 1968, fig. 14.5)

The measured variables in this diagram are birth weight
(B), gain to weaning (G), and their sum, weight at 33 days
(W), size of litter (L), and the interval (I) between litters
if 65-76 days, cases in which oestrus occurred immediately
after parturition. The correlation between this interval
(I), and the gestation period (A), was estimated to be 0.95.
Among hypothetical factors, fetal weight at 55 days is represented by E while the daily rate of gain from age 55 to
parturition is represented by F. Experiments by Ibsen (1928)
demonstrated that litter size has little effect on E, much on
F.

It should be noted that size of litter is almost wholly
determined at conception in guinea pigs as shown by the
slightness of the difference between the number of corpora
lutea and size of litter at birth. The situation is very
different in the much larger litters of mice in which prenatal
death and absorption are important.

Minot (1891) found that the birth weight of guinea pigs
showed a very strong inverse relation to size of litter. He
noted that this might be either a consequence of prenatal
competition or of a stimulus to early parturition from a
large litter. He found that the gestation period did, indeed,
tend to vary inversely with size of litter and that birth
weight tended to vary directly with the gestation period. He
concluded from these and other considerations that the effect
of litter size on gestation period rather than prenatal competition was the major explanation of the inverse relation of
birth weight to size of litter. I verified his observations
but came to the opposite conclusion from a path analysis
(Wright, 1921a). This conclusion was later verified by
Ibsen's direct observations.

Both of the possible paths of influence, $L \to F \to B$ and
$L \to A \to B$ are represented in Figure 11. The compound coefficient, $P_{BFL} = (-0.75) \times (+0.72) = -0.54$ is four times as
great as $P_{BAL} = (-0.53) \times (+0.25) = -0.13$ using the values from
a later study (Wright, 1960, 1968). It may be noted that
while the paths from L to F (competition effect) and from L
to A (effect on time of parturition) are causal, those from
F to B and from A to B are merely mathematical, birth weight
(B) being determined by the course of the late fetal growth
curve and the time at which this is interrupted by birth.

The relations between gain and factors A and B are more
complex but can be interpreted as meaning that relatively
advanced development and large weight at birth are favorable
to rapid growth thereafter. A large litter size implies

postnatal as well as prenatal competition but that after
birth tends to be reduced by death, M, of littermates. Mortality between birth and weaning was not introduced into the
calculations because of serious nonlinearity in its relations,
especially with size of litter. While mortality is increasingly severe in litters of more than 3, it is also relatively
severe for the usually very large singletons. Three was the
optimal size in the vigorous control stock, two in most of the
inbred strains. There was nonlinearity in the determination
of birth weight but this was relatively slight and could itself be treated as a factor (N).

The residual factors for early fetal growth (E), late
fetal growth (S), and postnatal growth (T), consisting principally of the condition of the dam in successive periods, are
undoubtedly correlated but only token values were used in the
calculations. An important factor back of littersize is not
represented. This was delay or absence of delay of conception
after birth of the preceding litter. Studies of crosses between inbred lines (Wright, 1977, pp. 51-53) indicated that
litter size was a purely maternal character as expected, but
regularity in producing litters depended twice as much on the
male as on the female. Inbred male by crossbred female produced only half as many litters as the reciprocal cross, and
about one third as many as cross bred x crossbred, but twice
as large litters as inbred x inbred. Thus delay was favorable to large size of litter.

HOG AND CORN CORRELATIONS

The most extensive etiologic study by path analysis has
been on the relations among various aspects of corn and hog
production over the period between the Civil War and World
War I, stimulated by membership in a committee of the Animal
Husbandry Division concerned with maintenance of hog production during the war (Wright, 1925).

The corn variables studied consisted of adjusted
estimates of acreage, yield, crop (the product of the preceding) and Dec. 1 price for the years 1870 to 1915. The hog
variables consisted of the pack of western markets in summer
(March to October) and in winter (November to February), the
average live weight in these periods (summer only from 1889
to 1915), the product of the preceding and the average prices
per 100 pounds (summer only from 1880 to 1915).

Trends were fitted twice by eye and averaged. The
deviations from these trends were the variables studied.

More than 500 correlation coefficients were calculated. Each corn variable was correlated with the corn variables for the two preceding years, the same year and the two following years, and with the hog variables for the summer and winter seasons of the preceding year, the same year and the three following years. Thus the hog variables of each season were correlated with the corn variables of three preceding years, the same and the following year. They were correlated with the hog variables of each season of the two preceding years, same and two following years.

The summer and winter hog pack were very different in character. The winter pack was relatively homogeneous, consisting mainly of the main pig crop. The summer pack varied greatly in its age composition from year to year. For various reasons, the summer live weight must have been a remarkably good indicator of the amount of breeding during the year.

The corn crop showed a correlation of +0.87 with yield but only +0.49 with acreage showing the much greater importance of the former. The December price showed a correlation of -0.80 with the crop as estimated. Since neither showed much correlation with any preceding variable, it seemed best to treat the corn crop as an independent variable.

The first attempts to construct an etiological diagram for the hog variables were unsuccessful. It became evident that attention had better be focused on the variables that entered into the highest correlations. These consisted largely of the prices of the summer and winter packs, the corn price, and the summer live weight which in conjunction with the closely correlated winter pack of a year and a half later ($r = +.78$) was taken as an indicator of amount of breeding. The observed prices and the hypothetical factor, amount of breeding, were adopted as a central system and arranged after considerable trial and error in the pattern shown in Figure 12. Path coefficients were arrived at by trials at intervals of .05 until all of the observed correlations were approximated reasonably well, including the two indices of amount of breeding. Table 9 shows the path coefficients arrived at for this central system.

The principal other variables were then represented as functions of the corn crop of the same and two preceeding years and of the amount of breeding of the same and three preceding years with path coefficients calculated to the nearest .05 by repeated trial. Summer pork production was assigned a path from summer pack (coefficient 0.95) and one from summer live weight with coefficient 0.20. The corresponding path

coefficients for winter pork production and its factors were
0.95 and 0.25.

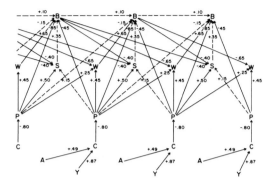

Figure 12.   Path diagram illustrating the system of inter-
             actions among corn crop (C), corn price (P),
             the summer price of hogs (S), the winter price
             of hogs (W), and an unmeasured variable (B), the
             amount of breeding, which has been found most
             successful in accounting for observed deviations
             from the trends during the period between the
             Civil War and World War I. (Wright, 1925, Fig. 27)

The values expected from these path coefficients agreed
with the 510 observed correlations as well as could be expected. Figures 13 to 15 show the expected values as dotted
lines in comparison with the observed values as solid lines
for the correlations with three of the variables, corn crop,
summer and winter pork production. The agreement in the
cases of the prices (fitted first), live weights and pack,
were at least as good.

The general conclusion was that the dominating features
of the hog situation were certain effects of the corn crop
and price and an innate tendency of the hog variables to fall
into a cycle of successive overproduction and underproduction,
two years from one extreme to the other.

The amount of breeding at a given time was determined
largely by the profits from hog raising during the preceding
year which depended on the ratio between the price the

TABLE 9

Path coefficients for amounts of breeding;
summer and winter prices of hogs over the
period between the Civil War and
World War I. Primes indicate preceding years

Factor	Price		
	Breeding	Summer	Winter
Corn price	−0.45	+0.15	+0.45
Corn price'	−0.85	+0.50	+0.25
Corn price''	−0.15		
Breeding'	+0.10	−0.40	−0.65
Breeding''		−0.40	
Summer hog price	+0.35		
Winter hog price'	+0.65		

TABLE 10

Path coefficients for summer and winter live weights
of hogs and for the summer and winter pack over the
period between the Civil War and World War I

Factor	Summer Weight	Winter Weight	Summer Pack	Winter Pack
Corn Crop		+0.65	−0.25	−0.20
Corn Crop'			+0.55	
Corn Crop''			−0.10	
Breeding	+0.80	+0.35	−0.10	
Breeding'	+0.30		+0.45	+0.85
Breeding''	−0.15		+0.35	+0.35
Breeding'''			+0.35	+0.15

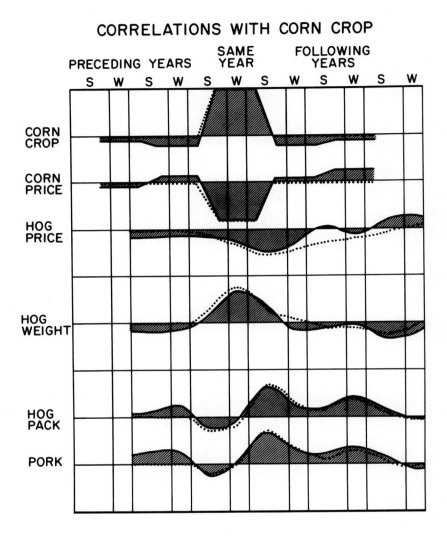

Figure 13.   The correlations between deviations from trend
              in the corn crop with those of other variables
              in preceding, same and following years in the
              period between Civil War and World War I.   The
              solid lines connect the observed correlations,
              the dotted lines, those expected from the system
              of deduced path coefficients.   (Wright, 1925,
              fig. 16)

CORRELATIONS WITH SUMMER PORK PRODUCTION

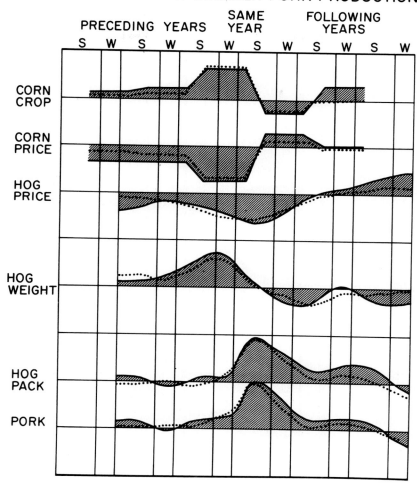

Figure 14.   The correlations between deviations from trend
in summer pork production with those of other
variables in preceding, same and following
years in the period between the Civil War and
World War I.   The solid lines connect the
observed correlations, the dotted lines, those
expected from the system of deduced path coefficients.   (Wright, 1925, fig. 24)

CORRELATIONS WITH WINTER PORK PRODUCTION

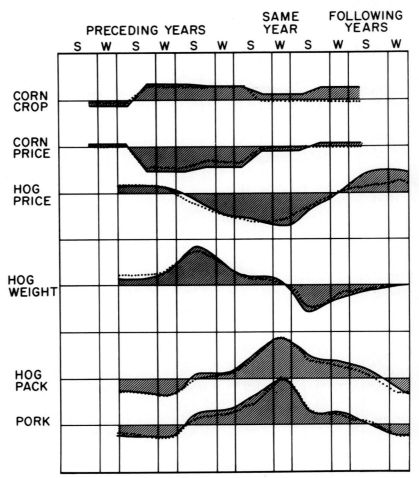

Figure 15.   The correlations between deviations from trend
            in winter pork production with those of other
            variables in preceding, same and following
            years in the period between the Civil War and
            World War I.   The solid lines connect the
            observed correlations, the dotted lines those
            expected from the system of deduced path co-
            efficients.   (Wright, 1925, fig. 25)

packers pay for hogs and the price of corn during the period in which they were raised and finished. The peak effect on breeding occurred from half a year to a year after the hog-corn price ratio had reached its peak and begun to decline. The result was a surplus of hogs a year or more later, low prices and losses. Breeding, however, did not reach its low point until some time after the hog-corn price ratio had begun to rise. A swing to underproduction was the consequence. Thus any cause which led to unusual profits or losses tended to set up oscillations in the hog population, four years from crest to crest.

RECIPROCAL INTERACTION

None of the path diagrams considered so far have paths that return on themselves as indicated by the arrows. It is sometimes useful in path analysis, however, to represent reciprocal interaction between variables (Wright, 1960b, 1968) by separate arrows from each of two variables to the other or by compound paths around a circle.

The basic equations $r_{AB} = \Sigma P_{Ai} r_{iB}$ and $r_{AB} = \Sigma P_{Bi} r_{iA}$ still hold and yield two independent equations for each correlation in ·systems involving a reciprocal interaction. The usual analysis of correlations into contributions from compound coefficients for each connecting path breaks down, however, under the proviso that there shall be no passage through the same variable twice in the same path. Valid equations can, nevertheless, be written for each correlation by step by step analysis in terms of the basic equation.

It is not practicable to go into details here, but I will give an illustration of such a diagram. J. S. Haldane and J. G. Priestley (1905) made experiments on themselves on the relations between CO_2 concentrations in respired air (A), and in samples taken after respiration to nearly the greatest possible extent (C), corrected for residual nonalveolar air as an imperfect estimate of the concentration in the alveolar air in the lungs (Y); and depth (D) and frequency (F) of respiration. Z is the unknown amount of CO_2 released into the blood by metabolism.

All possible correlations were obtained among variables A, C, D, and F in each subject.

In the case of JGP the virtual absence of correlations between estimates of CO_2 in the alveolar air (C) and the other

TABLE 11

Statistics from experiments on control of respiration
by Haldane and Priestley (1905)

Variable	Subjects			
	JSH		JGP	
	Mean	σ	Mean	σ
% CO_2 in respired air (A)	3.052	1.350	3.507	1.348
% CO_2 in alveolar air (C)	5.767	.478	6.568	.241
Depth of respiration(cc)(D)	1200	358	794	214
Frequency of respiration (F)	15.21	2.203	17.60	2.161
Correlations	r_{CA}	.823	.093	
	r_{DA}	.979	.710	
	r_{DC}	.772	.015	
	r_{FA}	.501	.779	
	r_{DF}	.530	.416	
	r_{CF}	.354	-.067	

variables and the high mean and low standard deviation suggest an overcorrection for nonalveolar air, making these
correlations unusable. I will give the final diagram arrived
at in the case of JSH and that for JGP on substitution of certain ones from JSH.

The homeostatic regulation of alveolar CO_2 by effects
on depth and frequency of respiration were evidently very
different in the two subjects.

The occurrence of path coefficients far in excess of 1
in some cases, is characteristic of homeostasis.

It may be seen from these illustrations that path
analysis has been used for etiologic interpretation in a
great variety of situations leading to a great variety of
patterns.

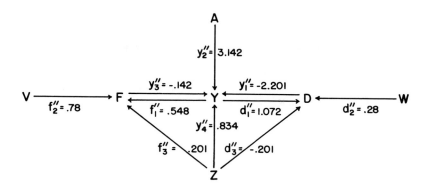

Figure 16. Path diagram of relations of CO_2 concentration of respired air (A), estimated CO_2 concentration of alveolar air (Y), depth (D) and frequency (F) of respiration, hypothetical CO_2 released into blood by metabolism, and residual factors (U,V) in subject J.S.H. (Wright, 1960b, fig. 15 data of J.S. Haldane and J.G. Priestley, 1905)

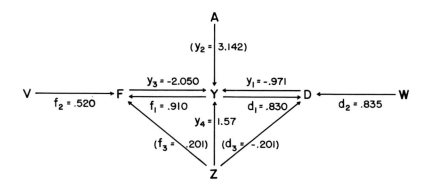

Figure 17. Path diagram similar to that of Figure 16 (and partially borrowed from it) for subject JGP (Wright, 1960b, fig. 16, data of J.S. Haldane and J.G. Priestley, 1905)

REFERENCES

Burks, B.S., in "27th Yearbook of the National Society for the Study of Education," Vol. 1, pp. 219-316. Public School Publishing Co., Bloomington, Ill., 1928.

Castle, W.E., "The Nature of Size Factors as Indicated by a Study of Correlation," Publ. no. 196, pp. 51-55. Carnegie Institution, Washington, 1914.

Dunn, L.C., Storrs Agr. Exp. Sta. Bull. 52, 1-112 (1928).

Fisher, R.A., Trans. Roy. Soc. Edinburgh 52, 399-433 (1918).

Haldane, J.S., and Priestley, J.G., J. Physiol. 32, 225-266 (1905).

Hotelling, H., Psychometrics 1, 27-35 (1936).

Ibsen, H.L., J. Exp. Zool. 51, 51-91 (1928).

Minot, C.S., J. Physiol. 12, 97-153 (1891).

Pearson, K., Phil. Mag., Series 5, 50, 157-175 (1900).

Sinnott, E.W., Genetics 20, 12-21 (1935).

Spearman, C., Amer. J. Psychol. 15, 201-292 (1904).

Thurstone, L.L., Psychol. Rev. 39, 406-427 (1931).

Wright, S., J. Washington Acad. Sci. 7, 532-535 (1917).

Wright, S., Genetics 3, 367-374 (1918).

Wright, S., Proc. Nat. Acad. Sci. U.S. 6, 320-332 (1920).

Wright, S., J. Agr. Res. 20, 557-585 (1921a).

Wright, S., Genetics 6, 111-178 (1921b).

Wright, S., U.S. Dept. Agric. Bull. no. 1121 (1922).

Wright, S., U.S. Dept. Agric. Bull. no. 1300 (1925).

Wright, S., J. Amer. Stat. Assoc. 26 Suppl., 55-163 (1931).

Wright, S., Ann. Math. Stat. 5, 161-215 (1934).

Wright, S., in "Statistics and Mathematics in Biology" (O. Kempthorne, T.A. Bancroft, J.W. Gowen, and J.L. Lush, Eds.), pp. 11-33. Iowa State Univ. Press, Ames, Iowa, 1954.

Wright, S., Biometrics 16, 189-202 (1960a).

Wright, S., Biometrics 16, 423-445 (1960b).

Wright, S., J. Cell and Comp Physiol. 56 Suppl. 1, 123-151 (1960c).

Wright, S., "Evolution and the Genetics of Population," Vol. 1. University of Chicago Press, Chicago, 1968.

Wright, S., "Evolution and the Genetics of Population," Vol. 2. University of Chicago Press, Chicago, 1969.

Wright, S., in "Genetic Structure of Populations" (N. E. Morton, Ed.), pp. 3-25. University of Hawaii Press, Honolulu, 1973.

Wright, S., "Evolution and the Genetics of Population," Vol. 3. University of Chicago Press, Chicago, 1977.

Wright, S., "Evolution and the Genetics of Population," Vol. 4. University of Chicago Press, Chicago, 1978 (in press).

FAMILY RESEMBLANCE

Path analysis is appropriate to pairs of relatives, and segregation analysis to nuclear families and pedigrees. Much attention has been given to cognitive performance because of the unusually varied data, its central role in an ideological controversy, and to illustrate that behavior genetics, to the extent that it deals with health-related traits, is an aspect of genetic epidemiology.

Segregation analysis leads to genetic counseling, a transaction in which data on a unique pedigree of interest are exchanged for a specific recurrence risk. This application of complex segregation analysis avoids the crude approximation and nonspecificity of empirical risks. Precision of risk is the sine qua non for control of disease by reproductive choice and preventive therapy.

PROGRESS OF THE KINSHIP CORRELATION MODELS

Ching Chun Li
Graduate School of Public Health
University of Pittsburgh, Pittsburgh PA 15261

I cannot help feeling we have come a long way since
Weinberg (1909, 1910) first calculated the genetic correlation between relatives in a random mating population.
A decade or so later, the monumental works of Fisher
(1918) and Wright (1921) appeared, both dealing with, a-
mong other things, correlation between relatives under a
wide range of conditions other than random mating. In
particular, they investigated the effects of inbreeding
and assortative mating on the kinship correlations. More
recently, in studying certain human quantitative traits,
special attention has been directed to the nature of environmental effects on the development of a phenotype and
on the kinship correlations. This communication traces
very briefly the progress made in constructing the correlation models, from the simple core to the more complicated ones, and discusses some of the problems involved.
Detailed historical descriptions of the progress must be
left to the students of history of science. Here we
merely indicate the main features of some basic correlation models. In order to save space, we shall dispense
with the random mating populations and begin with the
situation in which the parents are correlated, at least
phenotypically.

THE GENETIC CORE

Disregarding the effects of dominance and environment for
the moment, let us first treat the case of additive gene effects. Let L denote such a linear value (Fig. 1) of individuals, and $m = m_L = r_{PP}(L,L)$ be the correlation coefficient between the L's of the two parents. From Fig. 1 we see that
each parent-offspring pair is connected by two chains, yielding the parent-offspring correlation $r_{PO} = 1/2 + m/2$. The
pair of sibs is connected by four chains, yielding the sib-sib

correlation $r_{00} = \frac{1}{2}(\frac{1}{2}) + \frac{1}{2}(\frac{1}{2}) + \frac{1}{2}(m)\frac{1}{2} + \frac{1}{2}(m)\frac{1}{2}$. These results are summarized as follows:

$$r_{PP}(L,L) = m$$

$$r_{PO}(L,L) = \frac{1}{2}(1 + m) \qquad (1)$$

$$r_{00}(L,L) = \frac{1}{2}(1 + m)$$

where (L,L) reminds us that these correlations are calculated from the linear (or genic) values of the parents and their offspring. We note that although $r_{PO} = r_{00}$ in such a case, they assume the same value for different reasons. These two correlations would not be equal in a more general situation.

Fig. 1 and results (1) constitute the genetic core for all kinship correlation models. I know of no controversy about the core model, as it is a direct consequence of mendelian inheritance and path analysis.

If the mating is at random with respect to the trait under consideration, then $r_{PP} = m = 0$, and $r_{PO} = r_{00} = 1/2$. In studying the total ridge counts of human fingers, this is precisely what Holt (1968) found, as the number of ridges is genetically determined (without dominance) and is not influenced by any known environmental agents.

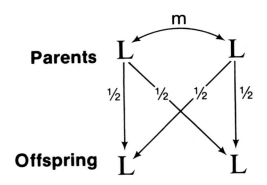

Fig. 1. The genetic core of all kinship correlation models. L = linear value = value determined by additive gene effects; m = correlation coefficient between the L values of the two parents. See (1) in text.

The genetic core (Fig. 1), though true, is of limited application. It covers only the simplest genetic traits. However, it forms the foundation upon which more elaborate models may be built.

THE REVERSE OF A PATH

As we shall have occasion to use a reverse path in subsequent sections, we digress for a moment to investigate this situation. Suppose that we take the standardized linear regression of Y on X, i.e. treating X as a cause and Y as an effect. Let U denote the residual (deviations from linearity), and let x and u be the respective path coefficients from X to Y and from U to Y. Then X and U are uncorrelated; and x = r(X,Y) and u = r(U,Y). Further, $x^2 + u^2 = 1$ for the complete determination of Y.

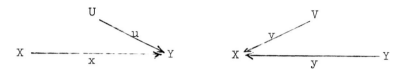

Now, let us reverse the process, taking the standardized linear regression of X on Y, with V as the residual uncorrelated with Y. Then, y = r(X,Y), v = r(X,V), and $y^2 + v^2 = 1$ for the complete determination of X. From these results we see that the path coefficient from X to Y is the same as that from Y to X, as x = y = r(X,Y) which does not change with the structure of a path diagram. It also follows that $u^2 = v^2$; that is, the fraction of determination by residuals also remains the same in both regressions. It may be shown that the two series of residuals, U and V, are correlated to the same degree as X and Y but with sign changed; that is, r(U,V) = - r(X,Y). In subsequent paragraphs we have occasion to make use of the fact that x(path from X to Y) = y(path from Y to X).

DOMINANCE AND GENOTYPE VALUE

Deferring environmental effects to the next section, we shall now introduce dominance and examine its effects on kinship correlations. Let Y be the (average) measurement of a genotype. For example, the average diastolic blood pressure of the genotypes NN, MN, MM, are Y = 85.3, 84.6, 81.7 mm Hg., respectively, among the Easter Islanders (Cruz-Coke, Nagel, & Etcheverry, 1964). Since the gene effects are not additive, the genotype values will not be linear and thus we write Y = L + D, where D represents dominance deviation; that is, deviation from linearity in the context of linear regression. Whatever the mating system practiced by a population, the least-squares fitting procedure always makes L and D uncorrelated, being a requirement of the normal equations. Hence,

$\sigma_Y^2 = \sigma_L^2 + \sigma_D^2$. The path coefficients from L to Y and from D to
Y are, respectively:

$$g = r(L,Y) = \sigma_L/\sigma_Y, \qquad d = r(D,Y) = \sigma_D/\sigma_Y$$

and
$$g^2 + d^2 = 1 \qquad (2)$$

for the complete determination of Y.

The kinship correlations may be read off Fig. 2, making
allowance for dominance effects (no environmental effects
yet). It is noted that the central portion of Fig. 2, consisting of the four L's, is the genetic core in Fig. 1. In
expanding the diagram from the core, several features should
be noted. First, we have assumed assortative mating; that is,
the primary correlation between parents is via their genotype
values Y, denoted by $m_Y = r_{PP}(Y,Y)$ at the top of Fig. 2. Then
the correlation between the parental L's, denoted by $m = m_L$,
is a consequence of the primary m_Y (Li, 1968). Second, we
note that the path is from Y to L for the parents because of
the primary nature of m_Y, while the path is from L to Y for
the offspring. In either case, the path coefficient involved
is $g = r(L,Y)$, as explained in the previous section on the reverse path. Combining these two features, we have

$$m = m_L = g(m_Y)g = g^2 m_Y \qquad (3)$$

The kinship correlations with respect to the genotype values
with dominance are (by summing all the connecting chains in
Fig. 2):

$$
\begin{aligned}
r_{PP}(Y,Y) &= m_Y && = m/g^2 \\
r_{PO}(Y,Y) &= \tfrac{1}{2}(1 + m_Y)g^2 && = \tfrac{1}{2}(g^2 + m) \\
r_{OO}(Y,Y) &= \tfrac{1}{2}(1 + m_L)g^2 + \tfrac{1}{4}d^2 &&= \tfrac{1}{4}(1 + g^2 + 2mg^2)
\end{aligned}
\qquad (4)
$$

When there is no dominance ($g = 1$, $d = 0$), then $m = m_L = m_Y$,
and this set of expressions becomes identical with (1). When
there is dominance ($g^2 < 1$, $d^2 > 0$), the relative magnitudes
of these correlations are no longer as simple as before. The
parent-offspring and sib-sib correlations are equal only when
$m = m_L = 1/2$. In most practical situations (even when m_Y
$= r_{PP}(Y,Y)$ is high), the genetic correlation between mates m
$= m_L$ is smaller than 1/2, and thus $r_{PO} < r_{OO}$. That is, dominance makes the sib-sib correlation higher than the parent-
offspring correlation under the usual condition $m < 1/2$.

Clearly, at the Y level (without environmental effects),
g^2 is a type of heritability and, indeed, it is in the true
sense of that term. We recall that L and D are uncorrelated

in determining the genotype value Y = L + D. In sexual reproduction, only the genes in the gametes are transmitted from
parents to offspring. The genotype of an offspring is formed
anew in each case, and is <u>not</u> inherited from his parent.
Translating this biological fact to statistical consequences,
we see that only the L values (of the genes) are transmitted
from parents to offspring (as shown in the genetic core of
Fig. 1), but the D values are not transmitted. They appear
anew as the genotype of an offspring is formed. In short, L
is heritable and D is not. In genetic literature there is no
particular name for g^2, although Fisher (1918) called d^2
$= 1 - g^2 = \sigma_D^2/\sigma_Y^2$ the "dominance ratio". For these reasons, we
may aptly call $g^2 = \sigma_L^2/\sigma_Y^2$ the <u>dominance heritability</u> (Li, 1975,
p. 254) to describe the effects of dominance on kinship corre-
lations. (Note: g^2, due to dominance only, is neither the
"broad" nor the "narrow" heritability to be discussed after
introducing the environmental effects.)

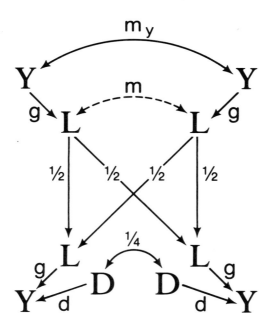

Fig. 2 Correlation when there is dominance between the
alleles of the same locus. Y = genotype value, D = dominance
deviation, and Y = L + D. At top, m_Y = correlation between the
Y values of the two parents. See (4) in text.

The only remaining feature of Fig. 2 that needs comment
is that the D values of full sibs are correlated to the degree
1/4. That this is true for random mating populations may be

easily demonstrated. Fisher's original treatise (1918) is abstruse, but apparently in his particular model and with his particular assumptions, he arrived at the result $r(D,D) = 1/4$ for full sibs in assortative mating populations as well. Further clarification on this point is overdue.

ENVIRONMENTAL EFFECTS AND PHENOTYPE

Environment refers to the aggregate of all the external conditions and influences affecting the life and development of an individual, resulting in his phenotype. Our surroundings are much varied. If examined in finest detail, the environment of no two individuals would be identical. By the same token, if the state of thousands of loci were considered simultaneously, the genotype of no two individuals would be identical. Such complexity would be unmanageable, and we would have no science of genetics. Science does not attempt to find out all the facts and laws of the universe at once, but proceeds piecemeal, working out one limited case after another, stating hypotheses that are subject to modification or rejection in the light of new knowledge gained by further studies. It is in this spirit that we shall first study the simplest type of environmental effects on kinship correlations.

The problem of directly measuring the totality of an environment is insurmountable and we are forced to construct some crude indices for certain aspects of the environment; this will be discussed later. For the time being, the magnitude of environmental effects on the formation of a phenotype may be estimated indirectly by studying the relative magnitude of the kinship correlations. This indirect method works reasonably well when we deal with random environmental effects on the phenotype. It is, therefore, the random environmental effects we shall study first.

We continue to use Y as the genotype value. Now let E be the random environmental effects on the measurement (Z) of the phenotype so that $Z = Y + E$, where Y and E are uncorrelated, and $\sigma_Z^2 = \sigma_Y^2 + \sigma_E^2$. By analogy with (2), we have the path coefficients from Y to Z and from E to Z, respectively:

$$h = r(Y,Z) = \sigma_Y/\sigma_Z, \qquad e = r(E,Z) = \sigma_E/\sigma_Z$$

and
$$h^2 + e^2 = 1 \tag{5}$$

for the complete determination of the phenotypic value Z. For such random environmental effects on phenotype, the kinship correlations may be read from Fig. 3, which is an extension of Fig. 2, which in turn is an extension of Fig. 1. Since E is uncorrelated with Y, it does not contribute to the kinship cor-

relation.   The primary correlation now is that between the
phenotypes of the parents, $r_{PP} = r_{PP}(Z,Z) = m_Z$, as shown at
the top of Fig. 3.   Then the genetic correlation (at the L
level) between the parents is $r_{PP}(L,L) = m = m_L = gh(r_{PP})hg$
$= g^2h^2m_Z$. The parent-parent, parent-offspring, and sib-sib
phenotype correlations (at the Z level) are, from Fig. 3,

$$r_{PP}(Z,Z) = m_Z = m/g^2h^2$$

$$r_{PO}(Z,Z) = \tfrac{1}{2}(1 + m_Z)\ g^2h^2 \qquad\qquad (6)$$

$$r_{OO}(Z,Z) = [\tfrac{1}{2}(1 + m)g^2 + \tfrac{1}{4}d^2]\ h^2$$

$$= \tfrac{1}{4}(1 + g^2 + 2mg^2)h^2$$

These are the classic results given by Fisher (1918), in which
$\mu = r_{PP}(Z,Z) = m_Z$, $c_1 = h^2$, $c_2 = g^2$, and $A = c_1c_2\mu = h^2g^2\ r_{PP}$
$= m_L = m$.   Thus, Fisher's results (6) are compatible with this
diagrammatic representation (Fig. 3).   Most of his other formulations of kinship correlation may also be represented by
path diagrams (Li, 1968).

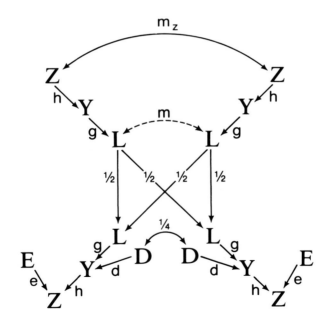

Fig. 3.   Correlation when there are both dominance and environmental effects (E) on phenotype (Z), but genotype and environment are not correlated.   See (6) in text.

As a parallel with the dominance heritability $g^2 = \sigma_L^2/\sigma_Y^2$ discussed previously, we may call $h^2 = \sigma_Y^2/\sigma_Z^2$ the environmental heritability, which depends only on the magnitude of the E effects on the phenotype and has nothing to do with dominance. In genetic literature, h^2 is called the "broad" heritability and $g^2h^2 = \sigma_L^2/\sigma_Z^2$ is called the "narrow" heritability. These terms do not distinguish the very different meaning of g^2 and h^2 and obscure the nature of the product g^2h^2.

Given a set of observed numerical values of r_{PP}, r_{PO}, r_{OO}, it is easy to solve (6) for the three unknowns: m, g^2, h^2. Then $e^2 = 1 - h^2$ gives us an indirect measure of the random environmental effects on the phenotype. The expressions (6) take no account of environmental effects other than random ones. When the sib-sib correlation is higher than the parent-child correlation, as is the case in most empirical studies, the solutions of (6) would yield a high value of h^2 (strong heredity) and a low value of g^2 (strong dominance), because only such conditions can make sib-sib correlation greater than parent-offspring correlation within the normal range of observations. In studying IQ test scores, Burt and Howard (1956) employed Fisher's correlation models (6); it is not surprising that high heritability and strong dominance are the two major findings of their studies. Jensen (1969 and later) seems to take the same tack, without realizing that these findings are direct consequences of the correlation models (6). However, the observation that $r_{OO} > r_{PO}$ may result from factors other than dominance. We shall investigate the simplest alternative in the next section.

COMMON FAMILY ENVIRONMENT

When a quantitative trait is assumed to be influenced by a large number of loci the importance of possible dominance of genes is not as great as in single locus traits, because in the case of multifactorial inheritance each allele is postulated to contribute a small quantity to the measurement of the phenotype. If we ignore dominance in the Mendelian sense and assume Y = L and D = O, so that g = 1, and d = 0, the higher value of the sib-sib correlation may be attributed to common family environmental conditions, a variable that is missing from the expression (6).

There is yet another reason to ignore dominance and adopt a strictly linear model with additive gene effects. It is the complicated nature of the inheritance of the dominance deviations D. Fisher's results show that the D's of full sibs are correlated to the degree 1/4 but L and D are not correlated for any pair of relatives, just as in random mating populations. This is a pleasingly simple result, but the precise

relationship may be more complicated in the presence of assortative mating. Wright (1952, p. 18) observes: "Assortative mating introduces a correlation between dominance deviations of parents and offspring and between dominance deviations of either and additive deviations of the other. Accurate
deduction of heritability thus becomes practically impossible
if there is appreciable assortative mating in the presence of
dominance." In view of this complication we should probably
limit ourselves to the case of no dominance in assortative
mating populations, at least for the time being.

Now we let g = 1, that is, Y = L and D = 0 (Fig. 4). In
contradistinction to the random elements E of the environment,
we use Γ to designate the systematic elements of the environment that exist in the common home of full sibs. It is these
systematic elements of the home environment that contribute to
the correlation between full sibs. In Fig. 4, γ is the path
coefficient from common environment Γ to phenotype Z, so that
the contribution of Γ to the sib-sib correlation is γ^2. Then
the three main kinship correlations are (Fig. 4):

$$r_{PP} = m_Z = m_o/h_o^2$$

$$r_{PO} = \tfrac{1}{2}(1 + m_Z)\, h_o^2 \qquad\qquad (7)$$

$$r_{OO} = \tfrac{1}{2}(1 + m_o)\, h_o^2 + \gamma^2$$

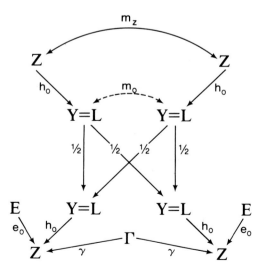

Fig. 4. Correlation when there is no dominance (L = Y),
but there are common elements (Γ) in the home environment contributing to the correlation between sibs. See (7) in text.

where $h_o^2 + e_o^2 + \gamma^2 = 1$ for the complete determination of
phenotype Z. The subscript (o) attached to h, e, and m in
expressions (7) serves to remind us they refer to Fig. 4
(with Γ). In general, when a new variable is added or deleted
from a path diagram all the path coefficients in that diagram
will be affected. The introduction of a separate factor
(called Γ here) for elements common to full sibs is not new,
and was employed by Wright in 1921 (p. 116).

Note that we have preserved the original meaning of E,
the random elements of the environment uncorrelated with genotype Y or with E of another individual in both Fig. 3 and Fig.
4. Some investigators prefer to use E to denote all environment elements, random as well as systematic. In such a case,
the contribution of the common elements of the family to sib-
sib correlation would be $e^2 \cdot r(E,E)$.

Both (6) and (7) can accommodate the observed fact r_{OO}
> r_{PO} reported in many studies. It would not be fruitful to
debate which model is closer to the true biological situation
(which is unknown) although Li (1975, pp. 323-324) applied (7)
to Jencks' data (1972, Appendix A).

However, we can examine the relationships between models
(6) and (7). Given a set of observed values of r_{PP}, r_{PO}, r_{OO},
all at the Z level, we will find that the genetic correlation
between parents remains the same in both models; that is,
$m_o = m = m_L$. The relationships between the other components
are:

$$h_o^2 = g^2 h^2, \qquad e_o^2 = \tfrac{3}{4} d^2 h^2 + e^2, \qquad \gamma^2 = \tfrac{1}{4} d^2 h^2 \qquad (8)$$

so that $h_o^2 + e_o^2 + \gamma^2 = (g^2 + d^2)h^2 + e^2 = h^2 + e^2 = 1$. The
relations (8) represent the shuffle of the various components
between the correlation models (6) and (7). First, we note
$h_o^2 < h^2$, because $g^2 < 1$. That is, model (7) always yields a
lower environmental heritability than model (6). Second,
$e_o^2 > e^2$; that is (7) allows for a greater role of the random
environmental effects. Finally, the "dominance effect"
$\tfrac{1}{4} d^2 h^2$ of (6) is construed as common family environmental effects γ^2 in the model represented by equations (7). The practical implications of the results of the two sets of estimates
of environmental and genetic effects on the phenotype could be
profoundly different. Investigators should be very clear a-
bout the capabilities and limitations of each model in interpreting the results of their analysis.

CORRELATION BETWEEN HALF-SIBS

The study of half-sibs correlation is scarce, but the situation may change in the near future. With early marriage, ear-

ly divorce, and early remarriage, there are a large number of
half-sibs in the population. The half-sibs are closely related in the genetic sense and may be reared either apart or together. They are unlike adopted children who are subject to
selection bias in the adoption process. The half-sibs will be
a potential source of material for the study of general and ⸻
special home environmental effects.

From (6) we may solve for g^2, h^2, and m; and from (7) we
may solve for γ^2, h^2, and m. If we wish to include both dominance (g^2) and common home environment (γ^2) in the study, then
we need a fourth equation based on the correlation between
some other relatives. The correlation between half-sibs will
provide the needed fourth equation, thus enabling us to separate the effects of dominance and common home environment (Li,
1977), which are usually confounded in the evaluation of sib-
sib correlations (Wright, 1952, p. 18).

Fig. 5 shows the relationship between half-sibs reared
together by the common parent L_0 (mother, say). The phenotypes of the three parents are not shown in the diagram, because only the genetic correlations (m = m_L) between the parents are needed to derive the half-sib correlation. It is also to be noted that the two fathers (L_1 and L_2) are assumed to
be correlated to the same degree m as the mates are. This is
equivalent to assuming that there is no change in the mating
behavior of the common parent, her two mates being chosen from
the same assortative group (subpopulation). Any two individuals of the same assortative group are correlated to the same
degree, and this correlation does not depend on sex or marriage. More complicated models may be constructed so that the
correlation between the two fathers may range from m to m^2

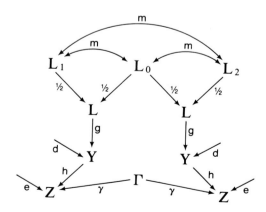

Fig. 5. Half-sib correlation. Dominance deviation D and
random environment E are not shown, as they do not contribute
to half-sib correlation. See (9) in text.

(Wright, personal communication), depending on the extent to
which the common parent changes her mating selection. In this
communication, without further empirical information on the
correlation between successive parents, it is reasonable to
assume $r(L_1, L_2) = m$, concurring with Rao, Morton, & Yee
(1974). From Fig. 5, we obtain

$$r_{0'0} = \tfrac{1}{4}(1 + 3m)\ g^2 h^2 + \gamma^2 \qquad\qquad (9)$$

where the subscripts 0'0 indicate half-sibs. This equation,
together with the three of (6), adding the term γ^2 to r_{00},
will yield estimates of the four parameters (m, g^2, h^2, γ^2).

In empirical studies it is perhaps worth noting that the
half-sibs should be chosen from the same population as the
other pairs of relatives, so that they have the same genetic
and environmental parameters. It is possible sometimes to
have the half-sibs from the same group of families, as a family may have both full sibs and half-sibs.

It is important to avoid bias in selecting the half-sibs
for study. Nichols (1970, cited by Loehlin, Lindzey &
Spuhler, 1975, p. 119) reported that the correlation between
full sibs with respect to height is 0.25 and that between
half-sibs is 0.43. This is not understandable on either genetic or environmental grounds, and can only be explained by a
sampling procedure that favors similar half-sibs or neglects
similar full sibs.

GENOTYPE-ENVIRONMENT CORRELATION AND CONSTANT h/e RATIO

Apparently different investigators have different definitions of environment. In the previous sections of this communication we have used E to denote those random elements of the
environment uncorrelated with the genotype or with each other,
and Γ to denote those systematic elements in the home environment being shared by the full sibs reared together. Of
course, there are many other kinds of elements in the environment that may affect the phenotype. Our main difficulty in
dealing with environment seems to be our inability to identify
and distinguish the relevant elements from the irrelevant
ones.

In most physical traits (e.g. height) which have a genetic component we may assume that environment and the genotype
are uncorrelated, as we can hardly claim that potentially tall
individuals tend to be born into homes with good nutrition.
In behavioral traits, however, the situation is more complicated. Certain behavioral traits can be directly learned from
parents and relatives (we cannot learn to be tall). When the

trait under consideration happens to be IQ test scores, many
investigators believe that the environment and genotype are
correlated to begin with in producing the phenotype. That is
to say, the individuals with the potential ability to achieve
high scores in tests tend to be born in better homes where
the child can learn more and earlier. Now we shall examine
the consequences of such an assumption.

The phenotype model is still $Z = Y + E$, but now Y and E
are assumed to be correlated to the degree $s = r(Y,E)$. Then,
for the complete determination of the phenotype we have, in
lieu of (5),

$$h^2 + e^2 + 2\,hse = 1 \tag{10}$$

Since $s < 1$, the direct effects of genotype and environment
($h^2 + e^2$) are always greater than their joint effect ($2hse$) on
the phenotypic variation. If heredity and environment act on
the phenotype the same way whether Y and E are correlated or
not, then the ratio of their respective path coefficients to
Z should remain the same whether Y and E are correlated or
not. That is, h/e will remain a constant, and so will h^2/e^2,
with varying values of s. Statistically it may be shown that
this is the case for two systems with the same ordinary multiple linear regression equation. The principle of constant h/e
ratio was employed by Wright (1931) when he formulated a new
equation for one system by "borrowing" the ratio of two path
coefficients of another system.

Rewriting (10) as $h^2 + e^2 = 1 - 2hse$ and dividing both
sides by $1 - 2hse$, we obtain

$$\frac{h^2}{1 - 2hse} + \frac{e^2}{1 - 2hse} = 1 \tag{11}$$

which attains the form $(h')^2 + (e')^2 = 1$ for uncorrelated Y
and E. Rao, Morton, & Yee (1974, 1976) have also assumed the
constancy of the ratio h/e without saying so explicitly. In
their notation, $\theta = 1/\sqrt{1 - 2hse} > 1$, so that $h' = h\theta$, e'
$= e\theta$, and $h'/e' = h/e$. In brief, the existence of $s = r(Y,E)$
will decrease the values of h^2 and e^2 but will not change
their ratio. In view of these considerations it seems that
the ratio h^2/e^2 is probably a better index to measure the relative hereditary and environmental influences, as it is independent of the genotype-environment correlation.

Since the existence of $s = r(Y,E)$ will decrease the value
of h^2, one might think that this would lower the estimates of
heritability and thus lessen the importance of heredity. This
would be the case only if h^2 alone measures the importance of
heredity. But this is not the case in general. When $s = 0$,
$h = r(Y,Z)$ = genotype-phenotype correlation; thus, either h or

h^2 may serve as a measure of the importance of heredity. However, when $s > 0$, the genotype-phenotype correlation is $r(Y,Z)$ = $h + se$ which in a sense measures the importance of heredity. Table I exhibits some numerical values of h^2, e^2, $2hse$, and $r(Y,Z)$ for various values of s with constant h^2/e^2 ratio It is seen that as s increases, h^2 and e^2 decrease and the joint term $2hse$ increases. The last column of the table shows that $r(Y,Z)$ increases with s despite the decrease of h^2. In summary, the existence of the genotype-environment correlation would increase the genotype-phenotype correlation.

Table I Fractions of Determination of the Phenotype
Variance and the Genotype-Phenotype Correlation for
Various Degrees of Genotype-Environment
Correlation. Upper Portion: $h^2/e^2 = 1$.
Lower Portion: $h^2/e^2 = 3$.

$s = r(Y,E)$	h^2	e^2	$2hse$	$r(Y,Z) = h + se$
$s =$ .00	.500	.500	0	.707
$s =$ .10	.455	.455	.091	.742
$s =$ .30	.385	.385	.231	.806
$s =$ .50	.333	.333	.333	.866
$s =$ .70	.294	.294	.412	.922
$s =$ 1.00	.250	.250	.500	1.000
$s =$ .00	.750	.250	0	.866
$s =$ .10	.690	.230	.080	.879
$s =$ .30	.595	.198	.206	.905
$s =$ .50	.523	.174	.302	.932
$s =$ .70	.467	.156	.377	.959
$s =$ 1.00	.402	.134	.464	1.000

Due to symmetry, the same conclusions hold with regard to the importance of environment. As s increases, the environment-phenotype correlation $r(E,Z) = e + sh$ also increases. That both $r(Y,Z)$ and $r(E,Z)$ increase with s reflects the fact that as s increases, Y and E gradually cease to be two distinct factors, as shown by the limiting situation $s = 1$ and thus $r(Y,Z) = h + e = 1$. This illustrates the meaning of joint determination. However, the point remains that the existence of genotype-environment correlation does not diminish the importance of heredity, nor of environment, but increases their correlations with the phenotype.

TENTATIVE MODELS

When genotype and environment are correlated, many different kinship correlation models may be constructed, depending on the assumptions, viewpoints, purposes, and available data of the investigator. The tentative models exhibited in Fig. 6 follow from the previous models discussed in this communication with the additional assumption that Y and E are correlated to the degree $s = r(Y,E)$. We continue to assume no dominance ($Y = L$ and $g = 1$) in the tentative models.

It may be reiterated that our assumption is assortative mating to be solely based on phenotypic resemblance. As to how the phenotype itself is determined, that is another question. Hence, the observed phenotypic correlation between the parents, $m_Z = r_{pp} = r_{pp}(Z,Z)$ shown at the top of Fig. 6, is the starting point of the correlation model. If the phenotype is partially determined by genetic factors, then the genes influencing the trait in the parents will also be correlated, albeit to a lesser degree. In other words, the genetic correlation $m = m_L = m_Y$ between the parents is a consequence of the primary phenotypic correlation m_Z.

With the basic assumption stated above, our first task is to find the path coefficient from parental phenotype to paren-

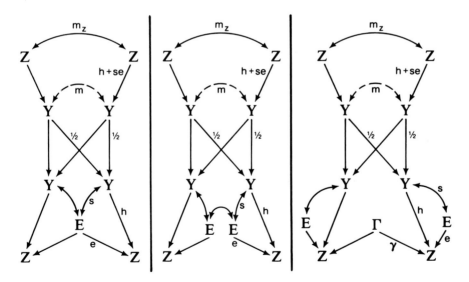

Fig. 6. Correlation when there is no dominance ($Y = L$), but there is genotype-environment correlation, $s = r(Y,E)$. Only half of the path coefficients are explicitly labelled on account of symmetry. See (14.0), (14.1), (14.2), (14.3) in text.

tal genotype; that is to say, we have to find the path from Z
to Y in the parent generation. We recall that $r(Y,Z) = h + se$.
The value of a correlation coefficient does not change with
the structure of a causal scheme. Now, in finding the reverse
path from Z to Y, we take the standardized linear regression
of Y on Z, as indicated in the following:

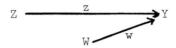

where W is the residual, uncorrelated with Z. Let the lower
case z and w be the path coefficients from Z to Y and from W
to Y, respectively. Then z is the correlation between Y and
Z. Hence,

$$z = r(Y,Z) = h + se \qquad (12)$$

as shown in the parental generation of Fig. 6. Since $z^2 + w^2$
$= 1$, we have from (12) and (10), $(h + se)^2 + w^2 = 1$, and w^2
$= e^2(1 - s^2)$. The genetic correlation between parents is thus

$$m = m_L = m_Y = (h + se)^2 m_Z \qquad (13)$$

The upper portions (up to offspring Y,Y) of the three diagrams
in Fig. 6 are the same. The lower portions are different, depending on how the environmental effects influence the full
sibs. In all three cases, however, the parent-parent and parent-offspring correlations are:

$$r_{PP} = m_Z = m/(h + se)^2$$
$$r_{PO} = \tfrac{1}{2}h(h + se)(1 + m_Z) \qquad (14.0)$$

The sib-sib correlations for the three cases vary with the al-
location of environmental effects. The expressions for such
correlations as well as that for complete determination of the
phenotype are as follows:

$$r_{OO} = \tfrac{1}{2}h^2(1 + m) + 2hse + e^2$$

Case (i). $\qquad\qquad\qquad\qquad\qquad\qquad\qquad\qquad (14.1)$

$$h^2 + 2hse + e^2 = 1$$

In this case the three observed kinship correlations (PP, PO,
OO) are sufficient to solve for the unknowns and there is no
need for the fourth correlation of half-sibs. In cases (ii)
and (iii), however, there is an extra parameter and a fourth

correlation is needed.

$$r_{00} = \tfrac{1}{2}h^2(1 + m) + [e^2 \cdot r(E,E)]$$

Case (ii). $\quad r_{0'0} = \tfrac{1}{4}h^2(1 + 3m) + [e^2 \cdot r(E,E)] \qquad\qquad (14.2)$

$$h^2 + 2hse + e^2 = 1$$

where $r(E,E)$ denotes the correlation between the E's of the two sibs.

$$r_{00} = \tfrac{1}{2}h^2 \quad + m) + \gamma^2$$

Case (iii). $\quad r_{0'0} = \tfrac{1}{4}h^2(1 + 3m) + \gamma^2 \qquad\qquad (14.3)$

$$h^2 + 2hse + e^2 + \gamma^2 = 1$$

Note that γ^2 is not equal to $e^2 \cdot r(E,E)$, as the expressions for the complete determination of a phenotype for the two cases are different.

It is a moot point to argue at this stage as to which model is closer to the true biological situation. Perhaps no single model can accommodate potentially very complicated and varying situations. We may note, however, that (14.1) corresponds to that given by Rao, Morton, and Yee (1976); while (14.2) involving $e^2 \cdot r(E,E)$ is somewhat similar to Wright's formulation (1969, Vol. 2, Chap. 11). In case (i), the entire environment E is assumed to be common to both sibs and this certainly exaggerates the environmental effects. The environments of two sibs would be regarded as the same only in terms of the crude indices for environment (see next section).

The only advantage of the tentative models suggested in Fig. 6 is that they involve a minimum number of parameters, the inclusion of s being compensated by the exclusion of g (no dominance). That the tentative models are inadequate to represent the true (unknown) biological situation goes without saying, but it is a step forward from Fig. 4.

ENVIRONMENTAL INDEX

There have been many other efforts to construct more realistic models for kinship correlations. Of these we shall discuss only one. Fig. 7 is a somewhat simplified version of that suggested by Rao, Morton, and Yee (1976, referred to as RMY subsequently) with some change of notation to render it roughly comparable to ours. In RMY's original diagram there are direct paths from parental E_1 and E_2 to child's E_0, which I omitted. Thus simplified, Fig. 7 becomes similar to that of

Jencks (1972, p. 268), except for the environmental indices.
The critical difference between Jencks' and our Fig. 7, however, is in the path coefficient from a parental genotype to
offspring's genotype. It may be shown that in an equilibrium
population that path coefficient is equal to 1/2 whether the
population practices random mating, inbreeding, or assortative
mating. Jencks assigns an independent parameter to that path
without obtaining a solution for it.

    We have noted in previous sections that the environment
consists of many different kinds of elements (random, systematic, general, special, etc.), the relevance or irrelevance
of which to the trait under consideration are essentially unknown. In fact, one of the purposes of study is to determine
which elements are relevant and which are not. The index for
environment is arbitrarily constructed, based on certain aspects of the environment that we thought might be a fair measure of the environment. Thus,

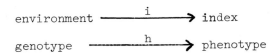

It is seen that the environment-index relationship is quite
analogous to the genotype-phenotype relationship. If we call
h^2 heritability, we may call i^2 measurability (of the environment). But their difference is equally important: a phenotype is observed while an index is constructed arbitrarily.
Different environmental scientists may construct different
indices for the same environment. The main contribution made
by the introduction of an environmental index is to clarify
our concept of the environment. What we have called the environment is not the true environment but merely a crude index for it. When an environment is said to be unimportant,
we may merely mean the index for it is poorly constructed.

    The practical consequence of introducing an environmental
index is that the correlations between two environmental indices and between an index and a phenotype may all be directly
observed. Statistically the introduction of additional parameters must be accompanied by additional observed correlations. The good intention of constructing a complicated model
is to try to represent the biological situation more closely,
but it often happens that our observations are so crude that
the data are fairly consistent with simple models but not with
complicated ones. Probably the basic difficulty is that the
manner in which the environmental elements affect the quantitative trait is not specifically known.

A CONTEMPORARY MODEL

Now we may turn our attention to Fig. 7, in which two parents (subscripts 1, 2) and one offspring (subscript 0) are shown. For each individual there are four variables (Z, Y, E, I), so there are twelve variables shown in that diagram. For each individual there are two observed variables: phenotype Z and environmental index I. Among these six observed variables there are altogether fifteen observed correlations. Among the four observed variables of the two parents, the six correlations are:

$$r(Z_1, Z_2) = h^2 m + e^2 u + 2\ hte$$

$$r(I_1, I_2) = i^2 u$$

$$r(I_1, Z_1) = r(I_2, Z_2) = i(e + sh) \tag{15}$$

$$r(I_1, Z_2) = r(I_2, Z_1) = i(th + ue)$$

We have introduced two simplifications to the original diagram. One is that the values of h and e are assumed to re-

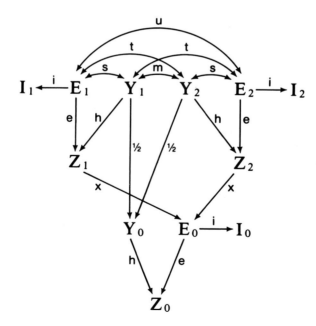

Fig. 7. Correlation model modified from Jencks (1972) and Rao, Morton & Yee (1976). I = index for environment E. No dominance (Y = L). See (15) and (16) in text.

main the same for the two generations in our Fig. 7, while in
the original diagram RMY allow for the possibility that they
may not. The second simplification is the omission of the direct paths from the parental E_1 and E_2 to the offspring E_0
mentioned above. E_1 and E_2 are childhood environments of the
parents. The childhood environment of the offspring, E_0, is
provided or at least influenced by the parental phenotypes,
but hardly by the childhood environment of the parents except
possibly by the atmosphere of some old furniture. Interestingly, RMY have designated this path coefficient by f. My
omission of f is to allocate more role to the people than to
the furniture.

Comparing the upper portion of Figs. 6 and 7, we see the
basic difference between the two models. It is not the presence of the environmental indices at all. In the former,
$m = m_L = m_Y$ is indicated by dotted line (redundancy, already
representated by $(h + se)^2 m_Z$), as it is a consequence of the
parental phenotypic correlation, $m_Z = r(Z_1,Z_2)$. In the latter,
$m = m_L = m_Y$ is an independent parameter (solid line) which
contributes $h^2 m$ to the observed $r(Z_1,Z_2)$. That is, the genetic correlation between the parents constitute a cause for the
assortative mating. The formulation of the parental relations
in Fig. 7 is analogous to the situation described by Wright
(1921, p. 151; 1969, Vol. 2, Chap. 11; also see Li, 1975, pp.
292-293), in which Y and E are uncorrelated ($h^2 + e^2 = 1$).

The remaining nine correlations involving the offspring
may also be obtained from Fig. 7. The correlations fall into
four pairs plus $r(I_0,Z_0)$. Consider $r(Z_0,Z_1)$. It must be the
same as $r(Z_0,Z_2)$ due to the symmetry of the relations of the
offspring with either parent. In tracing the connections between Z_0 and Z_1, it is best to proceed systematically. Z_0 is
connected with Z_1 either through Y_0 or through E_0. So the
connecting chains fall into two groups; each group of chains
may be traced out separately. Proceeding this way, we obtain

$$r(Z_0,Z_1) = r(Z_0,Z_2) = \tfrac{1}{2}h^2(1 + m) + \tfrac{1}{2}he(s + t) +$$
$$ex[1 + r(Z_1,Z_2)]$$

$$r(I_0,Z_1) = r(I_0,Z_2) = ix[1 + r(Z_1,Z_2)]$$

$$r(Z_0,I_1) = r(Z_0,I_2) = \tfrac{1}{2}ih(s + t) + iex(e + hs +$$
$$ht + eu)$$

$$r(I_0,I_1) = r(I_0,I_2) = i^2x(e + hs + ht + eu)$$

$$r(Z_0,I_0) = i(e + s_0h)$$

(16)

where

$$s_0 = r(Y_0, E_0) = hx(1 + m) + ex(s + t) = s \qquad (17)$$

assuming the s value remains the same in successive generations. These, (15) and (16), are the fifteen correlations directly calculated from Fig. 7.

In our simpler model (Fig. 6), s = r(Y,E) is an <u>unanalyzed</u> correlation which includes all causes, whatever they may be. In RMY's model (Fig. 7), the genotype-environment correlation s has a specified structure as shown in (17), from which we get

$$s = \frac{hx(1 + m) + ext}{1 - ex} \qquad (18)$$

Here s is not an independent parameter but a function of (m, h, e, t, x), another characteristic of RMY's model. It is not clear whether it is better to leave s unanalyzed and thus all inclusive, or to restrict the sources of the correlation to the few specified by the model.

The sib-sib correlation under model Fig. 7 could be complicated, but RMY assume one and the same E for both sibs, as indicated in case (i) of Fig. 6. Hence, the sib-sib phenotypic correlation given by RMY is the same as (14.1). We have already noted that this assumption exaggerates the influence of common environment, as no two individuals can have identical environments. If r(E,E) were introduced as in our case (ii) of Fig. 6, the sib-sib correlation would be much reduced. The correlation between half-sibs reared together by the common parent is very involved in RMY's model and we shall not reproduce it here. It becomes clear that RMY's model involves many parameters and requires many observed correlations for the unique solution of the simultaneous equations. Some of the algebraic difficulties we may encounter in solving such a system have been discussed by Goldberger (1977, and in this volume).

DISCUSSION

I have not intended this as a history of the kinship correlation models but have given a brief survey of such models, ranging from the genetic core to contemporary ones. Criticism may be raised against every one of them, including the genetic core. Obviously, the genetic core would not be true if sex-linked loci are also playing a role in the determination of the trait. However, every scientific formulation of a rela-

tionship between variables has its limitations and range of
validity. In spite of the many imperfections existing in the
kinship correlation models (as it is the case in all scientific models) I believe we have made some progress in constructing such models, although they are still far from the
truth. Much of this progress is due to criticism of the
existing ones; it is criticism that leads to the improvement
of models.

However, the difference between science and non-science
is not the "truth" contained in their statements. Science
often errs and non-science may stumble onto truth. A prediction made by an astrologer may turn out to be true.
According to Popper (1965, 1968) the demarcation between science and non-science is testability. The busy reader may
consult Magee (1973) for a summary of Popper's arguments.
Briefly, a scientific hypothesis must be capable of being
tested and thus refutable or falsifiable. That is to say, a
scientific hypothesis must be susceptible of being disproved
(Li, 1971, p. 178). If a proposal is couched in such flexi-
ble and vague terms that it can explain everything and whatever happens always confirms it, then it is not testable because there will never be any evidence against it.

Popper's demarcation between science and non-science has
many important implications. The criterion of testability
implies that a scientific hypothesis must have concrete and
informative content; otherwise there would not be anything to
be tested. From this view follows one of my pet phrases:
the usefulness of a wrong statement and the uselessness of a
correct one. Let me explain that immediately. Suppose that
sometime after lunch I asked you "What is the time?" and you
answered "Between 1:00 and 2:00". The answer turned out to
be wrong, as the true time happens to be 2:25. To avoid the
risk of being wrong you could have answered "Between 9:00 A.M.
and 9:00 P.M." which is certainly correct. But between these
two answers I prefer the wrong one, as it tells me something
about the time; the correct one tells me next to nothing.
The difference between these two answers is in their information content. "Between 1:00 and 2:00" is full of content and
thus has high refutability; while "between 9 A.M. and 9 P.M."
has hardly any informative content. A zero-content statement
carries no risk of being wrong.

The considerations above have immediate applications to
the controversy about heritability estimates derived from kinship correlations. If one claims that his data on a certain
trait yield an estimate of heritability of 75 - 80%, his
statement is concrete and informative, thus satisfying the
criterion of a scientific proposal, because it is fully exposed to the risk of being refuted and possibly replaced by a
better estimate. Even if the subsequent better estimate turns

out to be only 25 - 30%, the original (wrong) proposal has
played its role in the growth of knowledge. A statement of
that nature is to be preferred to a statement (or nonstate-
ment) such as "the heritability is between 0 and 0.99".

As a second example, suppose Dr. A claims: "Good environment can improve one's IQ". This statement has a low information content but it has enough to stimulate research
which may refute or enrich the statement with more substance.
Subsequently, Dr. B's research shows that "good environment
improves a child's IQ by one point per year" -- a statement
with more information and higher refutability than A's. This
is the way science progresses, replacing a low-content statement with a high-content one. Now, suppose Dr. A's reactions
are: "B's findings add no new knowledge; I knew it all the
time." Both sentences of A are false. B's findings do constitute new knowledge, especially to Dr. A, who did not know
that good environment improves IQ by one point per year. B's
claim, in turn, will be refuted, or corroborated, or modified,
or enriched with higher information content by future research.

In constructing kinship correlation models we realize
that the major difficulty is explicit description of the environmental effects on the phenotype and the various correlations. Naturally workers begin with simple models on the
principle of parsimony. In terms of Popper's philosophy,
this merely means that the simple models have the highest
refutability and we wish to get them out of our way first.
This, however, does not mean we should not use approximations
in practical work (which is a different thing from scientific
inquiry). Popper (1965, p. 56) says: ". . . from a prag-
matic point of view . . . false theories often serve well
enough: most formulae used in engineering or navigation are
known to be false, although they may be excellent approximations and easy to handle; and they are used with confidence
by people who know them to be false". Hence, if the presentations of the environmental effects in the correlation
models are wrong on theoretical grounds (and suppose they
are), our next question would be how good they are as approximations in practical work.

In formulating models describing environmental effects
on phenotype and kinship correlations we naturally look forward to having suggestions from the environmental scientists.
One of the more serious suggestions is "genotype-environment
interaction" which renders the simple models inadequate. The
interaction hypothesis is at the present time a low-content
statement with low refutability, as any two variables of any
system may be potentially interactive. The problem lies in
demonstrating its existence, in understanding its properties,
and in evaluating its importance. As a former plant breeder,

I have no doubt that genotypes and environment do interact
sometimes. Plant breeders can demonstrate by experiments that
certain varieties do not respond the same way to the same fer-
tilizer. In the field of behavior genetics, a modest beginning has already been made in studying genotype-environment
interactions with animal models (Cooper and Zubek, 1958) and
with simulated data (Rao and Morton, 1974). For a review see
Ehrman and Parsons (1976, especially p. 157). The point is
that the interaction hypothesis should be put in concrete
testable form and should not be vaguely stated as an escape
clause or as an explain-all.

Environmental scientists have many other conjectures and
hypotheses about the genotype-environment-phenotype relationship. Urbach (1974), in a long two-installment article, reviewed the arguments of the environmental scientists in great
detail; and showed that all the testable hypotheses are refuted. Although I disagree with Urbach on a number of points, I
think his main argument is well executed and scientifically
sound. His main criticism is that the arguments or counter
arguments offered by the environmentalists are mostly ad hoc
in nature, custom tailored for this or that particular case
only. A collection of ad hoc statements does not make a
science. Urbach (1974) calls this situation a "degeneration".
Urbach has apparently also been influenced by Popper who,
after having coined the word "ad hocness", says (1965, p. 61):
"the aim of science is to get explanatory theories which are
as little ad hoc as possible: a good theory is not ad hoc,
while a bad theory is".

Of course, nothing can be done about the non-testable
hypotheses, of which there are also many. With most of the
environmental hypotheses refuted (by Urbach), a non-testable
conjecture of extreme ad hocness arises, because it carries no
risk of being refuted. This remarkable conjecture says:
"One's environment is in his own head". Thus, one's environment is not his parents nor their income, nor his home, nor
his school or education, nor his neighborhood and friends, but
is something inside his head (just precisely where?). That
the "environment" is defined as the aggregate of all the external conditions surrounding us is conveniently forgotten.
With environment inside one's head, unique for each individual,
we can then explain every trait and every behavior of every
individual in terms of that inside environment, and indeed
explain nothing at all. We are·back to the zero-base again.

Recently statistical methods have been developed to test
whether the results of path analysis of kinship correlations
fit empirical observations. This is essentially a test of
goodness-of-fit by the chi-square criterion and is progress in
the sense that we have gained another tool with which to refute
certain hypotheses. If we use the statistical test as a tool

of refutation only, based on the badness-of-fit, we are probably on safe ground. But there always are people who take
"good fit" as evidence for the correctness, or at least for
the acceptability, of a hypothesis; and that is a very serious mistake in scientific inference. Only the falsity of a
theory can be inferred from empirical evidence. The truth,
being unknown, cannot be proved by empirical evidence. Neither confirmation (a little weaker situation) nor verification (a little stronger situation) by empirical evidence constitute a proof of the correctness of a theory. We merely
failed to disprove it. The same wrong undertakings will produce the same wrong results; and that is confirmation.

    The statistical test for goodness-of-fit, even when ex-
clusively used as a tool of refutation, is of low efficiency
in comparison with crucial and discriminating experimental
tests. A totally wrong theory may yield good fit with limited empirical observations by the criterion of chi-square. We
should continue to have attempted falsification of those models which have passed the goodness-of-fit tests. All interpretations based on such models, needless to say, are extremely fragile and tentative. Then, you may ask: "How about get-
ting more data?" That would help. But the growth of science
does not mean the accumulation of observations; it is an endless cycle of theory and observation followed by refutation.
The key of this vital process is refutation, without which
the process dies no matter how many observations may be accumulated.

    In the process of criticizing and refuting a scientific
hypothesis, it is immaterial as to who happens to be the author of that hypothesis. If the hypothesis happens to be
your own, you would spare no effort in the attempt to refute
or falsify it and be happy to see it replaced by a better one.
A scientist has no doctrine to preach, nor vested interest to
defend. He is a free man, completely liberated from the burden of any ideology or school of thought. This is not to say
that refuting one's own theory is easy, except for a few.
Thus, Albrecht Durer says: "But I shall let the little I have
learnt go forth into the day in order that someone better than
I may guess the truth, and in his work may prove and rebuke my
error. At this I shall rejoice that I was yet a means whereby
this truth has come to light." And John Carew Eccles says:
"I can now rejoice even in the falsification of a cherished
theory, because even this is a scientific success."

    In the discussions above I hope I have made it clear that
the successive refutations of scientific theories are not destructive forces but are stepping stones to progress and
growth of knowledge. If the existing theories on kinship correlations are not satisfactory (no existing theory is totally
satisfactory in any science), we have all the more reason to

intensify our attempt to refute them and replace them by more
satisfactory ones. There are, again, people who advocate
the complete cessation of research in this area, because they
feel there is no hope to reach a satisfactory model for kinship correlations. That comes close to nihilism.

In closing, I would like to answer one last question
that the reader may have in mind. If scientific progress
consists of a series of refutations and new conjectures, when
will it come to an end and reach the truth? It will not come
to an end. It is endless, because our ignorance is infinite.

SUMMARY

The models for kinship correlations under assortative
mating have been briefly reviewed and their characteristic
features have been pointed out. One major difficulty in constructing such models is to describe the environmental effects
on the phenotype. It is hoped that environmental scientists
would come up with concrete suggestions. It is emphasized
that criticism and refutation of existing models is a necessary step to obtain more satisfactory ones.

ACKNOWLEDGEMENT

I thank Professor Jerome H. Waller, my colleague at the
University of Pittsburgh, for reading the manuscript and making helpful comments. The nonsense that remains is mine.

REFERENCES

Burt, C. and Howard, M. 1956. The multifactorial theory of
    inheritance and its application to intelligence. Brit.
    J. Stat. Psychol. 8: 95 - 131.
Cooper, R. M. and Zubek, J. P. 1958. Effects of enriched
    and restricted early environments on the learning ability
    of bright and dull rats. Can. J. Psychol. 12: 159 - 164.
Cruz-Coke, R., Nagel, R. and Etcheverry, R. 1964. Effects of
    locus MN on diastolic blood pressure in a human popula-
    tion. Annals of Human Genetics 28: 39 - 48.
Ehrman, L. and Parsons, P. A. 1976. The genetics of behavior.
    Sinauer Associates, Sunderland, Mass.
Fisher, R. A. 1918. The correlation between relatives on the
    supposition of mendelian inheritance. Trans. Roy. Soc.
    Edinburgh 52: 399 - 433.

Goldberger, A.S. 1977. The non-resolution of inheritance by path analysis. Social Systems Res. Inst. Workshop Series 7709. U. of Wisconsin.

Goldberger, A.S. 1978. Models and methods in the IQ debate. This volume.

Holt, S. B. 1968. The genetics of dermal ridges. Charles C Thomas, Springfield, Illinois.

Jencks, C. et al. 1972. Inequality; a reassessment of the effect of family and schooling in America. Basic Books, New York.

Jensen, A. R. 1969. How much can we boost IQ and scholastic achievement? Harvard Educ. Rev. 39: 1 - 123.

Li, C. C. 1956. The concept of path coefficient and its impact on population genetics. Biometrics 12: 190 - 210.

Li, C. C. 1968. Fisher, Wright, and path coefficients. Biometrics 24: 471 - 483.

Li, C. C. 1971. A tale of two thermos bottles: properties of a genetic model for human intelligence. In Intelligence: Genetic and environmental influences (R. Cancro, Editor): 162 - 181.

Li, C. C. 1974. Assortative mating in man. Memorias de la II Reunion Nacional de la Sociedad Mexicana de Genetica: 48 - 108. Mazatlan, Mexico.

Li, C. C. 1975. Path analysis, a primer. Boxwood Press, Pacific Grove, CA. (second printing, 1977).

Li, C. C. 1976. First Course in population genetics. Boxwood Press, Pacific Grove, CA.

Li, C. C. 1977. Separation of common environment and dominance effects with classic kinship correlation models. Social Biol. 24: 259 - 266.

Loehlin, J. C., Lindzey, G. and Spuhler, J. N. 1975. Race differences in intelligence. W. H. Freeman, San Francisco.

Magee, B. 1973. Karl Popper. Viking Press, New York.

Popper, K. R. 1965. Conjectures and refutations; the growth of scientific knowledge. Harper & Row, New York.

Popper, K. R. 1968. The logic of scientific discovery. Harper & Row, New York.

Rao, D. C. and Morton, N. E. 1974. Path analysis of family resemblance in the presence of gene-environment interaction. Am. J. Human Genetics 26: 767 - 772.

Rao, D. C., Morton, N. E. and Yee, S. 1974. A linear model for familial correlation. Am. J. Human Genetics 26: 331 - 359.

Rao, D. C., Morton, N. E. and Yee, S. 1976. Resolution of cultural and biological inheritance by path analysis. Am. J. Human Genetics 28: 228 - 242.

Urbach, P. 1974. Progress and degeneration in the IQ debate. Brit. J. Phil. Sci. 25: 99 - 135; 235 - 259.

Weinberg, W. 1909. Uber Vererbunggsgesetze beim Menschen.
    Zeit. indukt. Abst. Vererbungs. 2: 276 - 330.
Weinberg, W. 1910. Weitere Beitrage zur Theorie der Verer-
    bung. Arch. Rassen-Ges. Biol. 7: 35 - 49; 169 - 173.
Wright, S. 1921. Systems of mating, I - V. Genetics 6:
    111 - 178.
Wright, S. 1931. Statistical methods in biology. Pro-
    ceedings Am. Stat. Assoc. 26: 155 - 163.
Wright, S. 1952. The genetics of variability. In Quantita-
    tive inheritance, pp. 5 - 41. Agric. Res. Council, Lon-
    don: Her Majesty's Stationary Office.
Wright, S. 1969. Evolution and the genetics of populations.
    Vol 2, The theory of gene frequency. U. of Chicago Press.

DISCUSSION

CHAKRABORTY: Dr. Li's comment on testability of models
calls for more research on power of resolution of genetic,
familial and environmental components of variation. It does
not simply constitute a mere estimation of these components
from a set of structural equations. The robustness of the
models is to be examined with data structures of different
kinds. For example, in the IQ research one must ask whether
any power is lost simply by extracting only the product-
moment correlations from the IQ scores and then building
models only on the basis of interdependence of these correlation coefficients. It may also be fruitful to examine the
adequacies of the alternate modes of analysis with the same
body of data.

RAO: This is a comment on the various ways of deriving
familial correlations for remote relatives involving multiple
spouses or spouses of sibs; each derivation makes certain
assumptions. To fix our ideas consider first cousins. Let
us restrict to genetic inheritance without the complication
of cultural inheritance (Figure 1). The correlational paths
with known values are curved downward in Figure 1 (e.g.,
genetic correlation between sibs = [1 + m]/2), whereas the
uncertain correlational paths are curved upward. For example,
the correlation $\rho_{G_1 G_{2S}}$ between the genotypes of ego (G_1) and
ego's sib's spouse (G_{2S}) is taken to be $\alpha(1 + m)/2$, where α

is arbitrary. Similarly, the correlation between spouses of sibs is

$$\rho_{G_{1S}G_{2S}} = \beta(1 + m)/2 \qquad (\alpha, \beta < 1)$$

Therefore the genotypic correlation between first cousins is

$$\rho_{G_X G_Y} = \tfrac{1}{4}[\frac{1 + m}{2} + 2\,\alpha(\frac{1 + m}{2}) + \beta(\frac{1 + m}{2})]$$

$$= \frac{(1 + m)(1 + 2\,\alpha + \beta)}{8}.$$

This general expression involves two unknowns, α and β. Fisher's result corresponds to $\rho_{G_X G_Y} = (\frac{1 + m}{2})^3$ which implies $1 + 2\alpha + \beta = (1 + m)^2$, or $\beta = m^2 + 2(m - \alpha)$. In particular, if $\alpha = m$, then $\beta = m^2$. Fisher seems to have accepted this without question, but it is only an assumption and not derivable mathematically. Nance and Corey (1976) wrongly inferred that the correlation between spouses of identical twins must be r^2, where r is the husband-wife correlation. Such multiplication of correlations is not admissible in path analysis.

Earlier we proposed $\alpha = \beta = m$ corresponding to population subdivision into strictly endogamous units (Rao et al., 1976) and therefore got

$$\rho_{G_X G_Y} = \frac{(1 + m)(1 + 3m)}{8} \text{ instead of } (\frac{1 + m}{2})^3.$$

On mathematical grounds neither result is more correct than the other: each involves an assumption. These uncertainties about the cross-correlations of the type $\rho_{G_1 G_{2S}}$ etc. do not arise if one restricts to nuclear families in which the marital parameters (m, u, s) are defined. It should be clear that Fisher's results, recent Birmingham models, and all other models involving spouses of relatives or multiple spouses are arbitrarily treated. Various models may be compared on data sets to see which assumption gives a better fit.

This complication in assortative mating is compounded with difficulties that arise through cultural inheritance in relationships more remote than nuclear families. Fortunately, nuclear families with indices are sufficient to determine the parameters of the general model (See Rao and Morton's paper in this book for details). Unusual and remote relationships provide additional tests of the model, but their special assumptions are not required for determinacy. It is fitting that nuclear families be the principal source of data, since they are the primary object of interest.

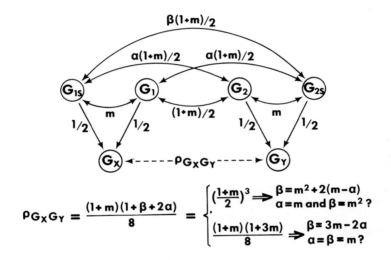

$$\rho_{G_X G_Y} = \frac{(1+m)(1+\beta+2\alpha)}{8} = \begin{cases} \left(\frac{1+m}{2}\right)^3 \Rightarrow \begin{array}{l} \beta = m^2 + 2(m-\alpha) \\ \alpha = m \text{ and } \beta = m^2 \, ? \end{array} \\ \\ \frac{(1+m)(1+3m)}{8} \Rightarrow \begin{array}{l} \beta = 3m - 2\alpha \\ \alpha = \beta = m \, ? \end{array} \end{cases}$$

Fig. 1. A path diagram for first cousins, showing all the relevant genotypes only. G_1, G_2 are genotypes of two sibs whose respective spouses' genotypes are G_{1S} and G_{2S}. G_X and G_Y are the genotypes of two first cousins. Here, α and β are arbitrary fractions.

REFERENCES

Nance, W.E., and Corey, L.A., <u>Genetics</u> 83, 811–826 (1976).
Rao, D.C., Morton, N.E., and Yee, S., <u>Am. J. Hum. Genet.</u>
    28, 228–242 (1976).

MORTON: In our work on path analysis we always assume a
residual environmental component (e) in addition to common
environment (our c, your γ). This is consistent with your
Figures 4 and 5, but not Figures 6 and 7 and the discussion
thereof. We never assume that the entire environment is
common to sibs unless this is required by a particular data
set as a logical constraint from the equation of complete
determination. Our experience supports deduction that
environmental indices with different values of i lead to the
same estimates of other parameters, notably c.
     I agree that the attempt to block research on family
resemblance "comes close to nihilism", in the Russian meaning
of <u>nigilizm</u> as a doctrine that conditions in the social
organization are so bad as to make destruction desirable for
its own sake, independent of any constructive program or
possibility. This is revolutionary propaganda masquerading
as peer review.

LI: It is difficult to establish exact correspondence
between your model (1976) and the ones sketched in my
communication. Strictly speaking, your model, though similar
to the one given by Jencks et al. (1972, p. 268) is <u>not</u>
assortative mating based on phenotypic resemblance only. For
instance, using your notation, if u = parental environmental
correlation and s = correlation between one parent's genotype
and the other parent's environment are both small, then the
correlation between parental phenotypes (P_F, P_M) will be

approximately equal to $(hz)^2 m$. Then, m = correlation between
parental genotypes will be <u>greater</u> than the correlation
between parental phenotypes, which is impossible for assortative mating based entirely on phenotypic resemblance. In
my model, I use $m = (h + se)^2 m_Z$ where m_Z is your $r(P_F, P_M)$.
This step is the same as that used by Jencks et al. (1972,
p. 273, 2(a)), although all other formulas are different.

SING: Path analysis is truly a remarkable example of the
development of a logical interaction between biological and
statistical analysis models. It is my reflection that
biological inferences from statistical analyses could be
greatly improved if we were to employ the path diagram and
its associated path model more often. In your opinion, what
are some of the more important reasons why path concepts have
been underutilized in biology? How does one handle the
situation where two a priori models seem appropriate? Is
there a goodness-of-fit test or other criteria?

LI: The path method has been "underutilized" in biology
(and in other fields), partly because we are overwhelmed by
the beauty and logic of formal statistical methods and partly
because we wish to be relieved of responsibility of using a
concept of our own. Consequently, many, if not most, of the
so-called "analyses" are simply based on pre-programmed
procedures, regardless of the particular meaning of each of
the variables under study, still less their possible step by
step relationships. When two or more tentative models are
equally consistent with observations, there is no immediate
way to distinguish them. Discriminating or crucial evidence
will have to come from further studies. This is the growth
of knowledge I discussed. Always keep in mind that there is
a strong possibility that further evidence may show none of
the models is correct. One of the points I emphasized here
is that goodness of fit does <u>not</u> prove the correctness of a
model, although a bad fit may help us to eliminate wrong
ones. Only the falsity of a theory can be inferred from
empirical evidence. Do not look for a miracle statistical
test that can prove the correctness of a theory.

MONOZYGOTIC TWIN KINSHIPS:

A NEW DESIGN FOR GENETIC AND EPIDEMIOLOGIC RESEARCH*

Walter E. Nance
Linda A. Corey
Joann A. Boughman

Medical College of Virginia
Richmond, Virginia

The greatest impediment to progress in the genetic analysis of quantitative inheritance in man has been the lack of a versatile genetic model for the resolution and estimation of relevant genetic and environmental variance components and not the absence of a theoretical basis for the interpretation of quantitative inheritance or a deficiency of suitable statistical procedures for the analysis of data. Classical twin studies and studies of nuclear family units simply do not provide a sufficient number of distinct relationships to permit an incisive resolution of the known causes of phenotypic variation. In order to estimate genetic and environmental variances from these data, it is frequently necessary to make assumptions which are untestable, implausible, or demonstrably false. For example, some investigators have tacitly assumed that the total genetic variances of monozygotic (MZ) and dizygotic (DZ) twins are equal despite marked genetic and ethnic difference in the frequency of DZ twins (1). Other

*This is paper #52 from the Department of Human Genetics and was supported by USPHS grants GM-21045 and HD-10291.

87

investigators have ignored the contribution of common environment to intrafamilial correlation or have assumed that
genetic effects in quantitative traits are invariably additive (2). When assumptions such as these are made repeatedly,
they acquire an aura of reality, and it becomes easy to ignore all evidence to the contrary or its logical consequences.
To circumvent these difficulties, the study of rare or abnormal relationships, such as MZ twins reared apart or adoptive
children, has frequently been advocated in the mistaken belief that only in this way could genetic and environmental
effects be unambiguously resolved. The investigation of separated MZ twins has recently become a topic that is of lively
historical interest (3), and the adoption paradigm will doubtless continue to provide useful information about foster parenting; but no serious investigator would deliberately choose
to draw inferences about normal individuals in the general
population from these relationships if similar conclusions
could be reached from studies of normal children raised in
their own homes by their biologic parents. Finally, the attempt to find truth by combining the results of independent
studies of different genetic relationships--behavioral studies which are separated in space and time by thousands of
miles and many decades--can only be likened to the alche-
mist's dream of converting lead into gold and should be rele-
gated to a comparable niche in the history of science(4).

I. DESCRIPTION OF MZ HALF-SIB MODEL

In 1972, we described a new model for the analysis of
quantitative inheritance in man which overcomes many of the
limitations of previous approaches (5). The method involves
the study of the families of identical twins: the twins
themselves, their spouses, and their offspring (Fig. 1). An
important advantage of the method is that each kinship contains individuals who share multiple unique relationships to
each other which can be exploited to resolve and estimate
many important genetic and environmental sources of variation,
thus avoiding the necessity of pooling heterogeneous bodies
of data. For example, the children of a twin are full-sibs
to each other but are also related in the same way as half-
sibs to the offspring of the co-twin. This remarkable relationship permits a clear resolution of additive and dominance
effects from observations on individuals who are members of
the same generation as well as the detection of epistatic
interactions. Maternal effects may be estimated by contrasting the analysis for male and female twins. To the extent
that maternal effects influence a trait, they will augment
the similarity of the offspring of female twins and increase

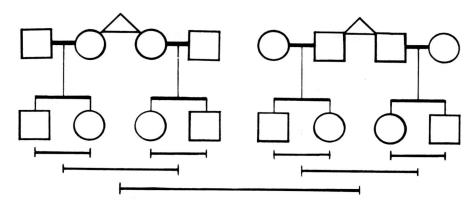

Fig. 1. Structure of data from monozygotic twin half-sibships. Lines below pedigree suggest how offspring data may be partitioned by a nested analysis of variance into among half-sibship, between sibship within half-sibship, and within sibship mean squares.

the differences between sibship means for the offspring of male twins whose mothers are genetically unrelated. Analysis of parental data permits resolution of the usually confounded effects of common environment and assortative mating, by comparing the husband-wife covariance with that observed between the spouses of the twins. Finally, in contrast to conventional half-sibships resulting from the death of a parent, divorce, or illegitimacy, there are no systematic parity differences between MZ twin half-sibs, and all of the parents are usually available for study.

Elsewhere we have described the model and the method of analysis in detail (6,7). Data from the offspring of male and female twins may be partitioned by a nested analysis of variance into among half-sibships, between sibships within half-sibships, and within sibships mean squares. These mean squares may in turn be expressed in terms of their constituent genetic and environmental variance components, providing a total of five distinct equations of estimation (Table 1). Additional equations can be derived from the parental data as well as from the multiple parent-offspring relationships. We have elected to solve appropriate sets of equations of estimation by an iterative weighted least squares procedure. If the original observations are normally distributed, the resulting solutions are regarded by many as being equivalent to maximum likelihood estimates (8). An important feature of our method is that the weighting matrix we use contains both diagonal weights and off-diagonal constraints, the latter to adjust appropriately for the non-independence of the interrelated

TABLE 1: Genetic Interpretation of Variance Components and Covariances Derived from the Children of Monozygotic Twins and Their Parents

Observed variance component or covariance		V_A	V_D	V_{AA}	V_M	V_{EH}	V_{ES}	V_{EW}
Offspring data								
[a] Among male half-sibships	$\sigma^2_{A\male}$	1/4	0	1/16	0	1	0	0
[b] Between sibships within male half-sibships	$\sigma^2_{B\male}$	1/4	1/4	3/16	1	0	1	0
[c] Within sibships	σ^2_W	1/2	3/4	3/4	0	0	0	1
[d] Between sibships within female half-sibships	$\sigma^2_{B\female}$	1/4	1/4	3/16	0	0	1	0
[e] Among female half-sibships	$\sigma^2_{A\female}$	1/4	0	1/16	1	1	0	0
Parental data								
[f] Among twin pairs	σ^2_{AT}	1	1	1	1	1	0	0
[g] Within twin pairs	σ^2_{WT}	0	0	0	0	0	1	1
[h] Husband-wife covariance	cov HW	0	0	0	0	1	1	0
[i] Spouse-spouse covariance	cov SS	0	0	0	0	1	0	0

Header span: "Genetic and environmental subcomponents" covers columns V_A through V_{EW}.

variances and covariances used in the analysis (9). With this procedure, estimates can be obtained of the additive genetic variance, V_A, the dominance variance, V_D, the additive epistatic effects, V_{AA}, the maternal effects, V_M, and three environmental components corresponding to sources of environmental variance acting among half-sibships, V_{EH}, between sibships within half-sibships, V_{ES}, and within sibships, V_{EW}.

The model permits the exploration of a broad range of alternative genetic explanations for a given data set. With seven available variables, 127 models of causation are theoretically possible for each set of equations selected for analysis. However, it is seldom possible to obtain valid simultaneous estimates of all seven parameters. Frequently, a particular model will yield negative variance component estimates for one or more variables, a finding which we interpret as an indication that the model does not fit the data. Other possible solutions can be rejected because they are inconsistent with the equations selected for analysis or are biologically implausible. For example, we are reluctant to place much reliance on solutions that do not include V_{EW} since most of the variables we deal with include experimental error or other sources of random variation. Similarly, we are a bit skeptical about solutions that include variables whose estimates are much smaller than their standard errors, even if these models fit the data well. Finally, if a univariate F-test of the mean squares from the offspring data gives evidence for a significant maternal effect, we are strongly biased towards models that include V_M. Our current practice is to attempt to fit genetic models to various combinations of equations in order to identify the biologically plausible solutions that lead to all positive variance component estimates. A choice between alternative models may then be made by comparing the χ^2 goodness of fit associated with each solution.

By partitioning the data from families of male and female twins into half-fraternities and half-sororities, we have shown how the model may be readily extended to separate the effects of X-linked and autosomal genes on quantitative traits (6). In this case, the offspring data alone yield 12 equations of estimation, and 15 additional functions may be derived from the parental data and the parent-offspring relationships. In general, we have tended to avoid the use of parent-offspring covariances in our estimation procedures because of our bias against the use of trans-generational comparisons in human quantitative genetics. Although the use of these relationships may be appropriate for some traits, such as total ridge count, one can think of many other traits in which qualitative changes in the environment may invalidate parent-offspring comparisons.

II. EXTENSION OF THE MODEL TO THE GRANDCHILDREN OF MZ TWINS

Corey, Nance and Berg have recently shown how the MZ half-sib model can be extended to include the F_2 generation (10). As shown in Fig. 2, the grandchildren of identical twins are related to each other in the same way as $1\frac{1}{2}$ cousins, and when all possible combinations of the sexes are considered, there are 20 distinct types of $1\frac{1}{2}$-cousin relationships. As in the

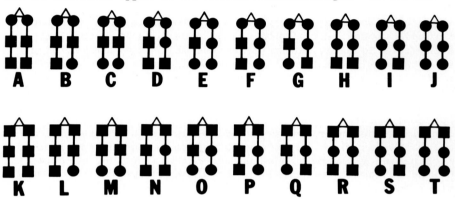

Fig. 2. Pedigrees showing twenty distinct $1\frac{1}{2}$-cousin relationships that exist among the grandchildren of monozygotic twins.

half-sib model, data from the grandchildren may be partitioned by a nested analysis of variance. However, in this circumstance there are four partitions of the data: among $1\frac{1}{2}$ cousibships, ak; between first cousinships within $1\frac{1}{2}$ cousinships, bc; between sibships within first cousinships, bs; and within sibships, ws. In conjunction with the previously described MZ twin half-sib relationships given by data from the parents and grandparents, observations on the grandchildren provide a powerful and definite set of equations for the analysis of quantitative inheritance in man. Of particular interest, the data on grandchildren permit a more detailed analysis of maternal effects, with resolution of variation arising from heritable cytoplasmic factors from that attributable to the additive or dominance effects of nuclear genes in the mother. In Fig. 2, for example, the covariance of matrilineal grandchildren of female twins (H,I,J) will include similarities attributable to both X-linked genes and cytoplasmic effects. The covariance of the offspring of women whose fathers are twins will include only the former effect (R,S,T), while the covariance of patrilineal grandchildren of male twins (K,L,M) will include neither of the effects. These relationships are reflected in Table 2, where the expected contributions of X-linked and autosomal genes as well as maternal, cytoplasmic, and environmental factors are given to the variance components derived from a nested analysis of variance of data from the grandchildren in 12 of the kinship types shown in Fig. 2. Equations derived from these relationships permit estimation of the additive and dominance effects of autosomal genes V_A and V_D, sex-linked genes V_{AX} and V_{DX}, and the maternal influences V_{AM} and V_{DM}, as well as cytoplasmic effects V_C and four environmental components, corresponding to sources of environmental variation acting among kinships V_{EK}, between first cousinships within 1½ cousinships V_{EC}, between sibships within first cousinships V_{ES}, and within sibships V_{EW}. Note that variation attributable to cytoplasmic effects appears in the among kinship component, σ_{ak}^2 for pedigree types H and J, in the between cousinships component, σ_{bc}^2 for pedigree types R and T, and in the between sibship component, σ_{bs}^2 for pedigree types A,C,K, and M. We do not claim that stable heritable cytoplasmic effects have been demonstrated in man. However, there are many aspects of the metabolic function of mito- chondria in fatty acid synthesis and energy transfer, for example, that could conceivably be altered by heritable cytoplasmic differences. Since maternal effects are known to influence a growing number of metric traits, the formal distinction between maternal and cytoplasmic effects has become an important issue. Consequently, we believe that the time has come to abandon the use of genetic models that offer no realistic hope of resolving genetic, environmental, and maternal sources of variation or of distinguishing between the nuclear and cytoplasmic effects of the maternal genome.

Other approaches to the analysis of data from these families are doubtless possible, including path analysis (4) and maximum likelihood estimation (11) and should lead to comparable results. Controversy over the relative merits of different analytic approaches is a matter for technicians to resolve and should not discourage widespread use of the model for genetic and epidemiologic research. It suffices to say here that we initially selected the weighted iterative least square approach because the data are highly structured and seemed to lend themselves so naturally to a hierarchical analysis of variance. In the half-sib model, this approach yields six mutually orthogonal mean squares from the offspring data which can be used to estimate unknown genetic and environmental variance components instead of the two full-sib and two half-sib correlations provided by the path analysis approach. We regard the inclusion of diagonal constraints in our weighting matrix to be a very important feature of our model. We do not believe it is proper to treat the multiple correlations derived from these data as if they were independent parameters, as Rao and Morton have done in their 1976 article

TABLE 2: Genetic Interpretation by Pedigree Type (see Fig. 2) of Variance Components Derived from Nested ANOVA of Data on the Grandchildren of Monozygotic Twins

Var. comp.	Genetic and environmental sources of variation										
	V_A	V_{AX}	V_D	V_{DX}	V_{AM}	V_{DM}	V_C	V_{EK}	V_{EC}	V_{ES}	V_{EW}
A σ^2_{ak}	1/16	0	0	0	0	0	0	1	0	0	0
σ^2_{bc}	1/16	0	0	0	0	0	0	0	1	0	0
σ^2_{bs}	3/8	1	1/4	0	1	1	1	0	0	1	0
σ^2_{ws}	1/2	1	3/4	0	0	0	0	0	0	0	1
C σ^2_{ak}	1/16	1/4	0	0	1/4	0	0	1	0	0	0
σ^2_{bc}	1/16	0	0	0	1/4	1/4	0	0	1	0	0
σ^2_{bs}	3/8	1/2	1/4	1/2	1/2	3/4	1	0	0	1	0
σ^2_{ws}	1/2	1/4	3/4	1/2	0	0	0	0	0	0	1
D σ^2_{ak}	1/16	0	0	0	0	0	0	1	0	0	0
σ^2_{bc}	1/16	3/8	0	0	1/4	1/8	1/2	0	1	0	0
σ^2_{bs}	3/8	5/8	1/4	0	3/4	7/8	1/2	0	0	1	0
σ^2_{ws}	1/2	1	3/4	0	0	0	0	0	0	0	1
E σ^2_{ak}	1/16	1/8	0	0	0	0	0	1	0	0	0
σ^2_{bc}	1/16	3/32	0	1/8	1/4	1/8	1/2	0	1	0	0
σ^2_{bs}	3/8	17/32	1/4	7/8	3/4	7/8	1/2	0	0	1	0
σ^2_{ws}	1/2	1/4	3/4	0	0	0	0	0	0	0	1
H σ^2_{ak}	1/16	1/4	0	0	1/4	0	1	1	0	0	0
σ^2_{bc}	1/16	1/2	0	0	1/4	1/4	0	0	1	0	0
σ^2_{bs}	3/8	1/4	1/4	0	1/2	3/4	0	0	0	1	0
σ^2_{ws}	1/2	1	3/4	0	0	0	0	0	0	0	1
J σ^2_{ak}	1/16	1/16	0	0	1/4	0	1	1	0	0	0
σ^2_{bc}	1/16	1/8	0	0	1/4	1/4	0	0	1	0	0
σ^2_{bs}	3/8	9/16	1/4	1/2	1/2	3/4	0	0	0	1	0
σ^2_{ws}	1/2	1/4	3/4	1/2	0	0	0	0	0	0	1

TABLE 2 (continued)

Var. comp.	V_A	V_{AX}	V_D	V_{DX}	V_{AM}	V_{DM}	V_C	V_{EK}	V_{EC}	V_{ES}	V_{EW}
K σ^2_{ak}	1/16	0	0	0	0	0	0	1	0	0	0
σ^2_{bc}	1/16	0	0	0	0	0	0	0	1	0	0
σ^2_{bs}	3/8	1	1/4	0	1	1	1	0	0	1	0
σ^2_{ws}	1/2	1	3/4	0	0	0	0	0	0	0	1
M σ^2_{ak}	1/16	0	0	0	0	0	0	1	0	0	0
σ^2_{bc}	1/16	1/4	0	0	0	0	0	0	1	0	0
σ^2_{bs}	3/8	1/2	1/4	1/2	1	1	1	0	0	1	0
σ^2_{ws}	1/2	1/4	3/4	1/2	0	0	0	0	0	0	1
N σ^2_{ak}	1/16	0	0	0	0	0	0	1	0	0	0
σ^2_{bc}	1/16	3/8	0	0	1/4	1/8	1/2	0	1	0	0
σ^2_{bs}	3/8	5/8	1/4	0	3/4	7/8	1/2	0	0	1	0
σ^2_{ws}	1/2	1	3/4	0	0	0	0	0	0	0	1
O σ^2_{ak}	1/16	0	0	0	0	0	0	1	0	0	0
σ^2_{bc}	1/16	7/32	0	0	1/4	1/8	1/2	0	1	0	0
σ^2_{bs}	3/8	17/32	1/4	1/2	3/4	7/8	1/2	0	0	1	0
σ^2_{ws}	1/2	1/4	3/4	1/2	0	0	0	0	0	0	1
R σ^2_{ak}	1/16	1/2	0	0	1/4	0	0	1	0	0	0
σ^2_{bc}	1/16	1/4	0	0	1/4	1/4	1	0	1	0	0
σ^2_{bs}	3/8	1/4	1/4	0	1/2	3/4	0	0	0	1	0
σ^2_{ws}	1/2	1	3/4	0	0	0	0	0	0	0	1
T σ^2_{ak}	1/16	1/8	0	0	1/4	0	0	1	0	0	0
σ^2_{bc}	1/16	1/16	0	0	1/4	1/4	1	0	1	0	0
σ^2_{bs}	3/8	9/16	1/4	1/2	1/2	3/4	0	0	0	1	0
σ^2_{ws}	1/2	1/4	3/4	1/2	0	0	0	0	0	0	1

ak = among kinship; bc = between first cousinships within 1½ cousinships; bs = between sibships within first cousinships; ws = within sibships. Letters at left refer to pedigree types shown in Fig. 2.

(12). In our judgment this "improvement" in our model is
like painting a dimple on the Mona Lisa or remodeling the
Pieta with a sledgehammer as a madman tried to do in Rome
several years ago.

Eaves (11) has recently shown how the maximum likelihood
algorithm proposed by Lange et al. (13) can readily be extended to permit the inclusion of dominance, common environmental effects and other sources of variation. It seems
likely that this method may be further extended to obtain
estimates of all the variables included in our MZ kinship
model. In essence, this approach involves the iterative pairwise comparison of every individual in the study. Although
elegant in concept and simplicity, the required computer time
will vary exponentially with the sample size and thus the
analysis of large bodies of data may become prohibitively
expensive or hardware-dependent, or both. In contrast, once
the relevant covariances and mean squares have been calculated,
sample size does not alter the length of time required for an
iterative, weighted least square analysis.

III. ADVANTAGES OF TWIN STUDIES

A compelling advantage of MZ twins as subjects for genetic
research is their cooperativity. Twins and their families
almost instinctively perceive the unique way in which twins
are "experiments of nature," and willingly participate even in
arduous protocols without monetary compensation. We recently
completed a five-month double-blind co-twin control study
which involved the twice daily administration of medication,
the daily filling out of a complex symptom diary by the mother
for both twins, and the biweekly collection of urine samples
(14). All 44 pairs of twins who entered into the protocol
completed the study, a compliance rate that astounded the
clinical pharmacologists with whom we were collaborating. In
an era of increasing concern about informed consent, it can
be argued with considerable cogency that for some types of
research, particularly epidemiologic studies involving the
sampling of large populations of normal individuals, studies
of MZ twins may offer the best possible strategy for obtaining
a truly random sample of genotypes in the population.

Twin studies have often been criticized because of the
rarity and the intrinsic biases that may be introduced by the
close relationship of monozygotic twins. The present model is
sufficiently over-determined that the equations derived for
the twin parents can be omitted if desired. Alternatively, as
we think appropriate, the parent-offspring equations may be
omitted. Even if both sets are omitted, a sufficient number
of equations remain to obtain useful estimates of many vari-

ables. With respect to their rarity, even though monozygotic
twins occur only once in about 240 births, we have estimated
that since 1915, when multiple births first began to be specifically recorded on vital records in Virginia, a total of
14,250 monozygotic twin births have occurred. If a mortality
rate of 0.3 in infancy and childhood is assumed, these data
suggest that about 19,950 monozygotic twin-born individuals
from this state have survived to adult life. Since about 76%
of the current adult population is native-born, we estimate
that we could ascertain 13,950 twin-born individuals in the
state through their birth certificates. Even for a relatively
rare trait such as diabetes, it should be possible to identify
at least 150 MZ twin pairs among current state residents
through vital records, one or both of whom have diabetes. In
a pilot study we found that 131 of approximately 7,600 infants
born in the state during the past decade could be successfully
linked to native-born parents who were twins. These observations suggest that at least 400 of the 70,000 infants born in
the state each year have a native-born parent who is an identical twin. In addition to providing a valuable population
based ascertainment source for MZ half-sib families, these
children constitute a subpopulation which could be used to
monitor reproductive variables in the population.

Traditionally, geneticists have been content with opportu-
nistic sampling strategies and have tended to view the epidemiologist's obsessional concern about randomization, matched
controls, response rates, and compliance levels with detached
amusement. For many purposes, such as genetic linkage or
segregation analysis, haphazard ascertainment through affected
probands may be an entirely adequate approach. However, as
soon as we begin to draw the kinds of inferences about normal
populations that are implied by the use of a heritability
ratio, we should become much more concerned than we have in
the past about sampling and the biases that can be introduced
by self-selection and various types of stratification. For
example, no one doubts that the striking association between
skin color and the sickle cell haplotype that has persisted
in this country for more than nine generations is a manifestation of racial stratification. However, stratification is
seldom even mentioned as a possible explanation for the bur-
geoning number of HLA-disease associations that are being
reported. With respect to twins, our experiences with contact-
ing probands ascertained through vital records have been illu-
minating. We have encountered some individuals who did not
know they were twins and others who had not seen their co-twin
in years and had no idea where they were. Based on previous
impressions derived from studies largely involving self-
selected volunteers, we would have regarded twin pairs such as
these as being virtually unheard of. These observations

emphasize the importance of using population based samples whenever possible for twin research. The recording of multiple births on birth certificates greatly facilitates the identification of such samples.

Finally, we are convinced the MZ kinship model can profitably be extended to qualitative traits such as birth defects. We have recently initiated a retrospective study of MZ twins in the Norwegian twin registry in which we hope to test critically the multifactorial model for the inheritance of certain birth defects and to measure the importance of maternal effects on fertility, pregnancy loss, and congenital malformation. A prospective design would obviously be superior, but at present, one can only imagine how much more we would know today about the cases of birth defects if the monumental study of Stevenson et al. (15) or the collaborative perinatal study (16) had been confined to the offspring of MZ twins!

IV. APPLICATIONS OF THE MZ HALF-SIB MODEL

A. Study Population

We have studied several variables with the MZ half-sib model using data collected at Indianapolis before and while the senior author was Principal Investigator of the Indiana University Human Genetics Center. Fertile adult MZ twins were ascertained through hospital records, advertisement, self-referral, and referral by other twins who had participated in the study. All available members of a kindred were generally studied on the same day in an outpatient clinic setting or occasionally at home. The sample included only Caucasian twins who were generally from middle-class backgrounds and cannot be regarded as a random or population based sample of MZ twins. The possible effects of self-selection or of stratification in distorting the range of genotype or environments sampled in the study should be borne in mind. On the other hand, there would seem to be few intrinsic biases in a sample selected through monozygotic twin probands, since, in contrast to DZ twins, MZ twinning does not appear to be influenced in a straightforward manner by genetic factors, race, maternal age, parity, or fertility drugs (17).

B. Blood Pressure (18)

Blood pressure measurements were made by trained technical and professional personnel with a mercury manometer using the fourth Korotkoff sound to define the diastolic pressure. Measurements were collected on 252 offspring of 43 female MZ

twins and 132 offspring of 26 male twin pairs, as well as the
twins themselves and many of the spouses, a total of 616 individuals in all. The offspring ranged from 3 to 31 years in
age and the parents from 25 to 59 years. In our sample there
was no significant sex difference in blood pressure, but the
data were adjusted by regression to remove the effects of age
prior to the analysis. The results of fitting four genetic
models to the data on systolic blood pressure are summarized
in Table 3. The simplest interpretation, in terms of a single
random environmental effect, yielded a poor fit (I). A full
environmental model gave a better but still inadequate fit
(II), as did a simple genetic model (III). However, when V_M

TABLE 3:   Systolic Blood Pressure:
Estimated Variance Components and Percent of Total
Variance Derived from Equations [a]-[g] in Table 1.

Var. Comp.	I Est. ± SE	I % Tot. Var.	II Est. ± SE	II % Tot. Var.	III Est. ± SE	III % Tot. Var.	IV Est. ± SE	IV % Tot. Var.
				Genetic Model				
V_A	–	–	–	–	100.8 ±15.2	59	82.0 ±22.4	47
V_M	–	–	–	–	–	–	17.7 ±15.6	10
V_{EH}	–	–	66.3 ±13.7	36	–	–	–	–
V_{ES}	–	–	10.7 ± 8.9	6	–	–	–	–
V_{EW}	155.2 ±10.0	100	107.1 ± 9.2	58	69.4 ± 9.7	41	73.7 ±10.9	43
χ^2	238.4		17.9		11.36		9.17	
df	6		4		5		4	
P	<0.001		<0.001		<0.05		>0.05	

was included in the genetic model, a satisfactory fit was
achieved (IV). Although the standard error of V_M was large
when it was estimated simultaneously with V_A and V_{EW}, an F-
test showed that the covariance of maternal half-siblings was
significantly greater than that of paternal half-siblings
($F = 2.14$, df 42,25,$P < 0.05$). The cause of the maternal effect is unknown. It could arise from prenatal maternal influences, as is true of birth weight (see below) or from some
postnatal aspect of the environment that is strongly influenced by the mother. The fact that a symmetrical increase was
not observed in the between sibship component for male twins
suggests that the effect may be more environmental (i.e., differing V_{EH}'s) than genetic.

The analysis of diastolic pressure leads to somewhat different results, as shown in Table 4. Again, a simple environmental model was rejected (I), but a full environmental model
yielded a remarkably good fit and cannot be excluded as an
explanation for the data (II). The simple genetic interpretation (III) actually yielded a poorer fit than the full environ-

TABLE 4:   Diastolic Blood Pressure:
Estimated Variance Components and Percent of Total
Variance Derived from Equations [a]-[i] in Table 1.

Var.	\multicolumn{8}{c}{Genetic Model}							
Var. Comp.	\multicolumn{2}{c}{I}	\multicolumn{2}{c}{II}	\multicolumn{2}{c}{III}	\multicolumn{2}{c}{IV}
	Est. ± SE	% Tot. Var.	Est. ± SE	% Tot. Var.	Est. ± SE	% Tot. Var.	Est. ± SE	% Tot. Var.
V_A	–	–	–	–	66.2 ±10.6	55	41.4 ±14.6	33
V_{EH}	–	–	34.6 ±7.9	28	–	–	20.8 ±9.5	17
V_{ES}	–	–	7.2 ±6.2	6	–	–	2.4 ±6.8	2
V_{EW}	118.9 ±7.4	100	83.2 ±6.3	66	53.8 ±7.3	45	60.5 ±9.1	48
χ^2	\multicolumn{2}{c}{109.7}	\multicolumn{2}{c}{7.8}	\multicolumn{2}{c}{9.9}	\multicolumn{2}{c}{1.4}
df	\multicolumn{2}{c}{8}	\multicolumn{2}{c}{6}	\multicolumn{2}{c}{7}	\multicolumn{2}{c}{5}
P	\multicolumn{2}{c}{<0.001}	\multicolumn{2}{c}{≈0.25}	\multicolumn{2}{c}{>0.10}	\multicolumn{2}{c}{>0.90}

mental model. However, as shown in IV, when V_A was added to
the full environmental model, a significant improvement in fit
was achieved. Based on the results in III, we might have been
led to conclude that the heritability of diastolic blood pressure was 54%. A similar estimate of about 60% has been reported by Feinleib et al. (19). However, when all relevant
sources of environmental variation were included in the model,
the relative contribution of genetic factors fell to about 33%.
Since the environmental variance measured by V_{EH} and V_{ES} would
both contribute to the correlation of full-sibs, failure to
estimate these components could falsely inflate the evidence
for a genetic effect obtained from an analysis of conventional
nuclear family units.

C.   Total Ridge Count

The dermal ridge patterns of the fingertips are laid down
during the first trimester of fetal life and remain unchanged
thereafter. Previous studies have suggested that many features of the dermatoglyphic patterns of normal individuals are
strongly influenced by genetic factors. In particular, the
total digital ridge count has long been considered a classic
example of a polygenic trait. Total ridge counts were measured according to the method of Holt (20) in 362 offspring of
30 male and 44 female twin pairs, as well as in the twins
themselves and 104 spouses, a total of 614 individuals in all.
Since males are known to have a higher ridge count than females, a linear adjustment in the scores was made to remove
the effect of sex prior to the analysis. Preliminary analysis
of the offspring data showed no hint of a maternal effect.
The results of fitting several alternative models to equations
[a]-[g] from Table 1 are summarized in Table 5. As shown in
I and II, the simple and full environmental models can be rejected, but a surprising number of alternative genetic hypotheses were found to be consistent with the data. The simple
additive model (V) gave an excellent fit, but bivariate models
that assumed dominance or epistasis (III, IV) could not be
rejected on statistical grounds although many would regard
them as being biologically implausible. However, we consider
Model VI, which includes both additive and additive epistatic
effects, to be a very attractive explanation for the data,
and, considering the extent to which V_A and V_{AA} are confounded,
the standard errors of the estimates are remarkably small.
Finally, Model VII also fits the data well but the standard
error of V_{EH} is large, and the assumption that among half-
sibship environmental factors contribute to a trait that is
determined during the first trimester seems a bit tortuous.
Other more complex solutions did not fit the data.
In an attempt to substantiate further the existence of

TABLE 5: Total Ridge Count:
Estimates of Genetic and Environmental Variance Components
Derived from Relations [a]-[g] in Table 1.

Genetic Model

Var. Comp.	I Est. ± SE	II Est. ± SE	III Est. ± SE	IV Est. ± SE	V Est. ± SE	V % of Tot.	VI Est. ± SE	VI % of Tot.	VII Est. ± SE	VII % of Tot.	VIII Est. ± SE	VIII % of Tot.	IX Est. ± SE	IX % of Tot.	X Est. ± SE
V_A	—	—	—	—	2040 ±164	95	1051 ±978	54	2007 ±513	92	533 ±727	31	1960 ±876	86	2107 ±927
V_{AA}	—	—	—	1609 ±135	—		775 ±783	40	—	—	1078 ±635	64	181 ±694	8	-624 ±685
V_D	—	—	1578 ±133	—	—		—		—		—		—		—
V_{EH}	—	2228 ±285	—	—	—		—		65 ±388	3	—		—		—
V_{ES}	—	501 ± 90	—	—	—		—		—		—		—		—
V_{EW}	1912 ±141	529 ± 91	104 ± 17	104 ± 17	107 ± 17	5	105 ± 17	6	107 ± 18	5	65 ± 40	4	144 ± 14	6	64 ± 35
χ^2	66.9	130.7	4.9	3.5	-0.84		1.84		1.75		0.98		1.04		0.81
df	6	4	5	5	5		4		4		3		3		3
P	<0.001	<0.001	>0.25	>0.5	>0.95		>0.75		>0.75		>0.75		>0.75		>0.75

additive epistatic effects on total ridge count, we rank-
ordered the kinships by twin pair means and partitioned the
data from the families of male and female twin pairs into
upper, lower, and middle thirds. The epistatic model was
then fitted to the subdivided data sets, and the results are
shown in VIII-X. Since the data were truncated by selection
through the twin pair means, the among twin pair equation was
omitted and the analysis was based only on the five offspring
equations and the within twin pair equation. Model VIII shows
that there was increased evidence for epistasis in the families of twins with low ridge count; in the families of twins
with intermediate ridge counts, there was reduced evidence for
epistasis (IX), while in the high ridge count families, the
model failed (X), providing no evidence for epistasis.

   We believe that epistasis has too frequently been ignored
as a potential source of variation in man by geneticists who,
like Lewontin (21), narrowly view quantitative genetic analysis solely as a means of predicting the results of selection
experiments. A much more important goal of human biometric
genetics is to explain extreme phenotypes such as high blood
pressure, high cholesterol, short stature or mental deficiency.
Extreme phenotypes such as these are of great medical significance, and the distinction between single and multi-locus   .
determination has important practical and theoretic implications. The results of our analysis of total ridge count suggest a way in which the half-sib model may be used to approach
this problem and raise the possibility that low total ridge
count may, in fact, represent an example of additive epistasis
in man.

D. Birth Weight

   Data were available on 339 offspring of 23 male and 39
female monozygotic twin pairs of unknown placentation type.
Because of the well-known effect of placental vascular anasto-.
moses in exaggerating the birth weight differences of mono-
chorionic MZ twins (22), we elected to base the study entirely
upon the offspring equations [a]-[e] (Table 1). Prior to the
analysis, the birth weights were adjusted for gestational age
and sex using the normative data of Lubchenco et al. (23). A
preliminary F-test comparing the sum of the mean squares
associated with relations [b] and [e] with those of [a] and
[d] provided evidence that either genetic or environmental
maternal effects have a significant effect on variation in
birth weight (F = 2.32, df 51,33 P < 0.01). The results of
fitting various genetic models are summarized in Table 6.
Solutions I and II show that both the simple and full environmental models could be rejected. As shown in III, when the
data for the male and female twin half-sibships were pooled,

TABLE 6: Birth Weight:
Estimates of Genetic, Environmental, and Maternal
Variance Components Derived from Offspring Equations.

Var. Comp.	I Est. ± SE	II Est. ± SE	III Est. ± SE	III % of Tot.	IV Est. ± SE	IV % of Tot.	V Est. ± SE	V % of Tot.	VI Est. ± SE	VI % of Tot.
V_A	-	-	25.1 ±4.6	99	25.2 ±4.5	99	4.9 ±5.5	19	-	-
V_{AA}	-	-	-	-	-	-	-	-	10.6 ±8.2	42
V_M	-	-	-	-	-	-	10.1 ±3.1	40	9.9 ±2.7	40
V_{EH}	-	4.4 ±2.3	-	-	-	-	-	-	-	-
V_{ES}	-	7.7 ±2.2	-	-	-	-	-	-	-	-
V_{EW}	24.6 ±1.0	12.4 ±1.2	.02 ±2.8	1	.03 ±2.8	1	10.3 ±3.3	41	4.6 ±6.6	18
χ^2	388	13.2	0.59		15.9		2.9		1.9	
df	4	2	1		3		2		2	
P	<0.001	<0.001	>0.25		<0.001		<0.10		<0.25	

yielding three equations, a simple genetic interpretation in
terms of additive genetic and environmental effects gave an
excellent fit. However, when these same two variables were
fitted to the full five equations that were capable of detecting a maternal effect (IV), a very poor fit was observed and
the solution could be rejected. Finally, when V_M was included
in the solution, two models, V and VI, gave an excellent fit,
and no further improvement could be achieved by the inclusion
of any additional genetic or environmental variables. Had the
anaylsis been based on conventional genetic relationships
(III), we would have been quite satisfied with the false conclusion that additive genetic effects acting in the fetus account for virtually all of the observed phenotypic variation

in birth weight, when, in fact, they almost certainly account
for less than half of the variation, and are probably a less
important source than maternal effects which account for about
40% of the variation. Whether the observed maternal effects
are nuclear, cytoplasmic, or environmental in origin remains
to be determined, but the results clearly demonstrate how
treacherous it is to draw genetic inferences from data that
do not permit the resolution of genetic, environmental, and
maternal effects.

E. Stature

The analysis of height was based on measurements from 436
offspring of 31 male and 53 female monozygotic twin pairs, the
twins themselves, and 120 spouses of the twins, a total of 742
individuals in all. The data were adjusted by regression to
remove the effects of age and sex prior to the analysis. As
shown in Table 7, neither random environmental factors nor
additive genetic effects alone could adequately account for
the variation seen in the offspring data (I and II). When
both variables were fitted simultaneously (III), a satisfactory fit was achieved, yielding a solution which suggested
that 81% of the total variation is attributable to additive
genetic effects, in close agreement with previous estimates
(24). However, as shown in IV, when a source of common environmental variation, V_{EH}, was included in the solution, a substantial improvement in the fit was achieved, and the heritability estimate fell to 45%, while the proportion of total
variance explained by V_{EW} increased to 37%. The within sibship environmental variation includes not only random environmental effects but also residual variation resulting from differences in the age and sex of the siblings. In an elegant
longitudinal twin study, Sharma (25) has clearly shown that
genetic factors influence not only the ultimate stature but
the timing and rate of the adolescent growth spurt. Thus a
fraction of V_{EW} can be considered to represent a form of Genetic X Environmental interaction where age is treated as an environmental gradient. With these considerations in mind, it
is not surprising that, when equations from the full-grown
twin parents are added to the model, poor fits result because
the estimate of V_{EW} provided by the within twin equation, 3.34,
is so much smaller than that derived from the offspring data,
61.93. The difference between these two estimates, 58.59, or
35% of the total variation, can be taken as a measure of the
variation within sibships in the timing of childhood growth, a
form of Genetic X Environmental interaction. These results
indicate that the genetic analysis of growth clearly warrants
a more sophisticated treatment than the mere calculation of a
heritability estimate. A deeper understanding of growth could

TABLE 7: Stature:
Estimates of Genetic and Environmental Variance
Components Derived from Offspring Equations

Var. Comp.	Genetic Model							
	I		II		III		IV	
	Est. ± SE	% Tot. Var.	Est. ± SE	% Tot. Var.	Est. ± SE	% Tot. Var.	Est. ± SE	% Tot. Var.
V_A	–	–	179 ±11	100	133 ±25	81	75.76 ±38.92	45
V_{EH}	–	–	–	–	–	–	29.97 ±18.25	18
V_{EW}	168 ± 7	100	–	–	31 ±17	19	61.93 ±23.96	37
χ^2	269		7.15		3.61		1.34	
df	4		4		3		2	
P	<0.001		<0.25		<0.50		<0.75	

be gained by the collection of longitudinal data from half-sib
families or by the inclusion of parameters which take into account the difference in age between each pairwise comparison
of the children within a kinship, as suggested by Eaves (11).
   Analysis of the parental data permits resolution of the
usually confounded effects of assortative mating and common
environment. The calculations involved in estimating r_A, the
phenotypic correlation resulting from genetic similarity, are
set forth in Table 8, where the genetic expectations and observed covariances for the husband-wife (HW), spouse-spouse
(SS), and twin-sibling-in-law (TS) relationships are given.
Note that cov SS includes r_A^2 in the last term while the two
other covariances are linear in r_A. This relationship can be
most easily understood by the path-analysis approach, from
which it is evident that the spouses are separated by three
steps associated with correlations r_A, 1, and r_A, respectively,
whereas the subjects involved in cov HW and cov TS are each
separated by one or two steps. The close agreement between
cov HW and cov TS suggests that V_{ES} is negligibly small, in
agreement with the offspring analysis. If the estimate of
V_{EH} derived from the offspring analysis is subtracted from
each of the covariances, r_A may be estimated from the residual

TABLE 8: Estimation of Correlation Attributable
to Assortative Mating (r_A) for Stature

| | Genetic Relationship | | |
	Husband-Wife cov HW	Spouse-Spouse cov SS	Twin-Sib- in-law cov TS
Number of pairs	120	60	120
Genetic expectation	$V_{EH}+V_{ES}+r_AV_T$	$V_{EH} + r_A^2V_T$	$V_{EH} + r_AV_T$
Observed covariance	38.17	30.69	37.30
V_{EH} (Est.)	29.97	29.97	29.97
Residual	8.2	0.72	7.33
V_T	91.58	76.59	91.58
Correlation			
Adjusted r_A	0.089	0.097	0.080
Unadjusted r	0.417	0.401	0.407

variance using the estimates of total variance, V_T, derived
from the individuals involved in the covariances. The resulting values are in remarkably close agreement and are substantially lower than the unadjusted correlations. The three estimates of r_A give a weighted mean value of 0.087 which may be
used to obtain adjusted estimates of the genetic and environmental variance components as described by Cavalli-Sforza and
Bodmer (26). The final partition of variance is summarized in
Table 9, with comparable data from Fisher's classical study.

Our conclusions differ substantially from those of R.A.
Fisher (27). When genetic effects were estimated from members,
of the same generation, we found no evidence that dominance
makes an added contribution to the genetic variance. In contrast to Fisher, we found substantial evidence for environmental variation which markedly reduced the proportion of the
conjugal correlations accounted for by assortative mating.
Finally, our analysis identified a major Genetic X Environmental interaction component which inflated the total phenotypic
variance of children to 167 and disappeared as adult stature
was achieved at which time the total variance was markedly reduced. These results illustrate the hazards of including parent-offspring relationships in biometric analysis and the in-
sidious way in which the use of correlations can conceal major
and important sources of phenotypic variation.

TABLE 9:   Partition of Variance for Stature:
Comparative Summary

Source of Variation	% of Total Variance	
	This study	R.A. Fisher (27)
Genetic		
Additive		
Expected with random mating	40.06	62
From assortative mating	1.50	17
Dominance	–	21
Environmental		
Among half-sibships	19.06	–
Within sibships	4.39	–
Genetic Environmental		
Interaction	34.99	–

F.   Serum Cholesterol

The analysis is based on the mean squares reported by
Christian and Kang (28) for 261 offspring of 49 female twin
pairs and 163 offspring of 34 male twin pairs. From a univariate analysis of the mean squares, these authors concluded
that maternal effects account for about one-fifth of the total
variance. In a separate analysis, the heritability (h^2) was
estimated from parent-offspring and offspring correlations,
giving values ranging from 0.52 to 1.34. The results of an
overall, weighted, iterated, least squares analysis of the
offspring data are summarized in Table 10.

As shown in I, random environmental effects could confidently be excluded as the sole cause for the observed variation in cholesterol levels, but the full environmental model,
II, gave a marginal fit and could not be excluded as an explanation for the data. Note that the standard errors of the
estimates in this model are small, since the variables are
unconfounded. As shown in III, the additive genetic, random
environmental model also gave an acceptable fit which was
significantly improved (P <0.05) by the inclusion of maternal
effects in IV. Finally, a small additional improvement in the
χ^2 was achieved by the addition of a second environmental component, V_{EH}, as shown in V, although the standard errors of
the resulting estimates are large because of confounding.
The results of the best fitting model indicate that, when all
of the data are considered simultaneously, random environmen-

TABLE 10: Serum Cholesterol:
Estimates of Genetic, Environmental, and Maternal
Variance Components from Offspring Equations

Var. Comp.	Genetic Model						
	I Est. ± SE	II Est. ± SE	III Est. ± SE	IV Est. ± SE	IV % Tot. Var.	V Est. ± SE	V % Tot. Var.
V_A	–	–	644 ±118	232 ±176	30	196 ±193	25
V_M	–	–	–	214 ±90	27	198 ±103	25
V_{EH}	–	187 ±60	–	–	–	34 ±100	5
V_{ES}	–	136 ±55	–	–	–	–	–
V_{EW}	778 ±34	453 ±41	127 ±79	334 ±105	43	354 ±116	45
χ^2	239	5.15	5.21	0.78		0.64	
df	4	2	3	2		1	
P	<0.001	>0.05	>0.1	>0.5		>0.25	

tal effects account for 45 percent of the total variation and common environmental factors for only 5 percent, while additive genetic effects account for 25 percent of the variation (h^2) as do maternal effects. Whether the observed maternal effect is genetic, environmental, or cytoplasmic in origin remains to be determined. Because the full-sibships are nested within half-sibships, it would clearly be inappropriate to estimate the full-sib correlation from the intraclass correlation coefficient. However, estimates of the full- and half-sib correlations can be obtained by dividing the predicted values of the relevant covariances by the total variance. When this is done, we can estimate that the full-sib correlation is 0.4224, the paternal half-sib correlation, 0.1061, and the maternal half-sib correlation, 0.3597. The inclusion of data from the parents would greatly strengthen the analysis. We suspect they were not reported because of differences in

the total variance of the parents and offspring. Although the
cause for differences in the total variance of unrelated
groups of individuals can never be inferred with complete certainty (1), as seen in the analysis of stature, differences in
the total variance of related individuals can be meaningfully
interpreted to obtain estimates of differential environmental
effects, Genetic X Environment interactions, or the Genotype
X Environmental covariance.

TABLE 11: Immunoglobulins:
Estimates of Genetic and Environmental Variance Components.

Var. Comp.	IgG Estimate ± S.E.	IgG % Tot. Var.	IgA Estimate ± S.E.	IgA % Tot. Var.	IgM Estimate ± S.E.	IgM % Tot. Var.
V_A	1.354 ±2.154	19	0.481 ±0.090	50	−	−
V_{AX}	−	−	−	−	0.100 ±0.039	13
V_D	0.834 ±6.910	12	−	−	−	−
V_{DX}	−	−	−	−	0.480 ±0.101	63
V_{AA}	0.180 ±7.442	3	−	−	−	−
V_M	−	−	0.046 ±0.079	5	−	−
V_{EH}	1.494 ±0.600	21	0.071 ±0.051	7	−	−
V_{EW}	3.212 ±0.461	45	0.363 ±0.049	38	0.179 ±0.059	24
χ^2	0.90		2.23		−3.36	
df	4		5		7	
P	>0.9		>0.75		>0.75	

G. Immunoglobulin Levels (29)

The radial immunodiffusion method (30) was used to measure the levels of IgG, IgA, and IgM in the parents and 210 offspring in the families of 57 MZ female twins and the parents and 233 offspring in the families of 36 male MZ twins. In agreement with previous studies (31), preliminary regression analyses showed a significant effect of age on IgA levels, which accounted for 9% of the total variation of the raw scores, and a significant sex effect on IgM levels, accounting for 6% of the total variation. After adjustment for these effects, the data were subjected to analysis, and representative solutions are shown in Table 11. The immunoglobulin results were unusual in that many alternative models fit the data well.

Previous studies have suggested that of the three immunoglobulin classes, IgG is the most variable and subject to environmental changes with infection. When all nine equations were included in the analysis, the random environmental model could be excluded, but both the full environmental and the additive genetic, random environmental models were marginally acceptable with χ^2's of 10.88 and 10.43, respectively. The assumption of non-additive genetic effects were readily accommodated by the data giving a marked improvement in the goodness of fit. In the model shown in Table 1, environmental factors account for two-thirds of the variation, and three sources appear to contribute to the genetic variation. Several even more complex models including maternal effect also fit the data, but the estimates of V_M were very small.

The results for IgA were also fitted to the full nine equations and yielded an intermediate level of genetic determination. In contrast to IgG, both the simple and full environmental models were rejected, but several additive genetic, environmental models yielded acceptable fits. In the solution shown in Table 11, additive genetic effects accounted for 50% of the total variation.

Previous studies have suggested that levels of IgM are influenced by genes on the X chromosome (32). To test this hypothesis, we partitioned the offspring data into half-fraternities and half-sororities and fitted models to the resulting ten equations using the genetic expectations given previously by Nance and Corey (6). Both the simple and full environmental models were rejected (χ^2 = 61.8 and 18.2) as was the random environmental, additive autosomal model (χ^2 = 17.2). The best fitting model was the one shown in Table 11 which suggests that 76 percent of the total variation is determined by X-linked genes. Attempts to fit both X-linked and autosomal genes simultaneously were unsuccessful. For those intent upon demonstrating the feasibility of detecting genetic linkage

with quantitative traits, the analysis of IgM, Xg^a, and other
X-linked markers in the families of identical twins would seem
to be a useful test system.

V. SUMMARY AND CONCLUSIONS

The MZ half-sib study design has not been completely evaluated, and its limitations and full potential have yet to be
defined. In particular, we lack hard data on the power of the
model in comparison with other designs (33), the cost effectiveness of sampling through monozygotic twins, and the possibility that some of the biases that plague the classical
twin model may have a lingering effect in the descendants of
twins.

On the other hand, the examples presented here clearly
demonstrate that even with relatively modest sample sizes, the
design permits the detection of unexpected sources of variation including maternal effects, non-additive genetic effects,
X-linked gene effects, and Genetic X Environmental interactions, as well as a resolution of the influence of assortative
mating and common environment. Although the design is ideally
suited to the genetic analysis of continuously distributed
metric traits in normal individuals, we also believe that by
extending the analysis to the grandchildren of twins, it will
be possible to apply the method to the study of qualitative
traits such as birth defects.

Following a description of the MZ half-sib model in their
1976 article on path analysis, Rao, Morton, and Yee concluded
that "Perhaps it is time to suggest that for its contribution
to biometrical genetics, twin research might profitably be
left to twins." We believe that quite the opposite is true
and that for many purposes the MZ kinship design offers the
very best approach currently available for disentangling the
effects of genes and environment on complex human traits.

VI.   ACKNOWLEDGEMENTS

We gratefully acknowledge the helpful advice of Dr. Lindon
J. Eaves, the aid of P. Winter, D. Huntzinger, and Drs. P.
Bader, G. Bingle, and J. Christian with the data collection,
and the assistance of W. Belanger, L. Ewell, and J. Crowder
in data processing, analysis, and typing of the manuscript.

VII.   REFERENCES

1. Nance, W.E., Am. J. Hum. Genet. 28, 297 (1976).

2. Morton, N.E., Am. J. Hum. Genet. 26, 318 (1974).

3. Jensen, A.R., Behav. Genet. 4, 1 (1974).

4. Rao, D.C., Morton, N.E., and Yee, S., Am. J. Hum. Genet. 26, 331 (1974).

5. Nance, W.E., Nakata, M., Paul, T.D., and Yu, P., in "Congenital Malformations: New Directions in Research" (D.T. Janerich, R.G. Skalko, and I.H. Porter, Eds.), p. 23. Academic Press, New York, 1974.

6. Nance, W.E., and Corey, L.A., Genetics 83, 811 (1976).

7. Nance, W.E., and Corey, L.A., Genetics 84, March (1977).

8. Hayman, B.I., Biometrics 16, 369 (1960).

9. Elston, R.C., Biometrika 62, 133 (1975).

10. Corey, L.A., Nance, W.E., and Berg, K., Birth Defects Orig. Art. Ser. (in press).

11. Eaves, L.J., in "Proceedings of the Second International Congress of Twin Studies" (W.E. Nance, G. Allen, and P. Parisi, Eds.) (in press) Alan Liss, New York, 1978.

12. Rao, D.C., Morton, N.E., and Yee, S., Am. J. Hum. Genet. 28, 228 (1976).

13. Lange, K., Westlake, J., and Spence, M.A., Ann. Hum. Genet. 39, 485 (1976).

14. Miller, J.Z., Norton, J.A., Wollen, R.L., Griffith, R.S., Rose, R.J., and Nance, W.E., JAMA 237, 248 (1977).

15. Stevenson, A.C., Johnson, H.A., Stewart, M.I.P., and Golding, D.R., Bull. World Hlth. Org. 34, suppl, 1 (1966).

16. Berendes, H.W., in "Research Methodology and Needs in Perinatal Studies" (S.S. Chipman, A.M. Lillienfeld, B.G. Greenberg, and J.F. Donnelly, Eds.), p. 118. Thomas, Springfield, 1966.

17. Benirschke, K., and Kim, C.K., New Eng. J. Med. 288, 276 (1973).

18. Ewell, L.W., Corey, L.A., Winter, P.M., Boughman, J.A., and Nance, W.E., in "Proceedings of the Second International Congress of Twin Studies" (W.E. Nance, G. Allen, and P. Parisi, Eds.) (in press) Alan Liss, New York, 1978.

19. Feinleib, M., Garrison, M.S., Borhani, N., Rosenman, R., and Christian, J.C., in "Epidemiology and Control of Hypertension" (O. Paul, Ed.) p. 3. Stratton, New York, 1975.

20. Holt, S.B., in "The Genetics of Dermal Ridges," Charles C. Thomas, Springfield, 1968.

21. Lewontin, R.C., Am. J. Hum. Genet. 26, 400 (1974).

22. Corey, L.A., Kang, K.W., Christian, J.C., and Nance, W.E., Exerpta Med. Int. Cong. Ser. 397, 175 (1976).

23. Lubchenco, L.O., Hansman, C., Dressler, M., and Boyd, E., Pediatrics 32, 793 (1963).

24. Smith, D.M., Nance, W.E., Kang, K.W., Christian, J.C., and Johnston, C.C., J. Clin. Invest. 52, 2008 (1973).

25. Sharma, J.C., in "Proceedings of the Second International

   Congress of Twin Studies" (W.E. Nance, G. Allen, and P.
   Parisi, Eds.) (in press) Alan Liss, New York, 1978.
26. Cavalli-Sforza, L.L., and Bodmer, W.F., in "The Genetics
   of Human Populations," p. 543. W.H. Freeman, San Francisco, 1971.
27. Fisher, R.A., Trans. Roy. Soc. (Edinburgh) 52, 399 (1918).
28. Christian, J.C., and Kang, K.W., Am. J. Hum. Genet. 20,
   462 (1977).
29. Escobar, V., Corey, L.A., Nance, W.E., Bixler, D., and
   Biegel, A., in "Proceedings of the Second International
   Congress of Twin Studies" (W.E. Nance, G. Allen, and P.
   Parisi, Eds.) (in press) Alan Liss, New York, 1978.
30. Mancini, G., Carbonara, A.O., and Hermans, J.F., Immuno-
   chemistry 2, 235 (1965).
31. Grundbacher, F.J., Am. J. Hum. Genet. 26, 1 (1974).
32. Rhodes, K., Markham, R.L., Maxwell, P., Monkjones, J.,
   Brit. Med. J. 3, 439 (1969).
33. Eaves, L.J., Psychol. Bull. 77, 144 (1972).

DISCUSSION

WAGENER: Half sibs are siblings of a proband who share one
biological parent with the proband, but not two. The half sib
may or may not have been brought up by both of its biological
parents. He may or may not have been brought up in the same
family group as the proband. The proband and the half sib may
or may not share a biological father. All of these variables
of family group structure allow for the analysis of familial
relationships with some genetic control of the homogeneity of
the population.

   The estimation of correlations from linear models of
familial structures (Morton, 1974; Rao et al., 1974) requires
that the data be based on an unbiased sample of the general
population. Such data may not always be available or it may be
impractical to collect. We therefore propose another epidemiological strategy, that of selected samples. In the following
we discuss the half sib model of probands, pointing out the
advantages and disadvantages of this model over other selected
samples such as twin or adoptive studies.

   The half sib model has been used for breeding and
hybridizing research. Falconer (1960) describes these models
in his textbook. Of course, in human genetics these strict
breeding protocols are impractical.

   For human research we may consider traits, including
behavioral or cultural traits, for which the development is a

continuing process taking place over a substantial period of the individual's lifetime. The developmental process of these traits is dynamic, involving not only the biological maturing of the individual, but also some degree of teaching by the family and society and learning by the individual. We will consider familial traits influenced by variables of common environment, midparental genotype, random environment, and segregation from midparental genotype. We also add the variable of different parenting influence. That is, for certain traits the father or the mother (including her intra-uterine environment) will have a stronger impression on the development of the trait. An even more general familial environment is expressed by the role models of other members within the family, such as older sibs (Zajonc, 1976).

The half sibling approach, as discussed in Rüdin (1923), has been subsequently mentioned in the literature, but not often used as a research tool in human genetics apart from the occasional case reports, for instance in research on homosex-uality (Lang, 1960; James, 1971). Penrose (1951) mentions half sibling research in his review of genetic methods for psychi-atry. Also Kallman (1953) uses half sibs of affected probands. But the use of this tool has been only the observation of global frequencies of affected states among half sibs, with the expectation that this frequency is lower among half sibs than among full sibs of the probands. Kallman in his book gives frequencies of half sibs with either manic-depressive psychoses or schizophrenia.

Falconer (1960) and Comstock (1955) describe the conventional half sib model for analysis of variance. Nance and Corey (1976) have made the additional useful observation that the half siblings can be further analyzed for inclusion of maternal effects in the model. For their analysis, they emphasize the use of offspring of monozygous twins, a popula-tion which is difficult to amass.

More recently, Schuckit et al. (1972) have used the half sibs of affected individuals in their study of alcoholism. They used alcoholic probands to ascertain half siblings who then were studied as a new population, more homogeneous genet-ically than the general population by virtue of the relation-ship of affected individuals. However, in their analysis no control was made for any of the genetic relationships between the half sibling population and the sib populations. Also, they did not control for whether or not the half sibs were raised by their own biological parents or adopted parents. These controls would be necessary when accounting for genetic and environmental interaction.

Among half sibs we have the advantage of a population which is genetically related to a group of probands, all with

some common trait. Of course, there are other populations who
are genetically related to the proband, such as parents, full
sibs, twins or adopted away siblings. However, in the United
States adopted siblings are virtually impossible to study.
The consideration of twins is always made immensely complicated
by their low frequency. Only in countries, such as the
Scandinavian countries, with comprehensive registers, is such
a study feasible.

   With regards to either parental or full sib populations,
the half sib population has two advantages. Firstly, the half
sibs have often been reared in different family environments
than the proband. For instance, in Schuckit et al.'s study,
47 percent of the half sibs were not raised with the proband,
while only 8 percent of the full sibs were raised apart from
the proband. Another advantage of the half sib population is
that the dominance variance does not affect the comparisons
of half sibs (see Mather and Jinks, 1971).

   The disadvantages of this particular research design are
that the offspring have a high incidence of having been reared
in broken homes. The experience of a broken home may be
substantial to the development of the trait. A further,
possibly major, disadvantage of this method is that the shared
parent is usually the mother. To compare maternal effects two
sets of offspring are used, offspring of families where the
mother is the common biologic parent and those where the
father is the common biologic parent. However, if the shared
parent is by and large the mother, ascertainment of larger
populations is necessary.

   We look at different family structures, ignoring families
in which one sib has been raised by two adopting parents.
When the half sibs are raised together, one of the half sibs
will be raised with an adopted parent. However, they share a
family environment. Half sibs may be raised apart, but nevertheless raised by a common parent. In this case there may be
quite a spread in age between the two sibs so that the family
environment is not the same. Half sibs may be raised apart by
different parents so that the common parent does not contribute
to the family social environment. With the increasing number
of single parent families in the United States, such family
groups may or may not include a second foster parent.

   We now consider threshold traits. Then imposed upon this
dimension of whether half sibs have been raised together with
one or more biological parents, we can add the dimensions of
whether one or more parents is affected. In Figure 1 we show
eight different relationships that may exist when one offspring
has been raised by a biological parent and a foster parent.
If the half sib has been raised by both of its biological
parents, there are three such relationships, namely, one, two

or none of the parents affected, denoted B1, B2 and B0.

In Figure 1, the various relationships between biological parents and a foster parent have been shaded to indicate special relationships between the offspring and its parents. The family structures therefore include variables relating to whether probands and half sibs have been raised together and whether they have been raised by their biological or foster parents. Also taken into account are the traits of the parents. The model depends not only upon the phenotypic state of the individuals, but also on the genetic relationships between individuals.

Because these families are ascertained through the proband, a correlational analysis would give estimates of coefficients which would be biased for affected offspring. Instead, by using multiple comparisons we estimate the presence or absence of the variables mentioned above in the determination of the phenotype. For instance, to estimate the genetic influence of an affected parent, we compare the frequency of affected biological parents for affected half sibs to that for probands. To estimate the environmental influence of an affected parent, we compare the frequencies, among affected half sibs, of groups 1 through 5 plus group 7 (Figure 1) with the frequency of this composite group for nonaffected half sibs. Holding the genetic load constant, we compare the following groups: 3+4+5+6+B1 (one biological affected) to 7+8+B0 (no biological affected) or 3+5+B1 (one biological and one foster affected) to 4+6 (foster not affected) or 7 with 8+B0.

Maternal and paternal half-sibships can be disaggregated to compare the frequency of affected individuals among the half sibs. If, for instance, a maternal effect is present, the frequency of affection among the proband's maternal half sibs will be greater, controlling for the phenotype of the other parent.

REFERENCES

Comstock, R., Quant. Biol. 20, 93-102 (1955).
Falconer, D.S., "Introduction to Quantitative Genetics,"
    Oliver and Boyd, Edinburgh, 1960.
Kallmann, F.J., "Heredity in Health and Mental Disorder,"
    W. W. Norton and Co., New York, 1953.
Lang, T., Acta Genet. Med. 9, 370-381 (1960).
Mather, K., and Jinks, J.L., "Biometrical Genetics, 2nd Edition
    Edition," Cornell Univ. Press, Ithaca, 1971.
Morton, N.E., Am. J. Hum. Genet. 26, 318-330 (1974).
Nance, W.E., and Corey, L.A., Genetics 83, 811-826 (1976).

Penrose, L.S., "Research Methods in Human Genetics. Congres
    International de Psychiatrie VI: Paris," Hermann and Cie,
    Paris, 1950.
Rao, D.C., Morton, N.E., and Yee, S., Am. J. Hum. Genet.
    26, 331-359 (1974).
Rudin, E., Z Ges Neurol. Psychiat. 81, 459-473 (1923).
Schuckit, M.A., Goodwin, D.A., and Winokur, G., Am. J. Psychiat.
    128, 1132-1136 (1972).
Zajonc, R.B., Science 192, 227-236 (1976).

FAMILY STRUCTURE FOR OFFSPRING RAISED BY ONE FOSTER PARENT

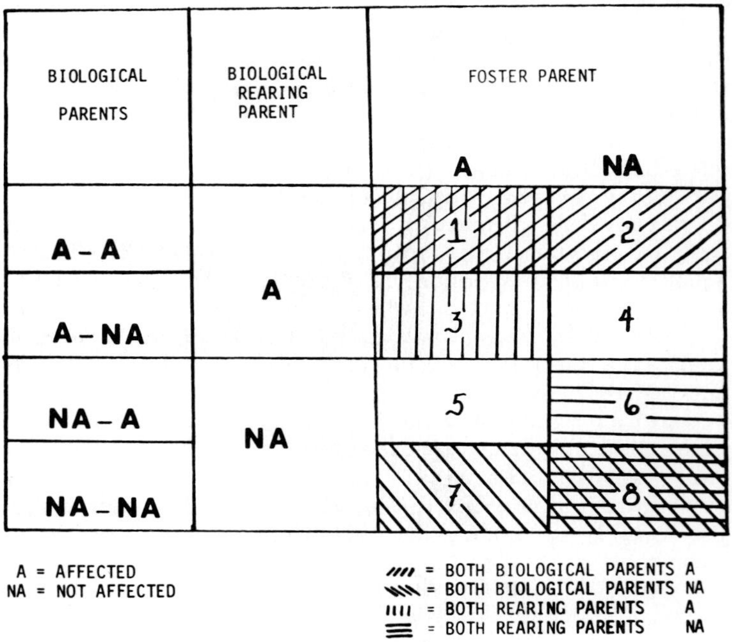

BIOLOGICAL PARENTS	BIOLOGICAL REARING PARENT	FOSTER PARENT	
		A	NA
A – A	A	1	2
A – NA		3	4
NA – A	NA	5	6
NA – NA		7	8

A = AFFECTED
NA = NOT AFFECTED

/// = BOTH BIOLOGICAL PARENTS A
\\\ = BOTH BIOLOGICAL PARENTS NA
|||| = BOTH REARING PARENTS   A
≡ = BOTH REARING PARENTS   NA

Fig. 1

NANCE: I agree completely with Dr. Wagener on the value of
the half-sib relationship for genetic analysis. However, as
a member of a Department of Psychiatry, she must certainly be
concerned about drawing inferences about normal individuals
from relationships that arise in broken homes caused by death,
divorce, or illegitimacy. Not only are there systematic
parity differences between half-sibs of this type, but all of
the relevant parents are seldom available for analysis.
Finally, there may be serious biases resulting from ethnic or
socioeconomic stratification. All of these problems can be

avoided by the use of MZ twin kinships, and there are many advantages of the design, some of which I enumerated in my paper. Wagener's objection to the use of MZ twins seems to be that she thinks twins are too rare. This is a common criticism of twin studies, but I have never heard anyone who has actually tried to find and study twins complain about their infrequency. All you have to do is hang a sign out and they will appear. In the city of Pittsburgh alone, there should be nearly 10,000 individuals who are twins and at least one in 50 individuals in the general population should have a grandparent who was an identical twin.

SING: What are the effects of correlations in the data between covariances? Does the unweighted ANOVA give unbiased estimates of variance components for each of the subsets of equations you select?

How do you see this design being used in epidemiology? Epidemiologists have identified twins and their relatives to be at higher risk for many diseases. I am concerned that your design does not overcome many of the problems faced by the geneticist in evaluating quantitative variables and I am skeptical that it will be any less troublesome for the epidemiologist. It is possible the use of the half-sib twin design to estimate simultaneously genetic and epidemiological parameters will lead to bias for both investigations.

Lastly, I am concerned about your strategy for model fitting and the consequences for the statements of type I error levels. Will you please tell us how you proceed through the model space to assure that your type I error rate is not inflated?

NANCE: As described more fully elsewhere (1), we do adjust for the correlation between covariances, using formulae pirated from the work of Elston (2). The ANOVA we use is weighted to account for variation in sibship size.

Presumably, the motivation for this conference is the existence of a set of problems that cannot be solved by genetic or epidemiologic methods alone. Our study design combines an incisive and homogeneous set of genetic relationships with many features that an epidemiologist would find attractive including a well-defined sampling frame, centralized recording of all potential subjects, randomness, high compliance, and statistical efficiency. Our model has many of the elements of a co-twin control design, and in the study mentioned in my paper, the co-twin control design was shown to be more than 10 times as efficient as the random block design for some

variables (3). If comparable efficiencies can be shown to be
associated with the MZ kinship model, the cost factor may be
another important advantage. Many of the most troublesome
epidemiologic biases of twin studies are associated with DZ
rather than MZ twins. My gut reaction is that for most
continuously distributed metric traits, the sampling of
families through MZ twin probands will not introduce important
biases and that even if there are biases in the MZ twin
relationship itself, they will be diminished or absent in the
children and grandchildren.

Our strategy for model fitting is not altogether different
from multiple regression where one can either start with a
complex model or build up from a simpler one. The criteria
we use for selecting solutions include the size of the standard errors in relation to the component estimates, the
magnitude and change in the goodness of fit χ^2 following the
addition of new parameters, the consistency of the solution
over data subsets, and the biological plausibility. We
attempt to minimize Type I errors by restricting our attention
to models we consider biologically plausible.

REFERENCES

1.   Nance, W.E., and Corey, L.A., <u>Genetics</u> 83, 811-826 (1976).
2.   Elston, R.C., <u>Biometrika</u> 62, 133-140 (1975).
3.   Miller, J.A.Z., Ph.D. thesis, Indiana University, 1977.

CHAKRABORTY: Dr. Nance, through his presentation, tried to
convince us that there are some virtues in MZ twin studies.
The examples he has chosen are really from a wide spectrum,
from stature to serum cholesterol level. What seems more
important is to show for some components of variation whose
resolution is possible by his design that this is not possible
by any other means. Probably other critics will raise some
biological issues, but let me briefly make some comments
relevant to statistical analyses of this paper.

First, I feel that it is not judicious to compare two
insignificant χ^2 values to claim that one model gives better
fit than the other, as this may simply occur by chance alone
in a given sample. Any such statement just reflects personal
bias towards a particular model at hand (as is done in
explaining Table 4).

Second, as we examine the various estimates more closely,
a systematic trend that appears in the tables (e.g., Tables
3, 4, 10, etc.) is that the standard errors of the variance
components are larger (at least in relative terms) more often
for the models which fit the data. Is this an artifact of

the "modest" sample size or the "improved" design?
     What is of more concern to me is the row described as χ^2.
Are these really distributed as chi-squares? If so, how can
they be negative? The authors went further to imitate the
Roman madman by putting probability statements on these
negative values as well.
     I, further, do not fully appreciate the comparability of
the data presented in Table 9. The two data sets are separated
in time and space. Are these sorts of comparisons meaningful?
Furthermore, to show that these are statistically different
one has to examine their sampling errors as well, which I
suspect would wash out much of the displayed differences.

NANCE: Dr. Chakraborty's comments are well taken, and I
appreciate the opportunity his question gives me to "explain"
the negative χ^2. In the current version of our computer
program, we use observed values for some of the covariances
which appear in the off-diagonal elements of the V matrix,
rather than employing estimates for all of the covariances in
an iterative manner. We believe this accounts for the negative
χ^2's. When we recalculated the χ^2 for IgM in Table 11,
setting all of the off-diagonal elements equal to zero, we
obtained a small positive, non-significant χ^2. As adumbrated
in our original description of this model in <u>Genetics</u>, it
seems likely that all of the covariances should be iterated.
     With regard to comparing non-significant χ^2's, I agree
that in general if a choice is made between equally well-
fitting models, it must be on biologic and not statistical
grounds. However, in Table 4, the loss of one degree of
freedom in the best fitting model was associated with a decrease
in the χ^2 of 6.4 and in this situation I feel there are some
grounds for claiming a significantly better fit.
     Our impression has been that the standard errors of our
estimates are more closely related to the number of variables
included in the model and the degree to which these variables
are confounded than they are to the χ^2 goodness of fit. The
inclusion of the within twin equation in any model also has a
potent influence on the error estimates and dominates the χ^2
to a remarkable degree.
     Fisher's data on stature are clearly not comparable to
ours. What we have done is to compare the conclusions drawn
from separate analyses of the two bodies of data and I would
readily acknowledge that we have not excluded the possibility
that temporal trends account for the observed differences.

MORTON: To avoid confusion we should distinguish data sets,
models, and analyses. The data set advocated by Nance, which

includes MZ twins, their spouses, and children, may be called
a <u>twin sector</u>. There is no limit to the number of models
(not necessarily determinate) that may be applied to any data
set. With colorful but imprecise rhetoric Nance advocates
one of the class of models in which cultural inheritance is
represented by a unique term for each relationship, then
realizes the futility of this approach and equates components
arbitrarily and, as we shall see, inconsistently. A more
economical and elegant class of model predicts cultural
inheritance for each relationship in terms of a small number
of transmission parameters, which may be represented as path
coefficients. Obviously this class of models is indefinitely
large. We may assume different kinds of assortative mating,
maternal effects, and so forth.

The model we prefer assumes social homogamy, in which
marital correlation is a consequence of group membership (1).
The environmental correlation of mates is u, and the path from
parent's to child's environment is f. Therefore f(1 + u)
plays the same role in this model for cultural inheritance as
(1 + m)/2 does in genetic inheritance. Although the two kinds
of inheritance are correlated, they are not confounded even in
nuclear families providing the appropriate observations,
including environmental estimates (called <u>indices</u>), are made.
Table 1 gives a special case of the model for 36 relationships,
of which 4 occur in nuclear families, 5 in half-sibships, 11
in twin sectors, 15 in regular pedigrees (without half-sibs,
twins, or adoptions), and 11 are unique to adoption studies.
In this special case there is no direct effect of parental
phenotype on child's phenotype (x = 0), but they are correlated
through both genotype and family environment. It is also
assumed that assortative mating is exclusively environmental
(m = 0): a corollary of these assumptions is that there is no
genotype-environment covariance. For simplicity maternal
effects are neglected here. These assumptions appear to hold to
a close approximation even for IQ; all the restrictions are
removed in the general model, which is less easily assimilated
but should be used in any analysis. Under the special case
the phenotypic correlation of two individuals, x and y, is

$$r_{xy} = h_x h_y M + c_x c_y U$$

where h_i^2 is genetic heritability and c_i^2 is cultural heritability. For all 36 relationships U depends only on two parameters
(f and u). It is the economy of this model which gives
goodness-of-fit tests power, compared with ad hoc models of
the type discussed by Nance.

Whatever model is chosen, the data may be represented by
variances, regressions, or correlations: bias-correction (if

appropriate) may or may not be made; the statistics may or may
not be normal in small samples. We have argued for bias-
corrected z transforms of correlations as opposed to variance
components, whose distribution is much further from normality
in small samples. Obviously the correlation of correlations
estimated from the same data set should be allowed for; this
is an entirely separate consideration from choice of a model.
Correlations are not appropriate for incomplete ascertainment
where path regression is suitable, nor for polychotomized data
where tetrachoric functions of correlations are applicable.

Studies of family resemblance require a well-designed
data set, a logically consistent, overdetermined model, and
valid analysis: if any of these is lacking, the conclusions
are unreliable. The studies of Nance and colleagues may be
faulted in all these respects.

First, they dismiss analytical problems as "a matter for
technicians to resolve". In their analysis they assume normal,
homoscedastic variables and indefinitely large samples, but in
practice their variables are not normal, their variance changes
dramatically with age, and the number of twin sets is small.
Careful workers would at least apply a normalizing transform
and use the logarithms of variances, which are much closer to
normality. Their neglect of such matters is not judgment, but
an indifference to the validity of their conclusions. Much of
the literature on variance components shows the same disregard
for statistical niceties, and I wonder how many of the conclusions (such as the low variance of cholesterol in MZ twins)
would survive fastidious analysis.

The model has multiple inconsistencies, as shown in Table
2. For example, V_{EH} is used for the environmental covariance
of spouses of MZ twins (i) and the variance of paternal half-
sibships (a), which are logically unrelated. Likewise $V_M + V_{EH}$
is given by the variances both among maternal half-sibs as
children (e) and among twin pairs as adults (f), which have
little in common. Many other logical inconsistencies may be
seen in Table 2.

This is not a consequence of the particular model we have
chosen: I defy Nance et al. to devise any model of cultural
inheritance compatible with their assumptions. In contrast,
our linear model gives a simple and logically consistent result.
Of course a goodness-of-fit test may show that our model is
untrue for a particular data set, but it beats any formulation
that is internally inconsistent. The examples of Nance et al.
are heuristic, but quantitatively meaningless.

This is not the end of difficulties with their approach.
Changes of variance with age are poorly handled by variance
components, since they cannot unambiguously be assigned to any
factor. Age effects of the kind clearly shown in Figure 1

should be interpreted as a succession of age-specific traits
(for example, birth weight and weight at maturity), not gene-
environment interaction for a single trait. In other words,
such age effects are a trivial consequence of failing to
measure all family members at exactly the same age, and really
have no bearing on gene-environment interaction.

Finally, the data set is no better than the analysis and
model. Common relationships, especially in nuclear families,
are of greatest interest for genetic counseling and formal
genetics, and relevance declines with rarity of the relationship. It makes no sense to dismiss parent-offspring
relationships because of self-admitted "bias against the use
of transgenerational comparisons" and in favor or rare
relationships rife with special problems of twin behavior.
If Nance and colleagues understood the demonstrated capability
of environmental indices to give full determinacy in nuclear
families, including maternal effects, I do not think they would
attempt their exercise on the children of identical twins.

If they want to extend their methods, they will find that
twin sectors give several additional relationships, besides
the 9 they recognize, as well as valuable information from
indices, all efficiently and consistently utilized by path
analysis, which takes as _its_ parameters the same paths as
determine nuclear families and therefore can predict
resemblance for relatives of any degree. They will then not
find it desirable to omit parent-child relationships, and may
even decide that changes in genetic and cultural heritability
at maturity are worthy of their interest. By isolating these
two types of heritability from the plethora of mechanically
defined variance components, they may come to some insight
into family resemblance in less peculiar relationships than
the children of twins.

Apart from the massive literature about effects unique to
twins, there is much evidence that children of sisters are
more likely to marry than are children of brothers. For
example, the ratios of these two types were 1.54 in Japan and
1.84 in Austria (2). Evidently sisters maintain closer
contact than brothers do, and this effect must be greatly
exaggerated if they are identical twins. When maternal effects
and common environment are estimated for such data, what are
they supposed to tell us about singletons, which to many of us
are the primary object of interest?

Nance has advanced the study of family resemblance by
drawing attention to an unusual data set that should be
considered as a supplement to nuclear families in studies of
common traits, providing its many assumptions unique to twins
can be validated. However, his contribution is obscured by
intemperate advocacy of an uninformative model and unreliable

methods of analysis. If the convention is established to
publish efficient estimates of actual variances, the data may
be examined more critically.

REFERENCES

1.   Rao, D.C., Morton, N.E., and Yee, S., Am. J. Hum. Genet.
     28, 228-242 (1976).
2.   Morton, N.E., Ann. Hum. Genet. 20, 116-124 (1955).
3.   Rao, D.C., MacLean, C.J., Morton, N.E., and Yee, S.,
     Am. J. Hum. Genet. 27, 509-520 (1975).

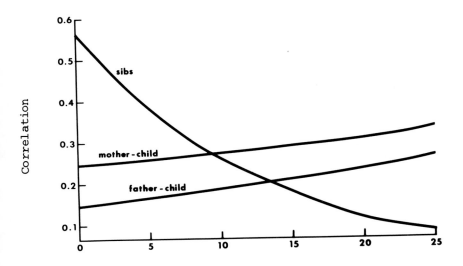

Age of child or age difference of sibs

Fig. 1.   Temporal trends in familial correlations for
normalized weight (3). The abcissa is the age of child (for
parent-child pairs) or absolute difference in age (for sibs).

TABLE 1

THE SPECIAL MODEL m=x=0 FOR 36 RELATIONSHIPS

Relation	Description	Genetic relationship M	Cultural relationship U
MZT	MZ twins reared together by parents	1	1
MZP	MZ twins reared apart, one by true parents	1	0
MZA	MZ twins reared apart by foster parents	1	0
MZF	MZ twins reared together by foster parents	1	1
FMT	father-mother at marriage	0	u
OPT	offspring-parent living together	1/2	$f(1+u)$
OPA	offspring-parent living apart	1/2	0
OFP	offspring-foster parent	0	$f(1+u)$
SST	full sibs reared together by parents	1/2	1
SSP	full sibs reared apart, one by true parents	1/2	0
SSA	full sibs reared apart by foster parents	1/2	0
HST	half-sibs reared together by parents	1/4	1
HSP	half-sibs reared apart, one by true parents	1/4	0
HSA	half-sibs reared apart by foster parents	1/4	0
HSS	half-sibs reared apart by own parents	1/4	$f^2(1+3u)$
FST	foster sibs reared together	0	1
FSP	foster sibs reared by parents of one	0	1
OET	offspring-excluded parent	0	$f(1+u)$
LIT	like in-laws (ego's spouse's sib's spouse)	0	$u/2$
UIT	unlike in-laws (ego's spouse's sib)	0	u
UNT	cognate uncle-niece	1/4	$f(1+u)$
ANT	affinal uncle-niece	0	$3uf/2$
FCT	first cousins	1/8	$f^2(2+5u)/2$
TUT	MZ twin and child of co-twin	1/2	$f(1+u)$
TAT	MZ twin's child and co-twin's spouse	0	$2uf$
TCT	children of MZ twins	1/4	$f^2(1+3u)$
GPO	grandparent-child	1/4	$f^2(1+u)^2$*
GGO	great grandparent-child	1/8	$f^3(1+u)^3$*
GUO	great uncle-child	1/8	$f^2(1+u)^2$*
FCR	first cousins once removed	1/16	$\cdot f^3(1+u)(2+5u)/2$*
SCT	second cousins	1/32	$f^4(1+u)^2(2+5u)/2$*
HIT	ego's spouse's half-sib, reared with spouse	0	u
HIA	ego's spouse's half-sib, reared apart by own parents	0	$uf^2(1+3u)$
MIT	MZ twin's and co-twin's spouse	0	u
MUT	spouses of MZ twins	0	u
PIT	parent and child's spouse	0	$u/2$

*This is approximate if $u \neq 0$.

TABLE 2

Expectations for Observed Environmental Variance Components of Nance et al.

Observed variance component	General expectation	Linear model $(m = x = 0)$	Expectations of Nance et al.
a) among paternal half-sibships	$\rho_{TCT(F)}$	$c^2 f_F^2 (1 + 3u)$	V_{EH}
b) between sibships within paternal half-sibships	$\rho_{SST} - \rho_{TCT(F)}$	$c^2 [1 - f_F^2 (1 + 3u)]$	$V_M + V_{ES}$
c) within sibships	$1 - \rho_{SST}$	$1 - c^2 - h^2$	V_{EW}
d) between sibships within maternal half-sibships	$\rho_{SST} - \rho_{TCT(M)}$	$c^2 [1 - f_M^2 (1 + 3u)]$	V_{ES}
e) among maternal half-sibships	$\rho_{TCT(M)}$	$c^2 f_M^2 (1 + 3u)$	$V_M + V_{EH}$
f) among twin pairs	$\rho_{MZT(A)}$	$c^2 y^2$	$V_M + V_{EH}$
g) within twin pairs	$1 - \rho_{MZT(A)}$	$1 - c^2 y^2 - h^2 z^2$	$V_{ES} + V_{EW}$
h) husband-wife	ρ_{FMT}	$c^2 y^2 u$	$V_{EH} + V_{ES}$
i) spouses of MZ twins	ρ_{MUT}	$c^2 y^2 u$	V_{EH}

127

TABLE 3

Variance Components for Singletons Reared by Own Parents

$(m = x = 0)$

Variance component	Children	Adults
maternal inheritance	$c^2\Lambda$	$c^2y^2\Lambda$
other cultural inheritance	$c^2(1 - \Lambda)$	$c^2y^2(1 - \Lambda)$
random environment	$1 - c^2 - h^2$	$1 - c^2y^2 - h^2z^2$

$$\Lambda = f_M^2 + f_F^2 + 2f_Mf_F(1 + u) - 2f_F^2(1 + u)$$

NANCE: Beneath the rhetoric and counter-rhetoric, there
are substantive differences between Morton's point of view and
ours. We favor designs in which each kinship contains all of
the relationships required for a detailed resolution of
genetic and environmental effects. Morton advocates pooling
data on multiple genetic relationships collected at different
times and places in separate studies by many investigators.
This kind of perfunctory concern for the niceties of study
design, sampling, and the comparability of data contributes to
the disaffection of epidemiologists and other scientists with
the methods of human quantitative genetics. To Morton's
demand that we show him where he has erred, I can say only
that a careful scientist would demur at pooling the results of
separate twin, adoption, MZA, half-sib, and nuclear family
studies in an overall analysis. Similar objections can be
raised to the use of parent-offspring regression in the analysis of psychological traits. Test scores in parents and
children may not be comparable even when administered at the
same age. A low parent-offspring correlation could simply
mean that previously hidden genes are being expressed, a
phenomenon which is dramatically illustrated by many pharmaco-
genetic traits. Morton's credibility is diminished by his
failure to acknowledge the advantage of basing a genetic
analysis on comparisons of individuals who are members of the
same generation.

Morton and I agree that, without the use of indices, his equations from nuclear families are indeterminate. In their paper, Rao and Morton also acknowledge that, even with the indices, the inclusion of dominance renders the equations indeterminate. A more important issue is the claim that the choice of an arbitrary environmental index does not influence the final parameter estimates. If this were true, random variables could be used instead of indices. In any case, I challenge Morton to show his estimates remain unchanged with different indices. If there is <u>any</u> change, how can it be claimed that the results have neither a hereditarian nor an environmental bias? In contrast, our design is sufficiently determinate to yield useful results without the use of ad hoc environmental indices.

We have made no attempt to study the transmission of environmental effects ("cultural inheritance"); our much more modest goal has been to develop improved designs for estimating genetic and environmental variance components. The most important tests of a biomathematical model are its utility, validity, and biologic plausibility and not its complexity, simplicity, or even its statistical elegance. We partitioned the environmental variance into three components because this treatment was consistent with the study design and because we could readily think of specific potential sources of environmental variation, such as endogamy, experimental error and dietary differences, among others, which would tend to be distributed among half-sibships, within sibships, or between sibships within half-sibships and would affect parents and offspring in a homogeneous manner. The formulae in Morton's Table 2 are clearly inappropriate. He gives $c^2f^2(1+3u)$ as the half-sib covariance, misdefining u as the correlation between mates, which does not even enter into the path diagram for half-sibs in our design, incorrectly equating the spouse-spouse and twin-spouse correlations, which do appear in our design, and erroneously fixing the correlation between the adult environments of MZ twins at unity. As we have previously noted, refinements of our model are possible, and the inclusion of a component to account for environmental differences between generations would appear to resolve many of Morton's objections to our present model (1, 2).

Morton assumes that martial correlations are entirely environmental in origin. Since fertile matings are almost invariably disassortative with respect to sex, his assumption leads to the startling conclusion that sex determination is environmental in origin! Morton further assumes the correlation between the spouses of twins is the same in sign and magnitude as the marital correlation, which is demonstrably false in the case of the phenotype sex. In contrast, our

model correctly predicts that the correlation between the
spouses of twins will be positive regardless of whether
matings are assortative or disassortative.

The concept that the relevance of a relationship declines
with its rarity is patently absurd. The relationship of rare
mutations to genetic disease has been of consuming interest
to geneticists and of importance to genetic counseling for
many decades. Among the creatures that inhabit the earth,
fruit flies are relatively rare and inbred mice are non-
existent in nature; nevertheless, experiments with these
organisms have made enormous contributions to formal genetics.
Progress in genetics has occurred in large measure through
the successive identification of unusual biological models
which permit new questions to be asked and answered. We
believe that the MZ kinship design is a model of this type.

In our analysis of stature, we adjusted the children's
heights to a constant age by regression prior to the analysis;
thus the increased variance we observed in the offspring cannot have been "a trivial consequence of failing to measure all
family members at exactly the same age." Since the excess
variance appeared primarily in the within sibship component,
we felt reasonably secure in attributing it to genetic variation in the timing of the adolescent growth spurt. Clearly,
changes in heritability that occur in response to an environmental gradient can provide a measure of genetic X environmental interaction. Our treatment of time as an environmental
gradient in our analysis of stature is of heuristic value in
suggesting a model for the genetic control of growth and a
method for estimating genetic X environmental interactions.
We think of growth as having a fixed genetic component and an
interaction component that varies with age, rather than
visualizing it as having a constantly variable heritability.
Our construct emphasizes the change in total variance during
growth, a feature that is not implied by the latter viewpoint.

Morton also seems to be confused when he wonders whether
the low variance of cholesterol in twins would survive
fastidious analysis. No twin mean squares were used in our
paper because none were given in the reference from which we
obtained the data for our reanalysis. If Morton has knowledge
of these data (3), perhaps he should publish the variances so
that they may be examined critically.

Because of the constraints of space and the suggestion of
the editor that we present results rather than models, we did
not give a full description of our study design, methodology,
or data set. However, we are aware that other relationships
exist within the design and have previously described 38
equations which can be derived from the X-linked and autosomal
models (1).

In my judgment, path analysis, maximum likelihood algorithms, and the iterative weighted least squares procedure we use are all valid approaches to data analysis. If this is true, the methods should lead to broadly similar conclusions when applied to the same body of data. When I stated that the differences between these approaches are a matter for technicians to resolve, I had in mind the recent attempt by Loehlin to reconcile the differences between the Hawaii and Birmingham solutions (5). Loehlin found that, when he made a few technical adjustments in the source data, corrected several errors in the Hawaiian equations, and included dominance in the model, the two solutions were in general agreement, showing evidence for dominance and no change in heritability between children and adults.

REFERENCES

1. Nance, W.E., and Corey, L.A., <u>Genetics</u> 83, 811-826 (1976).
2. Nance, W.E., and Corey, L.A., <u>Genetics</u> Letter to the Editor (1977).
3. Kang, K.W., Christian, J.C., Rao, D.C., and Morton, N.E., Abstract, <u>Am. J. Hum. Genet.</u> 29, 59A (1977).
4. Fulker, D.W., in Progress in Clinical and Biological Research: Twin Studies, W.E. Nance, G. Allen, and P. Parisi (Eds.), Alan R. Liss, Inc., New York (in press).
5. Loehlin, J.C., Ibid.

WORKMAN: Monozygotic twin families clearly provide a data base for genetic inference which has been neglected in past studies. There are, however, aspects of the biology of twinning, per se, which suggest that analytical inference should be generated with extreme caution. Developmental differences between monozygotic twins can be substantial and twins are well known to be at high risk epidemiologically just because of the embryogenesis of twins. Recent studies indicate that problems of lateralization following cleavage may also make twins unsuitable for many behavioral studies. These factors affect such measures as the correlation between mates, the amount and structure of phenotypic variation, and, in female twins, result in a confounding of developmental liability with maternal effects across maternal lines; this weakens the inference from twins to the non-twin population.
One would hope that other half-sib studies would indicate the degree of generality of results from the analysis of twin families; in any case the method may, by comparison with other studies, be a very important tool for understanding the nature of twinning and its biosocial consequences.

NANCE: I am aware of the biologic and epidemiologic
differences between twins and singletons (1, 2). However, the
fact that these differences may introduce a bias for some
traits does not imply that the results for all possible traits
would be similarly biased.   In our design this source of bias
can largely be avoided, whenever it is relevant, by omitting
the twin equations, as we did in our analyses of birth weights.
       For many traits, particularly behavioral traits, I would
have thought the potential biases imposed on conventional half
sibs by the death of a parent, divorce, illegitimacy or poly-
gamy would be far greater than those attributable to the fact
that a child's parent (or grandparent) is an MZ twin.
       Finally, with respect to lateralization in twins, when
this phenomenon is examined critically using objective morphologic traits, there is precious little evidence for enantio-
morphy in MZ twins (3).

REFERENCES

1.   Nance, W.E., <u>Medicine</u> 38, 403-414 (1959).
2.   Nance, W.E., <u>Birth Defects Orig. Art. Ser.</u> 13, 19-44 (1977).
3.   Potter, R.H., and Nance, W.E., <u>Am. J. Phys. Anthrop.</u>
     44, 391-396 (1976).

GENETIC EPIDEMIOLOGY

DYNAMICS AND STATISTICS OF TRAITS

UNDER THE INFLUENCE OF CULTURAL TRANSMISSION

L. L. Cavalli-Sforza
M. W. Feldman

Stanford University
Stanford, California 94305

ABSTRACT

We briefly describe previously published models in which a trait is determined not only by genetic but also by cultural inheritance. We exemplify two types of cultural inheritance. In one, the parents' phenotypes are imitated by the child (this is called phenotypic or F-transmission). In the other (E-transmission) the environment is transmitted by a "blending-type" inheritance and influences the phenotype. Transmission may be uniparental or involve both parents.

In the most complex model, E and F coexist as well as G (genetic transmission, which is assumed to be additive polygenic) and there is evolution under mutation and selection, as well as reciprocal developmental effects of phenotype and environment. Assortment for both phenotype and for environment is considered. Some expectations deduced under various models are indicated, with special attention to genotype-environment covariance and interaction.

The importance of using means, and not only covariances or correlations of adoptive children and parents in estimation of parameters is stressed. Biasses due to the selection of adoptive parents are pointed out. They tend to result in underestimation of the contribution of cultural inheritance from a study of correlation of adopted children and parents. Even after correction, there is poor agreement between the relative roles assigned to genetics and to cultural inheritance by second order moments, and by means from adoption data. Even after correction, second order moments tend to assign a lesser role to cultural inheritance.

133

I. MODELS FOR JOINT CULTURAL AND BIOLOGICAL INHERITANCE

     This paper is concerned with models of inheritance and
evolution of traits which depend, to some extent. at least, on
learning, being therefore under the influence of cultural
processes. We have suggested a number of different models
some of which introduce cultural transmission alone; others
involve the biological as well. When there is direct inheritance of non-biological factors affecting the phenotype of an
individual, such transmission is sometimes so heavily confounded with that of biological factors that a separation is
at best difficult. In the usual paradigm, according to which
the phenotype is determined by genotype and environment,
biological transmission is that of parent's genotype and
cultural that of phenotype and environment of parents to
phenotype and environment of child. Phenotypic and environmental transmissions should be kept distinct one from the
other for purposes of modelling, even though it may be difficult in practice to distinguish them.
     We have suggested a variety of models, which can be
classified according to whether the trait considered is continuous [1,2,4] or discrete [3], the number of loci involved
is one [1,3] or many [2,4] and the cultural transmission
considered is only phenotypic [1,3] or phenotypic + environmental [4].
     An analysis of cultural transmission prior to our at-
tempts was contained in a study of inheritance of IQ by path
analysis by S. Wright [5] in which parental environment was
transmitted over a generation. Jencks et al.[6], Rao, Morton
and Yee [7,8] have further developed S. Wright's analysis,
but never with an evolutionary motivation. The three models
employed in those studies are represented below, in a simplified form by indicating only one parent, and writing G for
genotype, E for environment and F for phenotype:

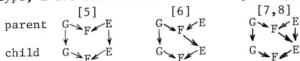

     A study by Conlisk [9] investigated models incorporating
the long term behavior of a simplified genotype and environmental transmission, both affecting phenotype. Another such
study was made by Eaves [10] and is included in our model
for one gene plus phenotypic transmission of a continuous
trait [1].
     We will limit our present review to methods suitable
for continuous traits, of which IQ is a typical example.

The models we consider are either of the phenotypic transmission type [1,2; see also 10], or phenotypic + environmental [5]. The superscript c stands for childhood and a for adult. We indicate only the simplest and the most elaborate considered.

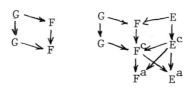

Considering both parents and the various possible modes of assortment and developmental patterns which were studied, there are up to 13 parameters to be estimated. The situation is simplified by assuming some of these parameters to be zero. This generates a number of simpler, closely related models. We can anticipate that the choice between them on the basis of real data is difficult. Moreover, we believe the most constructive way of reaching a satisfactory choice is not to test all models whose goodness of fit can be easily measured and choose the one with the lowest chi square. Rather than testing a number of models belonging in a restricted class and accepting the one which produces the lowest χ^2, it has been our approach to examine the consequences of a number of phenomena, the exact nature of which is often hard to model or quantify but whose importance is eminently plausible from a biological point of view. We feel that conclusions obtained can be reasonably trusted only if important alternatives have been adequately examined. Even if it is difficult to exclude some of them, for lack of data or relevant methodology, there is nothing to be gained by rushing into acceptance of one hypothesis whose major merit is to give superficially "good" chi squares, at a time when other important hypotheses are untested or untestable. Moreover, there is no practical or theoretical advantage gained by obtaining numerical estimates of heritability, or of fractions of variance determined by one or the other source, especially when the level of approximation is such that even the value of the first figure is uncertain. It seems, therefore, scientifically and politically unrewarding, even counterproductive, to give such estimates with two or three figure accuracy.

Among aspects to which, in our view, it is imperative to give adequate consideration before one speaks of "resolution of cultural inheritance" [8], one should consider the following, some of which we will briefly review in this paper:

1) model of assortative mating and its consequences
2) dynamic aspects of the system
3) genotype-environment covariance
4) variation of individual plasticity e.g., non-parallelism of the norm of reaction of different genotypes, which is potentially an important source of genotype-environment interaction
5) miscellaneous genetic problems (number of genes involved, distribution of their effects and their frequencies, dominance, epistacy) - these will not be discussed here
6) use of information from means and not only from variances and covariances
7) biasses intrinsic to the data and their consequences.

The simplest analytic models involve linear transmission. We assume the phenotype of child, f_{t+1}, will depend on the genotype of the child g_{t+1} which in turn depends on that of parents (g_t, g_t'), and on phenotypes and environments of parents (f_t, f_t') and (j_t, j_t') respectively

$$f_{t+1} = \gamma g_{t+1} + \delta_1 f_t + \delta_2 f_t' + \eta_1 j_t + \eta_2 j_t' + N(0,E) \qquad (1)$$

where $N(0,E)$ is a random variable (normal, for simplicity) of mean zero and variance E.

Phenotype transmission is contained in (1) and environment is transmitted as:

$$j_{t+1} = \alpha_1 j_t + \alpha_2 j_t' + N(0,V)$$

where j_t, j_t' are the parental values and $N(0,V)$ a normal random variable with constant variance. Genotype is transmitted according to the standard polygenic rule:

$$g_{t+1} = \frac{g_t + g_t'}{2} + N(0, V_{g,t}/2)$$

where g_{t+1} is the genotypic value of progeny, $N(.,.)$ is a normal random variable with mean zero and $V_{g,t}$ is the variance of the parental genotypic values.

When all relations are linear as above and the mating is not assortative, we are assured from previous work [2,4] and by an algorithm due to Karlin [unpub.] that except in certain degenerate cases [4] the system converges. Explicit equilibrium solutions are available, but the simplest way of obtaining them is probably numerical iteration of the generation recurrencies. Assortative mating introduces problems.

With a large or infinite number of genes – a truly polygenic system – expectations under assortative mating are only approximate [11]. When there is stabilizing selection, as is probably common [12], then there is no convergence problem. Without selection, we have no proof of convergence.

Even if the system has an equilibrium solution, an important source of uncertainty from applications to real data is generated by the dynamic aspects of the recursion system. Unless the system is at equilibrium, variances, covariances and correlations are continuously changing. The equilibrium solutions will be valid only if the environmental conditions and the transmission laws have remained stable for a long time. It would be very surprising if such stability were true of IQ.

Quite apart from the dynamic aspects of the system, which demand confidence that equilibrium has been reached, another type of constancy must be postulated: that of the assortative mating system. Here we encounter another major problem but we can at least supply a formal solution to the question of the consequences of the effects of various types of assortative mating.

II. ASSORTATIVE MATING AND GENOTYPE-ENVIRONMENT COVARIANCE

Call Σ the matrix of the population variances and covariances of genotypic values g, phenotypes f, environment j, θ that of correlations between spouses for the same variables. If one assumes that all the 6 correlation coefficients due to mating are constant as given, then θ is predetermined and there is no estimation problem. In the IQ case, however, it seems reasonable to assume that the assortment for genotype is secondary to that for environment and phenotype, so that the correlation for genotype, partialling out the other variables, is zero. Then:

$$\theta = \Sigma \begin{bmatrix} 0 & 0 \\ 1 & 0 \\ 0 & 1 \end{bmatrix} \begin{bmatrix} 1 & r_{fj} \\ r_{fj} & 1 \end{bmatrix}^{-1} \begin{bmatrix} a & c \\ c & b \end{bmatrix} \begin{bmatrix} 1 & r_{fj} \\ r_{fj} & 1 \end{bmatrix}^{-1} \begin{bmatrix} 0 & 1 & 0 \\ 0 & 0 & 1 \end{bmatrix} \Sigma$$

where $a = r_{ff'}$, $b = r_{jj'}$, $c = r_{jf'}$, the assortments for phenotypes of parents, their environments, and phenotype-environment, taken to be constant over time. Unfortunately, the only way to strengthen our confidence in this or any other models would come from a test of constancy with data from several generations. Incidentally, these conditions are not to be confused with the dynamics of the transmission system; assortative mating may be constant and the population variances and covariances keep changing.

It is of interest that the genotype-environment covariance is determined [4], given the transmission system, the development pattern, and the assortative mating. If its estimate is different from that expected on iteration of the system, either the system is not at equilibrium or the model is wrong. We predict that genotype-environment covariance will be slightly negative under stabilizing selection, and close to zero if selection is directional or absent. But if there is a partial effect of phenotype on environment (over generations, or during development) or if there is a phenotypic component of assortment, then genotype-environment covariance is positive and not negligible. The absence of positive genotype-environment covariance in one of the latest analyses by Rao, Morton and Yee [8] is therefore in disagreement with the expectations from equilibrium, as well as with these authors' earlier analysis [7].

III.   VARIATION OF PLASTICITY AND GENOTYPE-ENVIRONMENT INTERACTION

Genotype-environment interaction is another potential complication which is difficult to test. This important source of variation may be due to differences in individual norms of reaction, determined by genotypes. Any behavioral trait like IQ involves substantial learning; the models to which every individual is exposed, the teaching received, the motivation and the overall conditions in which training takes place vary considerably from one individual to the other. Every family, every social milieu must contribute a very different experience. It would be truly surprising if there were no genetic differences in the capacity to learn, and to react (which we call "plasticity"). What is inherited is probably plasticity; the final outcome will depend both on individual plasticity and the environment to which the individual is exposed. Variation in individual reactivity and in environment of exposure will probably lead to genotype-environment interaction. A dramatic example is that of PKU, in which a peculiar genotype may determine a normal IQ, or a very severely impaired one depending on a relatively simple change in nutrition. This is not a reactivity to a learning condition, but the principle should be the same. We considered a model [1] in which plasticity depends on genotype and involves a linear response to the environment (taken to be the parental phenotype). This is a phenotypic transmission scheme in which, unlike other models, the slope of the plasticity can also vary with the genotype. A further

characterization of this model and a search for conditions
of observation that would clearly discriminate this model
from the others would be valuable.

IV. THE MEAN IQ OF ADOPTED CHILDREN

Quantitative analyses of IQ are based on variances and
covariances, no attention being devoted to means. Valuable
information could be retrieved from means, in particular for
the estimation of parameters such as δ's amd η's in equation
(1). These questions are of more direct interest than the
fractions of variance which are usually estimated. They are
closer to intuition than fractions of variance, especially
for people who are not experienced in variance partition ·
techniques, and are perhaps more meaningful in general.
One of the most typical effects at the level of means
is that found in adopted children. In a summary of adoption
data [13], the mean IQ of adopted children averaged from
these classical studies is about 109. This is a conspicuous
increase over the population mean. The tendency among he-
reditarians is to dismiss this fact as uninteresting, or
easy to explain away, even if heritability is extremely high
[13,14]. The fact is that models involving only genetic
transmission do not supply the necessary algebra to evaluate
this effect, unless they are integrated with cultural transmission as in the models indicated in the first part of this
paper. There are various reasons for further study of means.
It is difficult to accept a theory which does not explain
them; after all, in means is concentrated an important part
of our practical interest. If IQ is at all important from a
social point of view, we cannot be insensitive to the fact
that mean IQ goes up or down. Moreover, means are statistically more informative being affected by a relatively smaller
standard error than variances or covariances. They may be
sensitive to biases, other than those affecting variances
and covariances. But they may, as we shall see, help us
study some of the biases affecting the second order moments,
which have previously passed unnoticed.
We will very briefly examine here how means of adopted
children can be predicted on the basis of a theory assuming
mixed cultural and genetic inheritance. A more sophisticated
treatment should involve joint estimation of all the parameters of the model using means and variances. We do not
believe presently available data lend themselves to a truly
satisfactory analysis. The great variety of sources and
nature of the data, the heterogeneity of populations involved
make it difficult to believe that the analysis of such a
diverse body of information is truly rewarding. If super-

ficially good fits are obtained this is probably more an
indication of the magnitude of the experimental error than
of the validity of the theories and uniformity of the data.
The following treatment should be viewed only as an indication that means can and should be used even if estimates
obtainable at present are not taken too seriously.

Using recent data on adoption [15] which are probably
more satisfactory than many earlier studies, we find white
children adopted in white families of the Northern States
have an average IQ of 106.2, while their adoptive parents
have an average IQ of 114.5. The authors give evidence that
these adopted children are not selected so that the IQ "genotypic" mean can be considered very close to the population
average.

We will first consider an FG model (genotypic plus phenotypic transmission only), i.e. $\eta=0$ in equation [1] and take
$\delta_1 = \delta_2 = \delta/2$. The expected phenotype of adopted children
will then be from [1]:

$$E(f_{t+1}^{(a)}) = \gamma\mu_{g,t+1}^{(a)} + \delta\mu_{f,t}^{(a)} \tag{3}$$

where $\mu_{g,t+1}^{(a)}$ is the genotypic mean of the adopted children,
and $\mu_{f,t}^{(a)}$ the phenotypic mean of their adoptive parents. In
the general population the mean of the phenotypic means of
the parents, $\mu_{f,t}$, is 100 and so is that of their children,
$\mu_{f,t+1}$:

$$\mu_{f,t+1} = \gamma\mu_{g,t+1} + \delta\mu_{f,t} \tag{4}$$

From what was said before, $\mu_{g,t+1}^{(a)} = \mu_{g,t+1}$. Taking the
expected means of $f_{t+1}^{(a)}$ equal to the observed values given
earlier, from the difference of (3) and (4):

$$\delta = \frac{E(f_{t+1}^{(a)}) - \mu_{f,t+1}}{\mu_{f,t}^{(a)} - \mu_{f,t}} = \frac{106.2-100}{114.5-100} = 0.43\pm.05$$

The standard error (S.E.) of δ given above is computed using
the approximate formula for the variance of a ratio, from the
S.E.'s of the observed means given in the original paper.
The value of γ can be expected to be equal to $1-\delta$, to permit
the phenotypic means to remain constant over generations at
equilibrium. The ratio of δ/γ is therefore close to unity.

This would indicate that the relative importance of genotype (γ) and parental phenotype (δ) in determining the child's phenotype are nearly equal.

An estimate of δ can be obtained also from variances and covariances. As shown in (1) in the absence of assortative mating (b in that paper = $\delta/2$) and in a paper in preparation for assortative mating ($\underline{a}$ = correlation between phenotype of spouses), the covariance between adopted offspring and adoptive parents is:

$$w_{APAO} = \frac{\delta}{2} (1+a) F,$$

where F is the phenotypic population variance, (F = 225 for IQ), or approximately $\delta = \frac{2 r_{APAO}}{1+a}$ (a better approximation will be given elsewhere). Unfortunately, however, the estimated value of r_{APAO}, 0.095 (namely the average for fathers and mothers) is biassed in the sample of adopted children, and so is that of the assortative mating of foster parents ($\underline{a}$ = 0.25 observed). The bias is due to the selection of adoptive parents, who have an abnormally high mean and low variance. It should be stressed that this bias almost always artificially reduces the correlation of adoptive children with foster parents. We suggest using a correction method based on the hypothesis that this selection is of gaussian type [16,17]. In the present case r_{APAO} is increased from 0.095 to 0.14, and $\underline{a}$ from 0.25 to 0.44. The estimate of δ is then 0.19±0.11, lower (t = 1.9, p around 5%) than that obtained from the means. Some further source of bias must be operating, or the transmission model is inadequate.

One possible source of error is that the correction for bias due to the selection of adoptive parents is inadequate. We have suggested that a test of the validity of our proposed correction method might involve checking if the distribution of IQ is normal among foster parents. Normality should be unaltered by the selection process envisaged. It was not altered in this sample of adoptive parents (S. Scarr, personal communication). We have proposed an alternative method of correction to be published in due course, for use when normality is altered.

This seems to dispose of a simple model of phenotypic and genotypic transmission. The test of the full model in equation (1) for δ, $\eta \neq 0$ is complex. If we try an alternative simplification ($\delta = 0$, $\eta \neq 0$ i.e. only genotypic and environmental transmission) we need, for analysis a good index of environment, which is of course difficult to obtain.

We take as a first approximation, education as such an index, and transform all variables to scales of unit standard deviation. We can obtain an estimate of η from the mean IQ of adopted children (which is 6.2/15 = 0.41 standard deviations above the general mean) and the average education of adoptive mothers, which is 0.74 standard deviations above the mean of the population:

$$\eta = 0.41/0.74 = 0.55 \pm 0.06$$

Again, η can be estimated also from correlations. A simplified formula is:

$$\eta = \frac{2r_{APAO}}{(1+a)r_{fj}}$$

where r_{fj} is the correlation between phenotype and environment index. This assumes the assortative mating is primarily determined by phenotype. The numerical estimate, $\eta = 0.30 \pm 0.24$, is not in disagreement with the estimate from means mostly because its standard error is very large. This unfortunate property of second moments does, of course, make estimates from means preferable, other things being equal. But an essential requirement is that both procedures of estimation, from means and from second order moments, give results in agreement. The indication from this preliminary analysis is that results from means make cultural inheritance about as important as genetics.

If the discrepancy between results from means and variances/covariances is real, it must be resolved before numerical conclusions can be trusted. If other sources of bias are responsible, they must be clearly sought and evaluated. If the discrepancy is not real, the inclusion of means in the process of estimation, and the correction of bias due to selection of adoptive parents will alter the estimates [7,8] of relative importance of cultural and biological inheritance. The former will be increased and the latter decreased. Inevitably, we feel that optimism [8] on the "resolution of cultural inheritance" is unjustified.

REFERENCES

1. Cavalli-Sforza, L.L. and Feldman, M.W. Cultural versus
    biological inheritance: phenotypic transmission from
    parents to children (a theory of the effect of parental
    phenotypes on children's phenotypes). Am. J. Hum. Genet.
    25, 618 (1973).

2. Feldman, M.W. and Cavalli-Sforza, L.L. The evolution of
    continuous variation II. Complex transmission and
    assortative mating. Theor. Pop. Biol. 11, 161 (1977).
3. Feldman, M.W. and Cavalli-Sforza, L.L. Cultural and
    biological processes, selection for a trait under complex
    transmission. Theor. Pop. Biol. 9, 238 (1976).
4. Cavalli-Sforza, L. L. and Feldman, M.W. Evolution of
    continuous variation III: Joint transmission of genotype
    phenotype and environment, (submitted to Genetics)(1977).
5. Wright, S. Statistical methods in biology. J. Am.
    Statist. Assoc. 26, 155 (1931).
6. Jencks, C. Inequality, Basic Books Inc., New York (1972).
7. Rao, D.C., Morton, N.E. and Yee, S. Analysis of family
    resemblance. II. A linear model for familial corre-
    lation. Am. J. Human Genet. 26, 331 (1974).
8. Rao, D.C., Morton, N.E. and Yee, S. Resolution of
    cultural and biological inheritance by path analysis.
    Am. J. Human Genet. 28, 228 (1976).
9. Conlisk, J. Can equalization of opportunity reduce
    social mobility? Amer. Econ. Rev. 64, 80 (1974).
10. Eaves, L. The effect of cultural transmission on continu-
    ous variation. Heredity 37, 41 (1976).
11. Crow, J.F. and Felsenstein, J. The effect of assortative
    mating on the genetic composition of a population.
    Eugen. Quart. 15, 85 (1968).
12. Haldane, J.B.S. The measurement of natural selection.
    Proc. 9th Int. Cong. Genetics, 480 (1953). Carylogia,
    vol. suppl., 1954).
13. Munsinger, H. The adopted child's IQ: A critical review.
    Psychological Bulletin 82, 623 (1975).
14. Jensen, A.R. Let's understand Skodak and Skeels, finally",
    Educational Psychologist, 10, 30 (1973).
15. Scarr, S. and Weinberg, R.A. The influence of "family
    background" on intellectual attainment; the unique
    contribution of adoptive studies to estimating environ-
    mental effects (MSSB Conference on Family Environment
    subsequent child development, CASBS, Stanford) (1977).
16. Pearson, K. Mathematical contributions to the theory of
    evolution. XI. On the influence of natural selection
    on the variability and correlations of organs.
    Philosophical Transactions 200, 1 (1903).
17. Cavalli-Sforza, L.L. and Bodmer W. The Genetics of Human
    Populations, W.H. Freeman & Co., San Francisco (1971).

IQ AS A PARADIGM IN GENETIC EPIDEMIOLOGY

D. C. Rao and N. E. Morton

Population Genetics Laboratory
University of Hawaii
Honolulu, Hawaii 96822

A general linear model with no environmentalist or hereditarian bias is presented here for the resolution of cultural and biological inheritance by path analysis. We place emphasis on tests of hypotheses about biological and cultural in-, heritance rather than mere estimation of variance components. The model is then applied to a large body of data on IQ. The lower part of the distribution of IQ is a medical as well as a social problem, the resolution of which is part of genetic epidemiology. Further, analysis of IQ data illustrates methods that promise to clarify the causes of family resemblance for other traits closely related to disease.

We believe that the methods are appropriate for a trait as complex as IQ; whether the available data are conclusive is another question. At best the IQ debate is solved; at worst a method is given for its solution if new data are required. In any case, a distinction must be made between a model with the capability to resolve cultural and biological inheritance and a data set which may or may not be adequate.

THE MODEL

In this paper variables are denoted by capital letters and parameters by lower case letters. The general model involves three unobserved variables as causes, and two observed

variables as effects: the causes are genotype (G), family
environment (C) and residual environment (E), and the two
effects are phenotype (P) defined by the quantitative trait
and an estimate of the family environment, called an index
(I), in which an individual was raised. Recent advances in
analysis of family resemblance depend critically on indices.
Figure 1 shows the path diagram describing our model, where
causes and effects are denoted by ellipses and rectangles
respectively.

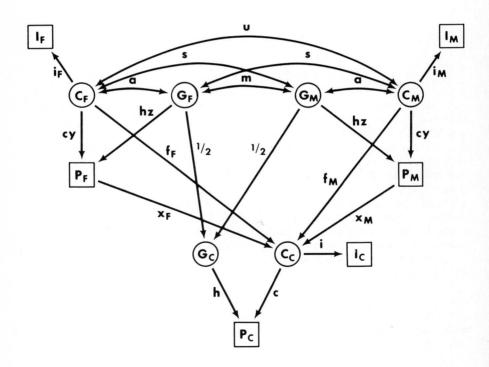

Fig. 1. General path diagram for nuclear families. The
subscripts F, M, C denote father, mother and child respectively. G is genotype, C is family environment with index I,
and P is phenotype. Each of the phenotypes and indices have
another path from an independent cause. These residual paths
are not shown since they do not contribute to family resemblance.

There are 14 functionally independent parameters in this model, defined in Table 1; as indicated at the bottom of the table, the parameter a, the correlation between an individual's genotype and family environment, is functionally dependent on the other parameters. Genetic and cultural effects are distinguished for children and adults: whereas h^2 and c^2 are the genetic and cultural heritabilities respectively for children, they are h^2z^2 and c^2y^2 for adults. Cultural is here used in the broad sense to include any aspect of family environment. Environment may be transmitted between generations either directly (f_F, f_M) or by an effect of parent's phenotype on child's environment (x_F, x_M): specific maternal effects are thus incorporated by subscripting the effects of parental variables on the children they raise. Subscripts F, M and C denote father, mother, and child respectively. The index may be of unequal precision for parents and children, and therefore we introduce separate indices for father, mother and children. An index is not assumed to be a perfect estimator of the relevant family environment: a path coefficient i (or i_F or i_M) measures the adequacy of I (or I_F or I_M) as an estimate of C (or C_F or C_M). The index of an individual may be created by regressing the phenotype on relevant observed variables which are not themselves products of the genotype. In the absence of maternal effects, $x_F = x_M = x$, $f_F = f_M = f$, and hence a = $[hzx(1 + m) + s(f + cyx)]/[1 - (f + cyx)]$.

Assortative mating is described by three marital parameters (m, u, s), and the correlation between mates is assumed to be independent of the duration of cohabitation. If this assumption is violated, the marital parameters would be overestimated. There are three natural constraints on the parameters. These arise through the total relative variances of child's phenotype ($\Sigma_{PC} + \sigma^2_{PC} = 1$), adult's phenotype ($\Sigma_{PA} + \sigma^2_{PA} = 1$) and child's common environment ($\Sigma_{CC} + \sigma^2_{CC} = 1$), where the σ^2's are residual components and

$$\Sigma_{PC} = h^2 + c^2 + 2hca$$

$$\Sigma_{PA} = h^2z^2 + c^2y^2 + 2hzcya$$

$$\Sigma_{CC} = f^2_F + f^2_M + x^2_F + x^2_M + 2(cy + hza)(x_F f_F + x_M f_M) \qquad [1]$$

$$+ 2(cyu + hzs)(f_F x_M + f_M x_F) + 2f_F f_M u + 2x_F x_M \rho$$

and ρ = expected phenotypic marital correlation. Therefore, the three constraints are

$$\Sigma_{PC} \leq 1, \Sigma_{PA} \leq 1 \text{ and } \Sigma_{CC} \leq 1.$$

TABLE 1

Path Coefficients of the General Model (Figure 1)

	Symbol	Definition
marital:	m	correlation between parental genotypes
	u	correlation between common environments of spouses
	s	correlation between common environment of an adult and spouse's genotype
environmental:	c	effect of common environment on child's phenotype
	y	ratio of the effects of common environment on adult's phenotype and on child's phenotype
	f_F	effect of father's common environment on child's common environment
	f_M	effect of mother's common environment on child's common environment
	x_F	effect of father's (adult) phenotype on child's common environment
	x_M	effect of mother's (adult) phenotype on child's common environment
genetic:	h	effect of genotype on child's phenotype (square-root of "heritability")
	z	ratio of the effects of genotype on adult's phenotype and on child's phenotype
indices:	i	effect of child's common environment on child's index (a measure of adequacy of the index)
	i_F	effect of father's common environment on father's index
	i_M	effect of mother's common environment on mother's index

derived:	a	correlation between individual's genotype and common environment

$$= [hz(1 + m)(x_F + x_M) +$$
$$s(f_F + f_M + cyx_F + cyx_M)]/$$
$$[2 - (f_F + f_M + cyx_F + cyx_M)]$$

ANALYSIS

The simplest sample design for this model is a collection of nuclear families. Phenotypes and indices of fathers, mothers and children generate 16 correlations. Therefore the general model is overdeterminate in nuclear families, leaving 2 degrees of freedom (d.f.) for testing goodness-of-fit of the model.

Methods for estimating the 16 correlations from nuclear families are described elsewhere (1), the corresponding expected correlations being derivable from Figure 1. The log-likelihood function is taken as

$$\ln L = -\chi^2/2 + \text{constant}$$

$$\chi^2 = (\underset{\sim}{z} - \overline{\underset{\sim}{z}})' \Sigma^{-1} (\underset{\sim}{z} - \overline{\underset{\sim}{z}}) \qquad \qquad \cdots \qquad [2]$$

where $\underset{\sim}{z}$ is the column vector of bias-corrected z transforms of the 16 observed correlations, $\overline{\underset{\sim}{z}}$ is the corresponding vector for expected correlations, and Σ is the covariance matrix of the z transforms (2, 3). Estimating all 16 correlations from the same set of data induces correlations between observed correlations. This aspect is incorporated into Σ following the result of Elston (4). The residual χ^2 after estimating κ parameters follows a chi-square distribution with $16-\kappa$ d.f. By specifying the expected correlations and hence $\overline{\underset{\sim}{z}}$ as functions of the parameters we make χ^2 a function of the parameters. Therefore, by maximising $\ln L$, or minimising χ^2, we estimate the unknown parameters and use the residual χ^2 for tests of hypotheses. If $\chi^2_{16-\kappa-\omega}$ is the value of χ^2 after estimating $\kappa + \omega$ parameters, and $\chi^2_{16-\kappa}$ is another value after estimating only κ of the $\kappa + \omega$ parameters, the other ω parameters being fixed under a null hypothesis, $\chi^2_\omega = \chi^2_{16-\kappa} - \chi^2_{16-\kappa-\omega}$ provides the likelihood-ratio test for the null hypothesis on the other ω parameters. The general model, in 14 parameters, is tested by the residual χ^2 with $16 - 14 = 2$ d.f. A computer program NUCVAR performs these analyses.

The most important underlying assumptions are: (1) a linear additive model, neglecting all interactions, and (2) the genotype-environment correlation a is in equilibrium. Violation of the first assumption has been shown to have no detectable effect on the estimates of genetic and cultural heritabilities (5). If the second assumption is false, the results are only approximate. The final word rests with the goodness-of-fit test.

EXTENSIONS OF THE MODEL

For a randomly adopted child G and C are not correlated
since G comes from the true parents whereas C comes from the
adoptive parents. The phenotypic variance of such children
is therefore reduced, and so correlations involving adopted
children are multiplied by θ or θ^2 depending on whether one
or both the individuals involved are adopted, where θ = ratio
of the two phenotypic standard deviations (2).

Models were presented (6) for a variety of other biological and social relationships such as twins, half-sibs,
foster children, uncle-niece and first cousins; these models
did not incorporate maternal effects nor different indices
for children and adults. Data on such relationships can be
added to data on nuclear families for tests of consistency
and increased power. If each correlation is estimated from
a different set of data, such estimates are independent,
leading to simplification of χ^2 in equation [2]. For m such
independent estimates

$$\chi^2 = \sum_{i=1}^{m} (z_i - \bar{z}_i)^2 / \sigma_{z_i}^2 \qquad \cdots \qquad [3]$$

where

$$\sigma_{z_i}^2 = \begin{cases} 1/(N_i - 3) & \text{if } i \text{ is interclass} \\ \\ 1/(N_i - 1.5) & \text{if } i \text{ is intraclass} \end{cases}$$

and N_i is the sample size. A variety of relationships have
been incorporated in a computer program NUVAR which uses
equation [3] for χ^2. If not all estimates are independent,
and not all are estimated from the same data, a combination
of equations [2] and [3] would yield the appropriate χ^2.

The most important underlying assumptions are: (1)
phenotypic similarity between twins due to common prenatal
and postnatal environment is no greater or less than for
ordinary siblings, and (2) adopted children are placed at
random and the true parents exert no influence on the children
either prior to or after the adoption. Violation of the first
assumption would overestimate heritability, whereas departure
from the second assumption would underestimate heritability.

However appealing a model may be, it is a simplification
of nature and may always be stigmatized as an oversimplifica-
tion (for example, by omitting gene-environment interaction,
dominance, epistasis, or environment specific to MZ twins).
To such criticism there is only one answer: a statistical
test of goodness-of-fit, which in samples of adequate size
and structure can rule out an inadmissible model. This was
the last aspect of path analysis to evolve.

ANALYSIS OF IQ DATA

Genetic epidemiology has an interest in resolving biological and cultural inheritance for IQ because the lower
part of the IQ distribution is by any definition a disordered
state of health. Analysis of IQ data encounters three major
difficulties: (1) the available data come from different
sources, mostly collected by psychologists and sociologists
for other purposes, and their quality and comparability are
questionable; (2) perhaps more than any other variable IQ is
subject to assortative mating and a presumption of gene-
environment covariance which require unfamiliar methods of
analysis; and (3) because IQ varies among socioeconomic
groups it arouses strong emotion. However, in compensation
for its thorns, IQ has two advantages at this stage of genetic
epidemiology: (1) it presents an unusual diversity of data
bearing on family resemblance and (2) it poses an analytical
problem whose solution cannot fail to be fruitful in studies
of blood pressure, glycemia, and other variables closely related to disease, both for understanding etiology and as a
predictor of recurrence risks in genetic counselling and
preventive medicine.

There is pronounced assortative mating for IQ and any
attempt to analyse IQ data should incorporate this aspect.
The simplest model of assortative mating is direct homogamy,
in which potential mates are assumed to assort on the basis
of inferred IQ independent of social contacts. As a more
realistic alternative, we suppose instead that individuals
are characterized by social homogamy H, which includes status,
tastes, contacts, and academic performance: assortative
mating for these factors leads secondarily to the marital
correlation for IQ. Specification of the causes of H is in
the domain of sociology: genetics is concerned with the
effects of H, which generates correlations between an individual's genotype and environment and those of his spouse
(figure 2). A simple model was used by Sewall Wright (7) for
mating on the basis of social class but is more general, since
it includes residence, schools, churches, jobs, and social
activities. In our notation social homogamy has a path coefficient $\sqrt{u}$ to environment and $\sqrt{m}$ to genotype. Therefore
the marital correlations are:

> m, between genotypes of father and mother
> u, between environments of father and mother
> $\sqrt{mu}$ between genotype and spouse's environment.

This generalization of homogamy is the special case $s = \sqrt{mu}$
of the general model presented in Figure 1. Also, since
maternal effects were ruled out for IQ in another

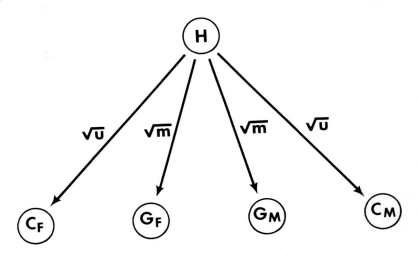

Fig. 2.   Primary marital correlations.   Social homogamy (H), genotype (G), family environment (C).   Subscripts F, M denote father and mother, respectively.   Residual paths are not shown.

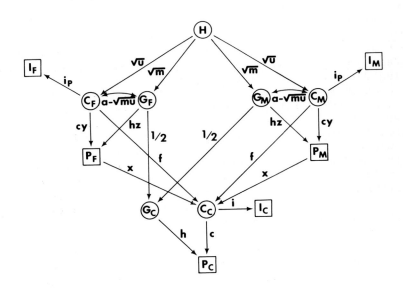

Fig. 3.   General model for the inheritance of IQ in nuclear families.   H denotes social homogamy and the subscript P denotes parent.

material (8), we propose to adopt the reduced model with $f_F = f_M = f$, $x_F = x_M = x$, and also $i_F = i_M = i_P$ ($\neq 1$) for the analysis of IQ data. Such a reduced model is presented in Figure 3 which contains only 10 functionally independent parameters. Ideally one would exploit the 16 correlations in nuclear families, leaving 16 - 10 = 6 d.f. for testing goodness-of-fit of the model. For immunoglobulin E (9) and lipoprotein concentrations (1) where data on nuclear families are available, we have successfully adopted that strategy. Unfortunately no single study on IQ collected such data. Therefore here we compile and analyse all familial correlations available for IQ that can be analysed by our methods.

To take advantage of goodness of fit tests we require more than 10 familial correlations. Except for the pioneer study of Wright (10), prior experience has been limited to phenotypic correlations (11), neglecting valuable information from correlations between indices or between phenotype and index (2), and using a model substantially different from ours.

To assemble a suitable data set is not easy. We seek a measure of IQ which is comparable to the Stanford-Binet or Wechsler test and an index comparable to the Duncan occupational scale. The population should be defined, and we choose Americans (predominantly white, non-farm) as providing the greatest amount of information. Less ample data are available for the normal populations of England and Russia. Because of the limited information in these sources, we shall use them mainly for tests of consistency with the American sample.

AMERICAN IQ: THE COMPLETE DATA SET

We found 65 estimates of 16 relevant correlations in samples which appeared representative of the white, non-farm American population (appendix). Any attempt to select data on family resemblance is liable to capriciousness, and so we have been inclusive: except through oversight no relevant data have been omitted, even though their comparability may be questioned. We are grateful to Prof. A. S. Goldberger for drawing our attention to several studies and for his important comments on others; however, we are responsible for any errors of omission or commission that remain. Better bibliographers would find other references. Having examined these data in many ways, we doubt that the conclusions can be altered by such perturbations.

Table 3 presents the heterogeneity χ^2's for multiple estimates of the same correlation. Total heterogeneity in this material due to differences in sampling and measurement

is highly significant (χ^2_{49} = 142.46). To offset this as well
as possible we have used σ^2 = 142.46/49 = 2.907 as the error
variance for tests of hypotheses and standard errors. Tests
of hypotheses are carried out in terms of F-ratios. If
χ^2_{m-k} and χ^2_m are the residual chi-squares under the model
(general) and a specific null hypothesis respectively, the F-
ratio on k and 49 d.f. for testing the null hypothesis is
calculated as

$$(\chi^2_m - \chi^2_{m-k})/k\sigma^2$$

Goodness-of-fit of a model is calculated as

$$\chi^2_{m-k}/(m-k)\sigma^2$$

on m-k and 49 d.f.

Since previous estimates of the genetic marital correlation (m) were not significant, we propose to work with
m = 0 as the general model for IQ, reducing the number of
functionally independent parameters to 9. Tests of hypotheses on American IQ data are summarized in Table 2. The
general model with m = 0 fits well ($F_{7,49}$ = 1.95, P > .05).
Thus there is no evidence for dominance, epistasis or gene-
environment interaction. The gene-environment correlation is
estimated as

$$a = \frac{hzx}{1 - f - cyx} = .013 \pm .045$$

which is surprisingly small. This illustrates how easily one
can incorporate gene-environment correlation into analysis of
family resemblance, contrary to the reservations expressed by
Moran (12). Tests of hypotheses on the significance of x and
f are also presented in Table 2. Parental environments contribute significantly to the environment of their children
($F_{1,49}$ = 18.75, P < .001). A simple hypothesis with x = 0 is
not rejected ($F_{1,49}$ = 0.03, P > .50), and therefore parental
phenotypes do not significantly affect the environment of
their children. We therefore take m = x = 0 as the parsimonious model for American IQ. Table 3 shows the fit of this
model to the 16 equations, and the last line in Table 5 gives
the variance components.

Except for three correlations involving adopted children
(FST, FSP and AMA), consistency over data sets is remarkable
(Table 3). These three observed correlations are elevated
due to assortative placement, and it is small wonder that
these correlations are under-predicted by our model. Hence,
these discrepancies do not constitute evidence against our
model for nuclear families. If desired, a nuisance parameter

TABLE 2

Tests of Hypotheses on American IQ data (m = 0)

Hypothesis	Residual		F-ratio	P
	χ^2	df		
general (m = 0)	39.74	7	1.95	> .05
m = f = 0*	94.26	8	18.75	< .001
m = x = 0	39.83	8	0.03	> .50

F-ratio is defined as the residual mean square divided by the error mean square, where the error mean square = average heterogeneity between estimates of the same correlation = 142.46/49 = 2.907. The associated df = 7,49 for the general model, and 1,49 for the other hypotheses.

*The unconditional solution yielded $\Sigma_{CC} > 1$. This solution is constrained to have $\Sigma_{CC} = 1$ (see text for Σ_{CC})

---

can be introduced to offset assortative placement. Wright (7) accepted the marital correlation as direct homogamy, used the culture index of Burks, assumed that i = 1, made no goodness-of-fit test, and dealt with a mathematically indeterminate model, yet his prodigious intuition led to essentially the same inferences as the much larger sample considered here. Even Jencks et al. (13), despite arbitrary assumptions and failure to recognize inter-generational differences, obtained estimates of h and c not too far from Wright and us. Rao et al. (2) applied a simplified model to data which depended critically on Burks' culture index, yet their estimates of c, h, y, and z agreed closely with Wright's earlier work and with the present paper. Supplementing Burks' culture index by a larger body of sociological data on occupational status eliminates the borderline significance for covariance between genotype and environment. The present material clearly establishes a causal path from parental environment to child's environment (f ≠ 0).

  Heritability and the effect of family environment in children are both somewhat greater than Wright estimated (Table 5). Like us he concluded that adults are sensitive to their childhood environment and that heritability is less than for children, "presumably because the leveling effect

TABLE 3

Heterogeneity in the American IQ data, and goodness of fit of the model $m = x = 0$

Relation	Heterogeneity χ^2	d.f.	Goodness of fit to pooled samples N	r	$\hat{r}$	χ^2	Expected correlation
FMTXY	17.10	7	1118	.511	.516	0.05	$c^2 y^2 u$
FMTIXIY	0	0	1165	.226	.206	0.48	$u i_p^2$
OPTXY	6.10	4	1310	.484	.500	0.59	$h^2 z/2 + c^2 y f(1+u)$
OPTXIY	10.05	3	1272	.570	.544	1.77	$f c y (1+u) i$
OPTXIX	0	0	887	.347	.347	0.00	$c y i_p$
OPTIXIIY	26.91	5	17432	.343	.344	0.04	$f(1+u) i i_p$
OPAXY	0	0	63	.407	.228	2.41	$h^2 z/2$
SSTXY	32.93	10	2467	.516	.502	0.96	$h^2/2 + c^2$
SSTXIX	9.79	3	4717	.304	.314	0.57	$c i$
SSAXY	0	0	125	.249	.345	1.34	$h^2/2$
MZTXY	10.71	2	421	.842	.846	0.09	$h^2 + c^2$
AMAXY	0	0	19	.679	.301	4.32	$h^2 z^2$
FSTXY	8.38	5	421	.360	.157	19.91	c^2
FSPXY	1.91	3	228	.283	.157	3.94	c^2
OFPXY	10.32	5	1181	.228	.272	2.62	$c^2 y f(1+u)$
OFPYIY	8.26	2	774	.286	.314	0.74	$c i$
Totals	142.46	49				$\chi^2_8 = 39.83$	

of the school system is replaced by varying stimulation in different occupations" (7). For m = x = 0 the proportion of sibling resemblance in childhood due to genotype is

$$G = \frac{h^2/2}{h^2/2 + c^2} = .69$$

At maturity h is replaced by hz and c by cy, giving G = .22. Thus genetic inheritance accounts for a substantial part of sibling resemblance in childhood, while resemblance of adult sibs is mostly cultural.

AMERICAN IQ: REDUCED DATA SETS

Data on certain uncommon relationships are difficult to collect and interpret. Such relationships include MZ twins (reared together or apart) and foster-children. Much of this material was compiled a generation ago when our society was more tolerant of research on human biology, and inevitably can be faulted now because of imperfections in the data or its analysis (14). The most rigorous solution is to determine all correlations in the same well-designed study. Failing that, it is instructive to examine reduced data sets selected to reveal possible biases (Tables 4 and 5).

Of the reported relationships three involving foster children (FST, FSP and OFP) are expected to underestimate genetic heritability, because of selective placement. However, their omission has no appreciable effect on any estimate, nor does omission of the correlations for identical twins (which may include their special environmental similarity). Clearly the rare relationships that have borne the brunt of published criticism have made no difference in the conclusions. Of the adoption studies, some are expected to overestimate the genetic component (AMA, OPA and SSA) and some to have the opposite effect (FST, FSP and OFP). Omission of these studies makes no difference. Omission of FST alone, the most discrepant equation, does not alter the results much. Removing all the significantly discrepant equations (FSP, FST, AMA) has no detectable effect. Replacing the observed marital correlation (FMTXY) by a much smaller value of .33 based on 1016 pairs (15) reduces the estimate of u drastically. Thus, the high estimate of u (.940) for the original data set may be reflecting partly the post-marital resemblance as well. Tables 4 and 5 present various other reduced data sets. It is remarkable how little the estimates change over various subsets. The conclusion that genetic heritability decreases and

TABLE 4

Goodness-of-Fit Tests for Various Subsets
of the American IQ data (m = x = 0)

Relationships deleted from the data	Heterogeneity		Residual			
	χ^2	d.f.	χ^2	d.f.	F-ratio	P
FST, FSP, OFP	113.58	34	11.74	4	0.88	> .25
FST, FSP, OFP, OPA, SSA	113.58	34	8.03	2	1.20	> .25
FST, FSP, OFP, MZT, AMA	102.88	32	6.23	2	0.97	> .25
MZT, AMA	131.76	47	34.54	6	2.05	> .05
MZT, AMA, OPA, SSA	131.76	47	29.93	4	2.67	< .05
All indices*	87.47	36	31.99	6	2.19	> .05
FST	134.08	44	17.90	7	0.84	> .50
FST, FSP, AMA	132.17	41	9.05	5	0.56	> .50
FMTXY	125.36	42	39.34	7	1.88	> .05
FMTXY replaced by .33** (N = 1016)	125.36	42	48.29	8	2.02	> .05
None	142.46	49	39.83	8	1.71	> .10

*Parameters are indeterminate in this data set, and there-
fore only h, c, y, z are estimated here, fixing f and u at
the values obtained for the entire data set (last line of
this table). See Table 5 for the parameter values.

**This solution is constrained to have $\Sigma_{CC} = 1$ since the un-
constrained solution yielded $\Sigma_{CC} > 1$.

cultural heritability increases with maturity is stable over
data sets.

ENGLISH IQ

A large material on family resemblance was collected by
English workers, nearly all by Sir Cyril Burt (Table 6).
After his death many puzzling inconsistencies and ambiguities
were discovered in the reported data (16) which were severely

TABLE 5. Variance Components as Fractions of Total Phenotypic Variance and Estimates of Other Parameters for Subsets of American IQ Data Considered in Table 4 ($m = x = 0$).

Relationships deleted from the data	Variance components				Estimates of other parameters			
	Children		Adults					
	h^2	c^2	h^2z^2	c^2y^2	u	f	i	i_p
FST, FSP, OFP	.712	.138	.357	.559	.925	.463	.833	.464
FST, FSP, OFP, OPA, SSA	.701	.148	.293	.560	.923	.483	.799	.464
FST, FSP, OFP, MZT, AMA	.760	.132	.324	.562	.921	.461	.841	.463
MZT, AMA	.710	.158	.257	.551	.936	.484	.785	.468
MZT, AMA, OPA, SSA	.716	.158	.234	.553	.934	.488	.781	.467
All indices*	.642	.198	.258	.523	.940	.478	–	–
FST	.713	.136	.365	.556	.929	.459	.835	.466
FST, FSP, AMA	.716	.135	.334	.559	.925	.463	.833	.464
FMTXY	.690	.157	.300	.553	.992	.464	.794	.466
FMTXY replaced by .33* (N=1016)	.687	.159	.316	.532	.681	.545	.790	.478
None	.689	.157	.301	.549	.940	.478	.792	.469
	±.035	±.024	±.122	±.086	±.158	±.043	±.066	±.037

Previous analyses:

Wright, 1931 (10)	.50	.07	.30	.36
Jencks et al., 1972 (13)	.45	.35	.45	.35
Rao et al., 1974 (2)	.75	.09	.12	.52
Rao et al., 1977 (32)	.71	.08	.32	.50

*See footnotes to Table 4

TABLE 6

English Data

Relation	r	N	Source
FMTXY	.379	95	Jensen, table IX (16)
OPTXY	.489	963	"　　　　"　　　"
UNTXY	.354	375	"　　　　"　　　"
FCTXY	.289	552	"　　　　"　　　"
OFPXY	.19	88	"　　　　"　　　"
SSTXY	.51	412	Jencks, table A-6 (13)
	.498	264	Jencks, table A-9
FSTXY	.252	136	Jencks, table A-9
SSAXY	.423	151	Jensen, table VII
MZTXY	.87	211	Jencks, table A-6
MZAXY	.86	53	Jencks, table A-12
	.77	38	"　　　"　　"

criticized (14). Even though the English data give a poor
fit to the American parameter values (Table 8), the fit
improves substantially when h and c are estimated (χ^2_8 = 12.84,

Table 7); the estimates of h and c do not differ much from
the American values (Table 8). The best fit is for extreme
values of u and f, with somewhat larger values of h and z and
smaller values of c and y. If England represents a more
stratified society, then such stratification appears to be
without important genetic consequences. Whether the errors
in Burt's material are trivial or profound, accidental or
systematic, the published results are not so discordant with
other evidence as to play any critical role in the controversy
over determination of family resemblance for IQ.

　　　Jinks and Eaves (11) used a different model for Burt's
data. Their estimate of heritability (including dominance)
was .83, compared with .68 for some American data. The
latter is not far from our estimates of narrow heritability,
but there is no exact correspondence between the models (see
discussion).

TABLE 7

Goodness of Fit of American Parameters to English Data
When h and c are Estimated (m = x = 0)

Relation	N	r	$\hat{r}$	χ^2
FMTXY	95	.377	.434	0.43
OPTXY	963	.489	.477	0.21
UNTXY	375	.354	.353	0.00
FCTXY	552	.289	.195	5.45
OFPXY	88	.189	.229	0.15
SSTXY	676	.505	.508	0.01
FSTXY	136	.251	.132	2.02
SSAXY	151	.422	.375	0.46
MZTXY	211	.869	.883	0.70
MZAXY	91	.824	.750	3.41
Total			$\chi^2_8 = 12.84$	

See second line of Table 8 for the estimates
used here.

RUSSIAN IQ

Halperin et al. (17) presented a twin study of intelligence in pre-war Russia, using a combination of the Knox
Cube Test and the arithmetic computation subtest of the
Stanford Achievement Test. Their data are in good agreement
with American values of h and c (Table 9). Family environment is actually estimated to have a somewhat greater effect
in the Soviet material (c = .455) than in the U.S. (c = .397).
Thus there is no evidence that the importance of cultural
inheritance is diminished in a purportedly more egalitarian
society.

We are not aware of data on Israeli kibbutzim, Hindu
castes, or segregated races where relative effects of biological and cultural inheritance on IQ may be different from
national populations. Such studies would be of both genetic
and sociological interest.

A twin study (19) suggests that family resemblance may
decline in underprivileged groups, but whether the effect is
on biological or cultural inheritance could not be determined
(2).

TABLE 8

Estimates and Tests of Hypotheses for English Data, Fixing Non-Estimated Parameters at the Corresponding American Values for m = x = 0

Parameters estimated	d.f.	χ^2	Variance components				Estimates of other parameters	
			Children		Adults			
			h^2	c^2	h^2z^2	c^2y^2	u	f
None	10	21.77	.689	.157	.301	.549	.940	.478
h,c	8	12.84	.750	.132	.328	.467	*	*
y,z	8	17.78	*	*	.389	.389	*	*
h,c,y,z	6	12.06	.745	.137	.400	.397	*	*
All**	4	10.58	.746	.136	.376	.368	1.000	.500
All (m ≠ 0)**	3	8.40	.712	.075	.301	.256	1.000	.500

and $\hat{m}$ = .035

*Value from American data (first row)
**Minimum chi-square solutions were obtained by fixing u = 1, f = .5

TABLE 9

Analysis of Russian Data

Parameters estimated*	d.f.	χ^2	h^2	c^2
None	2	2.50	.689	.158
h	1	2.46	.684	.158
c	1	2.50	.689	.158
h,c	1	1.34**	.632	.207

*Parameters not estimated are fixed at the American values (last line of Table 5).

**Unconstrained solution yields $\Sigma_{PA} > 1$. This solution is constrained to have $\Sigma_{PA} = 1$, hence leaves $\chi^2 = 1.34$ with 1 d.f.

SOCIOFAMILIAL MENTAL DEFECT

One subpopulation has received special attention: the families into which mentally retarded children are born. These probands may be divided into two broad categories: a megaphenic group due to single specific etiological agents (major genes, chromosomal abnormalities, gross brain disease, infections, intoxications, and traumas) and a microphenic group due to cumulative effects of small, unidentifiable causes which produce continuous variation in mental ability. The latter group has been called "physiological," "aclinical," "subcultural," "undifferentiated," and "familial," but we prefer the term sociofamilial. Following a suggestion by Tarjan (19) it is defined as follows:

Currently available biomedical technology cannot demonstrate significant physical or laboratory pathology; no single, specific etiological agent can be made convincingly accountable for the condition; diagnosis usually made after school entrance, and often disappears at young adult age; normal in physical appearance; mortality not much greater than the general population; retardation usually mild, with the difference between mean parental IQ and that of the patient frequently small; often from the socially, economically, and educationally underprivileged strata of our society.

In practice it is sometimes difficult to distinguish concomitants of central nervous system pathology from coincidental physical abnormalities which may favor medical attention and institutionalization but are not significant causes of retardation. Since diagnosis is made by exclusion of alternatives, the sociofamilial group has been the despair of classifiers. Only by modifying the AAMD code do most cases fall into the aclinical categories .8 and .9 (20). In a given population the sociofamilial category is of homogeneous etiology and so should be conserved, despite diagnostic difficulties. Our interest here is to ask how the familial pattern depends on biological and cultural inheritance.

In 1938 L. S. Penrose published "A clinical and genetic study of 1280 cases of mental defect" from the Royal Eastern Counties Institution, Colchester, England (21). Variables used by Penrose but not tabulated in his appendix were extracted from the original records. Using the method of criterion scaling (22) all variables were converted into estimates of patient grades and combined by the first principal component of their correlation matrix. This severity index (which depends on characteristics of the patients and their parents, but not sibs) was used to separate sociofamilial from biological and medical cases (20): the validity of this distinction was confirmed by segregation analysis (table 11 of ref. 20).

TABLE 10

Etiological Groups in the Colchester Survey

	Medical	Biological	Socio-familial
Per cent of cases	7	33	60
Per cent of incidence	6	19	75
Incidence/100,000 births	176	524	2056
Per cent normal parents	91	98	62
Per cent IQ < 50	57	77	36
Per cent AAMD codes .7 - .9	0	43	70
Polyfactorial heritability	.40	0	.80

For the present paper we first rejected cases classified as exogenous or Down's syndrome and then selected the 773 smallest values of the severity index, corresponding to the

60 per cent of cases calculated to lie in the sociofamilial group. Variables relevant to parental phenotype and family environment were criterion scaled by sibling grade, and a family index was created by regression (Table 11).

These data present several difficulties for path analysis. Intellectual grade is a discontinuous variate based on psychometrics for probands but on subjective judgment of a skilled investigator for parents and sibs. The families were selected through probands, whereas path analysis assumes normally distributed, unselected variables. We shall analyse the data with probands excluded, but shall otherwise neglect these distributional problems in the belief that path analysis is rather insensitive to them. A more worrisome deficit is that no data are given to construct indices of the family environments in which the parents were raised. The utility of such information was not evident at the time the Colchester survey was conducted, but it has become a powerful tool in path analysis of family resemblance (6).

These limitations reinforce the general rule that the analysis must provide a goodness-of-fit test as well as estimates of path coefficients. The four variables (father's grade, mother's grade, child's grade and child's index) generate 6 interclass correlations in addition to the sib correlation. These 7 correlations, estimated by maximum likelihood (1), are presented in Table 12. As in other material there is striking agreement between paternal and maternal correlations (8). American IQ data gives estimates of various ancillary parameters, leaving others to be estimated from the data. American parameters give a good fit when only h, c and i are estimated from the data (Table 13).

For this analysis we used the NUCVAR computer program, which allows for the correlations between observed correlations estimated from the same sample (1). For comparison with other populations the estimates of h and c should be corrected for the attenuation due to incomplete selection and polychotomization of IQ. The correction factor when h, c, i are estimated is,

$$\sqrt{\frac{H^2 + c^2}{h^2 + c^2}} = 1.299$$

where capitals denote population values (American IQ, Table 5) and estimates for sociofamilial mental defect are in lower case. Corrected estimates for mental defect are

$$h = .838 \pm .056$$
$$c = .379 \pm .025$$

TABLE 11

Criterion Scaling of Sociofamilial Probands. Unknown and Other Denoted by *

Variable	i	Scale (z_i)	σ_i	b_i
Grade of proband or sib	1	S → -200, N → 0, M_0 → 100, M_1 → 200, M_2 → 300, M_4 → 400	89	.
Grade of father	2	N → 34, M_0 → 66, M_1 → 125, M_2 → 200, * → 28	23	.
Grade of mother	3	N → 22, M_0 → 68, M_1 → 110, M_2 → 100, * → 37	31	.
Reliability	4	1 → 48, 2 → 40, 3 → 30	4	.51
Occupation of father	5	A_2 → 26, A_3 → 48, C → -29, D → 68, E_1 → 29, E_2 → 53, * → 36	13	.75
Rating of home	6	B → -3, C → 34, D → 62, E → 73, * → 29	17	.87
Rooms in home	7	R → 60 - 2.33R, * → 32	8	.
Illegitimacy	8	1 → 57, 0 → 45	1	.

The equation A → N signifies that probands in category A are assigned their mean severity N.

The family index is computed by regression as $Y = \sum_{i=4}^{6} b_i z_i$, with grade of sibling as the dependent variable (sample size = 2607). Correlation with grade of sib = .22.

TABLE 12

Observed Correlations (r) and Sample Sizes (N)
Estimated from Families with Sociofamilial Probands

Source	N	r
Father x mother	574	.274
Father x index	574	.279
Father x child	792	.289
Mother x index	574	.290
Mother x child	792	.346
Child x index	792	.218
Sib	1114	.296

Probands and sibships of size 1 were excluded. Sibships with n probands were enumerated n times, as in
the Weinberg method for multiple selection. The data
were analysed by the NUCVAR computer program, allowing
for correlations between correlations.

TABLE 13

Estimates and Tests of Hypotheses
for Sociofamilial Mental Defect. Parameters not
Estimated here are Fixed at the American Values
(last line of Table 5)

Estimated parameters	d.f.	χ^2	h^2	c^2	i
i	6	124.01	.689	.158	.416
h,c,i	4	6.35	.416	.085	.573

These agree closely with the American IQ data. Evidently
cultural inheritance is no more or less important for mental
defect in the Colchester sample than for IQ in the general
population. It remains a plausible but untested hypothesis
that mental defect in more stratified societies has a larger
cultural component. Estimation of genetic and cultural
heritabilities is the sine qua non for prediction of specific
recurrence risks in genetic counseling and preventive medicine (23).

DOMINANCE

     R. A. Fisher (24) founded a distinguished school of bio-
metrical genetics which still flourishes. It is characterized by emphasis on the role of dominance in family resemblance, neglect of environmental causes of the marital
correlation and of intergenerational differences in genetic
and cultural heritability, radical simplification of family
environment as unique to sibs or shared equally with sibs
and children (but no other relatives), omission of environmental indices, and use of large-sample theory for tests of
hypotheses (11). Only the emphasis on dominance is readily
defended. It has its roots in the controversy between bio-
metricians and Mendelists in the early part of the century.
Quantitative traits of complex inheritance do not show complete dominance, but Fisher demonstrated that dominance may
in principle be detected by its contribution to the correlation of bilateral relatives like sibs. He succeeded
brilliantly in his main endeavor, and thereafter biometrical
genetics had a Mendelian basis. However, Fisher's application of his model to height in man was an accidental conse-
qence of the fact that no such set of familial correlations
was available for other organisms. If he had intended a
serious analysis of human data his neglect of familial
environment would have been inexplicable.
     Fisher gave rise to two historical streams in bio-
metrical genetics. One fused with developments elsewhere,
largely due to Sewall Wright. This branch is represented by
Kempthorne (25) and Falconer (26). The other stream developed
in Birmingham under Mather, Jinks, and Eaves and is typified
by the book of Mather and Jinks (27). Through the interest
of the Birmingham group in behavior genetics the Fisherian
model was disseminated among psychologists. There is no
exact correspondence between their parameters and those of
path analysis. The two models are not readily compared by
goodness-of-fit tests, since the Fisherian model does not
incorporate indices and therefore gives no expectation for 6
of the 16 relations in Table 3. There is every reason to pay

tribute to that approach in any history of biometrical
genetics, but no reason to perpetuate it.

Family environment was controlled in principle by the
Birmingham school for diallel crosses of inbred lines, where
assignment of sibs to random locations and dates requires
fastidious replication that is rarely attempted. In man
these methods are not feasible, and so we should not estimate
dominance from the excess of the sib correlation over the
parent-offspring correlation. Sibs may resemble each other
more than their parents because contemporaries share more of
the environment than do members of successive generations.
Reduction of heritability with age may have the same effect.
There is little reason to hope that dominance can be resolved
in nuclear families except by demonstrating segregation of a
major gene (28).

Heritability is best defined narrowly in terms of
additive variance, as free as possible of contributions from
dominance, epistasis, and gene-environment interaction and
covariance. It is such narrow heritability which is predictive of recurrence risks and selection response and all
attempts to estimate broad heritability in man, depending as
they do on identical twins reared apart, are lacking in
credibility because of nonrandom adoption. The effort to
collect such data is disproportionate to its value.

It seems to us therefore that the attempt to estimate
from family resemblance a variance component due to dominance
for a trait like IQ is poorly motivated. We subscribe to
the view of Falconer (26):

> "The <u>additive</u> <u>variance</u>, which is the variance of
> inbreeding values, is the important component
> since it is the chief cause of resemblance be-
> tween relatives and therefore the chief deter-
> minant of the observable genetic properties of
> the population and of the response of the popu-
> lation to selection. Moreover, it is the only
> component that can be readily estimated from
> observations made on the population."

If this is true for the experimental organisms considered by
Falconer, it holds <u>a</u> <u>fortiori</u> for man. The concept of broad
heritability (which includes dominance and epistasis) has
attracted only human geneticists, who are least able to
estimate it. Instead, we prefer to elaborate cultural inheritance realistically even though in so doing we sacrifice
the estimate of dominance. In principle dominance should make
data on resemblance of foster children, half-sibs, and identical twins give a significantly bad fit, which conceivably
could be discriminated from other failures of the additive
model. It is convenient to have a single degree of freedom
testing for dominance: this may be done by introducing a

path coefficient which contributes d^2 to the correlation of
MZ twins, $d^2/4$ for sibs, and to no other relationship (3).
Power to test this null hypotheses requires MZ twins and/or
half-sibs. This diversion of effort to less common relationships is useful if dominance is important.

Tests of hypotheses on dominance (d) and intergenerational differences (y,z) are summarized in Table 14 for the
American IQ data. In the entire data set there is no evidence
for dominance (F-ratio = 0.00 on 1 and 49 d.f., P > .95),
whereas the hypothesis of equal heritabilities (y = z = 1) is
rejected outright (F-ratio = 55.27 on 2 and 49 d.f., P <
.001). Since u goes to the logical limit when y = z = 1, we
repeated the analysis by replacing the marital correlation
(FMTXY) with a smaller value of .33 (15) for reasons explained
before. Here the general model does not fit by the conventional criterion (F-ratio = 2.31 on 7 and 42 d.f., P close to
.04), but the general features remain unchanged. We also
repeated this analysis on the 10 phenotypic correlations only,
rejecting all the indices; the results on the nonsignificance
of d and the significance of intergenerational differences
are still preserved. Other investigators looking at dominance for IQ have ignored intergenerational differences rather
than test for their significance as we have done here. Only
a likelihood ratio test under a model that includes both
intergenerational differences and dominance is a valid test
of either; mere goodness of fit of a model with d > 0 and
y = z = 1 does not imply either significance of d or nonsignificance of intergenerational differences.

DISCUSSION

We have shown that genetic analysis of IQ data is
simple, determinate, and consistent over data sets. Results
are relevant to genetics, epidemiology, and sociology. To
extend these studies it would be desirable to have more
homogeneous samples that could be collected with less labor.
Nuclear families are the material of choice. Sixteen correlations are generated by observing phenotypes of children and
parents and the three corresponding indices, if one dis-
tinguishes parternal and maternal correlations but does not
observe sibs as adults. This is sufficient to fit all the
required parameters, without exploiting information from
twins, adopted children, and other relationships which provide an independent test of inferences from nuclear families.
Indices could be improved by including parental education as
well as occupation, combining these and other socioeconomic
indicators by regression with child's phenotype as the dependent variable. Like Burks' culture index this is likely to

TABLE 14

Tests of hypotheses on dominance and intergenerational differences

in American IQ data (m = x = 0)

Data set	Hypothesis	Residual				Variance components and estimates of other parameters						
		χ^2	d.f.	F-ratio*	p	h^2	c^2	h^2z^2	c^2y^2	d^2	f	u
Entire data (error variance = 142.46/49 = 2.907)	general	39.83	7	1.95	> .05	.686	.158	.302	.549	.003	.478	.940
	d = 0	39.83	8	0.00	> .95	.689	.157	.301	.549	0	.478	.940
	y = z = 1**	200.39	9	55.27	< .001	.266	.343	.266	.343	.231	.500	1.000
FMTXY replaced by .33 (N = 1016, error variance = 125.36/42 = 2.985)	general**	48.29	7	2.31	< .05	.685	.159	.317	.533	.003	.546	.677
	d = 0**	48.29	8	0.00	> .95	.688	.158	.317	.533	0	.546	.677
	y = z = 1**	137.89	9	15.01	< .001	.388	.289	.388	.289	.165	.500	1.000
Indices excluded† (error variance = 87.47/36 = 2.430)	general	29.68	5	2.44	> .05	.500	.224	.276	.515	.122	.478	.940
	d = 0	31.99	6	0.95	> .25	.641	.198	.257	.521	0	.478	.940
	y = z = 1	79.42	7	20.47	< .001	.248	.365	.248	.365	.244	.478	.940

*d.f. for the F-ratios are as follows: 7, 49 or 7, 42 or 5, 36 for the general hypothesis, 1, 49 or 1, 42 or 1, 36 for d = 0, 2, 49 or 2, 42 or 2, 36 for y = z = 1

**This solution is constrained to have $\Sigma_{CC} = 1$. The unconstrained solution yielded $\Sigma_{CC} > 1$.

†Parameters are indeterminate in this data set, and therefore f and u are fixed at the values obtained for the entire data set.

correlate highly with parental phenotype, but in a way that is accounted for by the estimate of i (with different values for parents and children if necessary), and does not disturb the rest of the analysis providing indices are determined in the same sample which gives familial correlations for IQ.

In any future study of family resemblance for IQ particular attention should be directed to parental indices and adult sibs, since genetic and cultural heritability are poorly determined for adults. If occupational choice is the principal mechanism for cultural inheritance of IQ, intervention strategies may be more successfully applied to vocational training than to pre-school enrichment.

This discussion illustrates that data on family resemblance for IQ can be analysed dispassionately and are not without scientific interest. So far the literature on inheritance has suffered from a high ratio of commentary to data collection and analysis. This was due to lack of an appropriate methodology, domination of the field by psychologists and sociologists with primary interests and competence outside genetics, and strong philosophical commitments of the more extreme protagonists. These problems now have only historical interest, since the present model has no hereditarian or environmentalist bias.

The "nature-nurture controversy" was partly an ideological confusion of individuals and populations, partly a methodological problem in distinguishing cultural and biological causes of family resemblance. As far as that problem has been formulated, it is solved. Methods here applied to IQ are being used to determine causes of family resemblance for other traits like blood pressure and glycemia closely related to disease (29,30). We may hope that well-designed studies on nuclear families will also be conducted for IQ so that polemics about determinants of family resemblance need not engage scientists.

The model presented here is not limited to quantitative traits under complete selection. Methods for the analysis of qualitative traits under complete and incomplete selection are developed in a separate paper (31). Incomplete selection for quantitative traits can be handled through path regressions: regression of various relatives on probands yields regression coefficients which are normally distributed under suitable assumptions; expected values of such regression coefficients are the same as expected correlations given by the present model.

SUMMARY

A general linear model is presented for path analysis of quantitative traits in nuclear families, which is also extended to relationships outside nuclear families. These methods are used to analyse data on family resemblance for IQ. American, English, and Russian IQ data are shown to be in quantitative agreement with a simple model, which also describes English data on sociofamilial mental defect. In these samples the relative variance due to genetic inheritance in children is $h^2 = .689$, and the relative variance due to family environment is $c^2 = .157$. For adults heritability is less and cultural inheritance is greater, as first shown by Sewall Wright. Presumably these shifts are mediated by occupational choice. Contrary to its marginal significance in a previous analysis of part of this material, gene-environment correlation does not approach significance. There is no evidence for dominance, epistasis, or gene-environment interaction.

REFERENCES

1. Rao, D. C., Morton, N. E., Gulbrandsen, C. L., Rhoads, G. G., Kagan, A., Yee, S., Ann. Hum. Genet., in press (1978).

2. Rao, D. C., Morton, N. E., Yee, S., Am. J. Hum. Genet. 26, 331-359 (1974).

3. Rao, D. C., MacLean, C. J., Morton, N. E., Yee, S., Am. J. Hum. Genet. 27, 509-520 (1975).

4. Elston, R. C., Biometrika 62, 133-140 (1975).

5. Rao, D. C., Morton, N. E., Am. J. Hum. Genet. 26, 767-772 (1974).

6. Rao, D. C., Morton, N. E., Yee, S., Am. J. Hum. Genet. 28, 228-242 (1976).

7. Wright, S., "Evolution and the Genetics of Population" Vol. 4, The University of Chicago Press, Chicago, in press (1978).

8. Freire-Maia, A., Freire-Maia, D., Morton, N. E., Behav. Genet. 4, 269-272 (1974).

9.   Gerrard, J. W., Rao, D. C., Morton, N. E., <u>Am. J. Hum.</u>
     <u>Genet.</u>, in press (1978).

10. Wright, S., <u>J. Am. Stat. Assoc.</u> 26, 155-163 (1931).

11. Jinks, J. L., Eaves, L. J., "IQ and inequality,"
     <u>Nature</u> 248, 287-289, book review (1974).

12. Moran, P. A. P., <u>Ann. Hum. Genet.</u> 37, 217 (1973).

13. Jencks, C., Smith, M., Acland, H., Bane, M. J., Cohen,
     D., Gintis, H., Heyns, B., Michelson, S., "Inequality:
     a reassessment of the effect of family and schooling
     in America," Basic Books, New York, 1972.

14. Kamin, L., "The Science and Politics of IQ," Eribaum
     Assoc., Potomac, MD., 1974.

15. Higgins, J. V., Reed, E. W., Reed, S. C., <u>Eugen. Quart.</u>,
     9, 84-90 (1962).

16. Jensen, A. R., <u>Behav. Genet.</u> 4, 1-28 (1974).

17. Halperin, S. L., Rao, D. C., Morton, N. E., <u>Behav.</u>
     <u>Genet.</u> 5, 83-86 (1975).

18. Scar-Salapatek, S., <u>Science</u> 174, 1285-1295 (1971).

19. Tarjan, G., in "Socio-cultural Aspects of Mental
     Retardation" (E. C. Haywood, Ed.), Appleton-Century-
     Crofts, New York, 1970.

20. Morton, N. E., Rao, D. C., MacLean, C. J., Bart, R. C.,
     Lang-Brown, H., Lew, R., <u>J. Med. Genet.</u> 14, 1-9 (1977).

21. Penrose, L. S., <u>Medical Research Council</u>, special
     report series No. 229 (1938).

22. Beaton, A. E., "Scaling Criterion of Questionnaire
     Items," Socio-Econ. Plan. Sci. Vol. 2, pp. 355-362.
     Pergamon Press, New York, 1969.

23. Lalouel, J. M., "Recurrence Risks as an Outcome of
     Segregation Analysis," presented at this conference,
     1978.

24. Fisher, R. A., <u>Trans. R. Soc. Edinb.</u> 52, 399-433 (1918).

25. Kempthorne, O., "An Introduction to Genetical Statistics," Wiley, New York, 1957.

26. Falconer, D. S., "Introduction to Quantitative Genetics," Oliver and Boyd, Edinburgh, 1960.

27. Mather, K., Jinks, J. L., "Biometrical Genetics," Chapman and Hall, London, 1971.

28. Morton, N. E., Rao, D. C., in "Yearbook of Physical Anthropology," in press (1978).

29. Morton, N. E., in "Proceedings of Symposium on Gene-Environment Interaction in Common Diseases" (E. Inouye and H. Nishimura. Eds.), 1977.

30. Morton, N. E., in "The epidemiology of prematurity" (D. M. Reed and F. J. Stanley, Eds.), pp. 213-230, Urban & Schwarzenberg, Baltimore, 1977.

31. Rao, D. C., Morton, N. E., Yee, S., in preparation (1978).

32. Rao, D. C., Morton, N. E., Yee, S., Am. J. Hum. Genet., in press (1978).

33. Burks, B. S., in "Yearbook of the National Society for the Study of Education," pt. 1, pp. 219-316, 1928.

34. Willoughby, R. R., Genetic Psychology Monographs II, 239-277 (1927).

35. Leahy, A. M., Genetic Psychology Monographs 17, 236-308 (1935).

36. Outhit, M. C., Archives of Psychology 149, 1-60 (1933).

37. Conrad, H. S., Jones, H. E., in "39th Yearbook of the National Society for the Study of Education," pt. 2, pp. 97-141, Public School Publishing Co., Bloomington, 1940.

38. Freeman, F. N., Holzinger, K. J., Mitchell, B. C., in "27th Yearbook of the National Society for the Study of Education," pt. 1, pp. 103-217, Public School Publishing Co., Bloomington, 1928.

39. Duncan, O. D., Featherman, D. L., Duncan, B., "Socio-economic Background and Achievement," Seminar Press, New York, 1972.

40. Duncan, O. D., Featherman, D. L., in "Structural Equation Models in the Social Sciences" (A. S. Goldberger and O. D. Duncan, Eds.), pp. 229-253, Seminar Press, New York, 1973.

41. Skodak, M., The Pedagogical Seminary and Journal of Genetic Psychology 77, 3-9 (1950).

42. Hart, H., School and Society 20, 382 (1924).

43. Madsen, I. N., School and Society 19, 559-562 (1924).

44. McNemar, Q., "The Revision of the Stanford-Binet Scale: an Analysis of the Standardization Data," Houghton-Mifflin, Boston, 1942.

45. Hildreth, G., in Contributions to Education, p. 186, Teacher's College, New York, 1925.

46. Schoenfelt, L., Measurement and Evaluation in Guidance 1, 130-140 (1968).

47. Newman, H. H., Freeman, F. N., Holzinger, K. J., "Twins: A Study of Heredity and Environment," Chicago University Press, Chicago, 1937.

48. Sims, V. M., "The influence of blood relationship and common environment on measured intelligence," J. Ed. Psych. 22, 56-65 (1931).

49. Scarr, S., Weinberg, R. A., "Intellectual similarities within families of both adopted and biological children," University of Minnesota, Jan. 1977 (unpublished manuscript).

50. Nichols, P. L., "The effects of heredity and environment on intelligence test performance in 4 and 7 years White and Negro sibling pairs," University of Minnesota doctoral dissertation, 1970.

APPENDIX

American Data on IQ. Codes are Described in Rao et al. (2,6)

Relation	First variable	Second variable	Code	r	N	Source	Comments
Marital (FMT)	P_F	P_M	FMTXY	.55	174	(33)	cf. Goldberger discussion
				.42	100	(33)	
				.40	141	(34)	
				.43	164	(35)	Jencks, Table A-1 (13)
				.61	174	(35)	
				.74	51	(36)	
				.52	134	(37)	
				.49	180	(38)	
	I_F	I_M	FMTIXIY	.226	1165	(39)	Table 7.3 FGMA data
Offspring-parent (OPT) together	P_F,P_M	P_C	OPTXY	.46	200	(33)	
				.51	366	(35)	
				.49	501	(37)	
				.58	102	(36)	Jencks, Table A-2 (13)
				.35	141	(34)	
	P_F	I_C	OPTXIY	.67	100	(33)	
				.71	105	(33)	
				.57	180	(38)	

P_F					
I_F	OPTXIX	.539	887	(40)	Corrected for part-whole correlation of Wechsler similarities subtest (dividing by .8)
		.348	887	(40)	
I_C	OPTIXIY	.371	9389	(39)	OCG Data
				Table A.2	Index is composite
		.328	4386	(39)	dominated
I_F				WISC Data	by occupation.
		.282	314	(39)	Table 6.8
		.297	1165	(39)	Table 7.3 FGMA Data
		.306	1013	(39)	Table 3.4 DAS Data
I_M		.260	1165	(39)	Table 7.3 FGMA Data
Offspring-parent living apart (OPA) P_M					
P_C	OPAXY	.41	63	(41)	
Full sibs together as children (SST) P_C					
P_C	SSTXY	.50	312	(37)	
		.45	399	(42)	Jencks, Table A-7 (13)
		.63	63	(43)	
		.53	384	(44)	
		.67	63	(36)	

	P_C		.63	450	(45)	Jencks, Table A-7 (13)
			.42	280	(34)	
			.54	156	(46)	Jencks, Table A-6 (13)
			.63	50	(47)	
	I_C	SSTXIX	.40	203	(48)	
			.42	107	(49)	with interracial adoptions
			.293	4386	(39)	Table 6.15 WISC Data
			.47	36	(38)	
			.45	194	(35)	
			.44	101	(33)	Cultural index
Sibs apart (SSA)	P_C	SSAXY	.25	125	(38)	
Identical twins together (MZT)	P_C	MZTXY	.89	50	(47)	Jencks, Table A-6 (13)
			.85	335	(46)	
			.62	36	(50)	
Adult identical twins apart (AMA)	P_C	AMAXY	.69	19	(47)	

		FSTXY			
Unrelated foster sibs together as children (FST)	P_C	P_C			
		.23	21	(33)	
		.40	93	(38)	⎫
		.12	10	(35)	⎬ Jencks, Table A-8 (13)
		.65	41	(41)	⎭
		.29	203	(48)	} Unrelated children closely matched (see Kamin, 14).
		.39	53	(49)	Interracial adoptions
		FSPXY			
Adopted-natural pairs (FSP)	P_C	P_C			
		.38	47	(38)	⎫
		.06	25	(35)	⎬ Jencks, Table A-8 (13)
		.21	22	(41)	⎭
		.30	134	(49)	Interracial adoptions

180

Offspring-foster parent (OFP)							
P_F	P_C	OFPXY	.07	178	(33)		
			.37	180	(38)		
			.19	178	(35)		Jencks, Table A-3 (13)
P_M	P_C		.19	204	(33)		
			.28	255	(38)		
			.24	186	(35)		
	I_C	OFPYIY	.37	394	(38)		
			.14	194	(35)		
P_C			.25	186	(33)		Cultural index

181

DISCUSSION

ANDERSON: One of the students at Minnesota, Ellen Barker,
has completed a Ph.D. thesis (1977) which involved a follow-up
of individuals identified in the larger Reed and Reed study of
mental retardation. She identified somewhat over 100 families
in which two or more children had been tested during their
school years. She then retested these individuals as adults.
The two sets of data are not strictly comparable since
different tests of intelligence and different modes of testing
were used. Nevertheless, it is clear that the sib-sib
correlations for adult pairs were lower (0.11 and 0.16 for two
different tests) than as school-age children (0.39).

Reference

Barker, E.B., unpublished Ph.D. Thesis, Univ. of Minnesota,
(1977).

MORTON: Table 5 predicts for all parameter sets a higher
correlation for adult sibs than for children. Studies on
adult sibs will be of critical value to improve these results.
It is of course essential that the tests administered to
children and adults be equivalent in content and reliability.
The effect of family environment on occupational choice and
subsequent test performance may be decreasing. If y were
abolished we would predict the correlation of adult sibs to be
only .15, but any residual value of y would raise this.
     Nuclear families may be augmented by sibs of parents to
form a pedigree sector in which adult sibs, uncle-niece, and
affinal pairs extend the power of nuclear families to resolve
genetic and cultural inheritance.

FAMILY STRUCTURE IN MODELS OF
CULTURAL INHERITANCE*

by

Theodore Reich, M.D.

C. Robert Cloninger, M.D.

Collins Lewis, M.D.

John Rice, Ph.D.

From the Department of Psychiatry, Washington University
School of Medicine and the Jewish Hospital of St. Louis
St. Louis, MIssouri 63110

In order to develop realistic models which depict
the effects of both genetic and cultural influences
on the transmission of psychopathological traits over
several generations, we have been investigating the
variation in family structure which occurs in different subcultures. Prior models of cultural transmission implicitly assume that both biological parents
are the only agents of cultural inheritance except
for specific separation and fostering experiences
which occur at random in a particular nuclear family.
A family is described here as an intact nuclear
family if the biological mother and father are both
present and the only parents-of-rearing. Non-nuclear
family structures include both "broken" homes and
also "extended" families in which both biological
parents and remote relatives live in the home and
each acts as a parent-of-rearing. Available data
support the following three observations about
family structure which will be described further
below: (i) both nuclear and non-nuclear family
structures are common; (ii) familial psychopathology is associated with variation in family
structure; and (iii) family structure may itself be

*Supported in part by U.S.P.H.S. grant AA-00209 and
 Research Scientiest Development Award MH-00048(CRC)

familial, that is, the composition of the family-of-rearing
of parents and that of their children are correlated, not
independent. If cultural factors are important in the
development of a trait, then these three observations
must be taken into account when the transmission of the
trait is analyzed. In particular, interactions between
psychopathology and family structure may well distort
and invalidate models which are based only on the
nuclear family. Some empirical data indicating the
practical importance of these considerations will be
presented here.

TABLE 1

DISTRIBUTION OF FAMILY SIZE AND STRUCTURE IN 1391 FAMILIES
(Adapted from Kellam and associates, 1977)

Number of parents of rearing

1			2			3+	
N			N			N	
Mother	517	37%	Mother-Father	483	35%	Total	124	11%
Other	37	3%	Other	202	15%			
Total	554	40%	Total	685	49%			

Kellam and associates (1977) examined the family structure of 1391 families of first grade students in Woodlawn, a poor innercity community in Chicago (1966-67). Personal interviews to determine family structure were undertaken. Some findings of this study are displayed in Table 1. These data indicate that the most common family structure was the single parent family in which children were reared by a mother living alone (37%). Although two parents of rearing was the most common arrangement (49%), only 35% of the entire sample of children were being reared by their biological mothers and fathers. A surprising total of 11% were being reared by 3 or more parents, and in only a minority of these were the biological mothers and fathers also present in the home. In this large sample, 81 different family structures occurred, and in a majority of these, related individuals other than the biological father and mother or the child were involved in child rearing. In this population, models for the transmission of behavioral traits should include children being reared by parents who contribute less than half their genes to the child, but who also contribute a large measure of cultural influence.

The Woodlawn sample is largely black so we attempted to obtain comparable data from a white population. The only relevant data available' is that collected in St. Louis by Cloninger, Reich, and associates in which the families of white convicted felons and alcoholic inpatients were examined. These data are displayed in Table 2. In constructing these tables, family structure is reported at age 10, at age 15, and during the period from 0-15 years. In the alcoholic sample (mean age 41 years), at age 10, 58% of the subjects were being reared by their biological father and mother and 12% were reared by three or more parents. At age 15, 48% were being reared by their biological fathers and mothers, 28% by a single parent, and 12% by three or more parents. Considering the entire period from 0-15 years, only 40% of the alcoholic patients had been reared by only their biological father and mother, and 42% were reared by three or more individuals (either consecutively or at one time).

TABLE 2A

STRUCTURE OF THE FAMILIES OF 50 ALCOHOLIC PATIENTS
(Mean Age = 41 years)

Number of parents of rearing

		1		2		3+
At age 10	Mother	8%	Mother-Father	58%		
	Other	6%	Other	16%		
	Total	14%	Total	74%	Total	12%
At age 15	Mother	12%	Mother-Father	48%		
	Other	16%	Other	12%		
	Total	28%	Total	60%	Total	12%
From 0-15			Mother-Fahter	40%		
			Other	18%		
	Total	0	Total	58%	Total	42%

TABLE 2B

STRUCTURE OF THE FAMILIES OF 50 FELONS
(Mean Age = 21 years)

Number of parents of rearing

		1		2		3+
At age 10	Mother	8%	Mother-Father	70%		
	Other	6%	Other	12%		
	Total	14%	Total	81%	Total	4%
At age 15	Mother	10%	Mother-Father	68%		
	Other	12%	Other	16%		
	Total	22%	Total	74%	Total	4%
From 0-15			Mother-Father	54%		
			Other	22%		
	Total	0	Total	76%	Total	24%

In Table 2B, similar data are displayed for the family structure of 50 felons (mean age 21 years) interviewed at the St. Louis County parole office. Although this sample contains a higher proportion of nuclear families than the alcoholic sample, only 54% of the felons lived in a nuclear family consisting of the proband, his siblings and a biological father and mother from the ages of 0-15 years. In both the alcoholic and felon samples, no proband was reared consistently by the same single parent from ages 0-15. Examining the data sets displayed in Table 2, family structure changed considerably during the formative years, and this change may exert considerable influence on subsequent psychopathology. It is possible that the fragmentation of the family may well be the consequence of psychopathology in the parents, but the exact relationship between the transmission of psychopathology and the presence of non-nuclear family structure is unknown.

The extent to which non-nuclear family structure is correlated with psychiatric illness is important in determining the kinds of cultural models which are appropriate. Some data is available from a study conducted in St. Louis by Drs. Guze, Cloninger, Woodruff, and Clayton, in which a random sample of 500 clinic outpatients was studied using systematic interviews. In Table 3 the diagnosis of these patients is compared with their divorce rate. Since parental divorce is an important element in generating non-nuclear families of rearing for the children, groups with a high divorce rate can be expected to produce families where non-nuclear structure is common. It can be seen that the divorce rate is high in patients with homosexuality, drug dependence, alcoholism, hysteria, sociopathy and sexual deviation. By contrast, patients with unipolar primary affective disorder and anxiety neurosis have lower rates which are similar to those in the general population. The large group of undiagnosed psychiatric illnesses were generally patients with depression who had insufficient symptoms to meet criteria for

TABLE 3

DIVORCE AND DIAGNOSIS*

Diagnosis	Total Patients N	Ever Married N	Marrieds ever divorced %
Homosexuality	12	5	80
Drug dependence	13	12	67
Alcoholism	70	59	49
Hysteria	36	30	47
Sociopathy	35	24	46
Secondary affective disorder	95	75	43
Sexual deviation (other)	9	7	43
Mental retardation	16	11	36
Bipolar primary affective disorder	19	17	35
Anxiety neurosis	62	53	34
Schizophrenia	22		
Undiagnosed psychiatric illness	140	108	30
Unipolar primary affective disorder	139	105	26
Organic brain syndrome	10	9	22
Obsessional neurosis	3	3	0
Epilepsy	6	0	—

*Adapted from Woodruff and associates, 1972

primary affective disorder. These data indicate that
models for the transmission of disorders such as alcoholism (population prevalence approximately 6%) and
sociopathy (population prevalence approximately 3%)
should allow for variable family structure. It is important to note that the disorders associated with a
high rate of divorce usually have their onset prior to
divorce and frequently occur prior to marriage, so that
it is not plausible to consider divorce the primary
cause of the association with psychopathology. However,
both alcoholism and antisocial personality are strongly
familial and the relationship between divorce and the
severity or onset of these disorders in the offspring
is poorly understood and requires further study.

TABLE 4

DIVORCE IN PARENTS OF MARRIED, SEPARATED AND DIVORCED
PSYCHIATRIC PARENTS

(Adapted from Woodruff and associates, 1972)

Patients	N	Divorce in Parents	"Reared by Relatives or friends"
Divorced or separated at least once	121	23%	23%
Married, never divorced	251	13%	14%

Since divorce leads to variation in family structure, some light on the transmission of family structure may be cast by examining the frequency of divorced individuals who have been reared by parents other than their biological ones. Such data has been collected in the St. Louis Clinic study referred to above and is displayed in Table 4. Of 121 patients who have been divorced or separated at least once, 23% came from homes in which their parents were divorced and 23% were reared by relatives or friends. These groups largely overlap. By contrast, patients who are married and never divorced had lower rates of divorce in their parents and were less frequently reared by relatives or friends. Although we are unable to determine whether or not non-nuclear family structure is familial when psychiatric illness in the parents is controlled, this question must receive careful attention before realistic models for the multigenerational transmission of psychopathology can be described. Specific separation and fostering experiences obviously change the proportion of phenotypic variance due to cultural factors in a particular individual, and this is most simply treated if such variation in rearing experience is independent of the trait in question. As shown here, available data cast doubt on these simplifying assumptions.

It seems clear that cultural factors are an important feature of the transmission of behavioral traits from parent to offspring. Each family or class of families, acts as a subculture in which child rearing practices, social attitudes, and maladaptive behavior can be transmitted by cultural mechanisms. The parents of rearing may vary in their ability to transmit these factors, in contrast to genetic transmission where each biological parent transmits precisely 1/2 of his genes. Moreover, fathers and mothers may transmit different characteristics to varying degrees. With respect to cultural transmission the coefficient of relationship between a parent and offspring is not necessarily one half.

If traits were entirely due to cultural or entirely due to genetic factors, then models of transmission would be relatively simple (Rice, 1977) It is likely, however, that the etiology of psychiatric disorders is due to both cultural and environmental factors which interact. Unfortunately, the effects of these interactions are made more complex by phenotypic assortative mating which is observed

to a high degree in behavioral traits. As a consequence
of assortative mating, parents of rearing and biologically
unrelated children not only have non-genetic correlations
between them, but may also have genotypic correlations
which should be considered. Fortunately, these complexities appear to be tractable using available methods and
are currently receiving careful attention (Cloninger et al,
1978 a & b).

SUMMARY:

In constructing models which include both cultural
and genetic modes of transmission, non-nuclear family
structure appears to be common and should be taken into
account when multigenerational models are constructed.

Family structure and psychiatric disorder are not
independent so that the children of affected individuals
are often reared by friends and relatives.

Family structure itself may be familial, although
whether or not this occurs only as a consequence of
parental psychopathology is unknown.

Models which include both genetic and cultural modes
of transmission are made more complex by a large degree
of assortative mating which is frequent in behavioral
traits. Phenotypic assortative mating for traits which
are transmitted by genetic and cultural mechanisms induces
complex genotypic and cultural interactions which must be
included in realistic models.

References

1. Kellam, S.G., Ensminger, M.E., and Turner, R.J. <u>Arch.</u>
    <u>Gen.</u> <u>Psychiat.</u> 34, 1012-1026 (1977).

2. Woodruff, R.A., Guze, S.B., and Clayton, P.J. <u>Brit.</u> <u>J.</u>
    <u>Psychiat.</u> 121, 289-302 (1972).

3. Rice, J., Cloninger, C.R., and Reich, T. "Multifactorial
    Inheritance with Cultural Transmission and Assortative
    Mating: I. Description and Basic Properties of the
    Unitary Models", (in preparation).

4. Cloninger, C.R., Rice, J., and Reich, T. "Multifactorial
    Inheritance with Cultural Transmission and Assortative
    Mating: II. A General Model of Combined Polygenic and
    Cultural Inheritance", (in preparation).

5. Cloninger, C.R., Rice, J., and Reich, T. "Multifactorial
    Inheritance with Cultural Transmission and Assortative
    Mating: III. Family structure and the Analysis of
    Separation Experiments", (in preparation).

MORTON: Unusual relationships are interesting in their own
right and to extend tests on nuclear families. However, they
introduce additional assumptions which are not required for
nuclear families. I prefer the pedigree sector, which involves
only nuclear relationships.

GOLDBERGER: It would be a mistake to accept Rao and
Morton's American data set as definitive. Readers who compare
the listing of 65 correlations in the Appendix with Jencks's
(1) compilation and then with the original studies will find
some slippage. For example, the sample sizes have been
reversed in the first two items in the FMTXY collection. In
the FSTXY collection, Burks's 21 cases reappear in Freeman's
93 cases. In the FSTXY collection one figure is spurious: no
unrelated foster sibs raised together can be found in Sims'
study. Readers will also note that the vast majority of the
figures come from studies undertaken before 1940, and that
over half of the 65 figures come from adoptive families and

matched controls, a demonstrably nonrepresentative group.

It would be a mistake to use Rao and Morton's calculations on the English data set as evidence for the quality of Cyril Burt's data. They arbitrarily treat Burt's uncles as cognate rather than affine; a rough calculation indicates that doing the opposite would raise the Table VII chi-square by about 4 points. For the key MZAXY kinship, they pool Burt's figure with Shields's; a rough calculation indicates that not doing so would raise the Table VII chi-square by another 2 points. Furthermore, they totally ignore several kinships for which Burt's figures can be found in Jensen's (2) tables: e.g., grandparents, second cousins, parent-as-child, biological siblings adopted together.

References

1. Jencks, C., Smith, M., Acland, H., Bane, M.J., Cohen, D., Gintis, H., Heyns, B., Michelson, S., "Inequality: a Reassessment of the Effect of Family and Schooling in America", Basic Books, New York, 1972.

2. Jensen, A.R., Behav. Genet. 4, 1-28 (1974).

MORTON: Perhaps no two investigators agree on the best data set for IQ. It is our contention, based on much experience, that perturbations of our data set have only trivial effects on the estimates. Only by rejecting most of the evidence can substantially different estimates be obtained.

The composition of Sims' study is given as a comment in the appendix. It was drawn to our attention by Leon Kamin (1), who claims that it throws new light on foster children. Examination of the FST data in the appendix shows that its inclusion has no appreciable effect on the estimates.

Our analysis of the English samples does not address the quality of Burt's data, merely its close similarity to other evidence. Our methods permit extension to distant relationships but because the expected correlations are small, random sampling impractical, and the effects of assortative mating uncertain, there is little point in including remote relatives.

Reference

1. Kamin, L., "The Science and Politics of IQ", Eribaum Assoc., Potomac, MD., 1974.

GENETIC EPIDEMIOLOGY

PITFALLS IN THE RESOLUTION OF IQ INHERITANCE

Arthur S. Goldberger

Department of Economics
University of Wisconsin
Madison, Wisconsin

I. INTRODUCTION

As a social scientist with no training in genetics, I am grateful for the opportunity to discuss the resolution of IQ inheritance at this conference. I am filled not only with gratitude but also with trepidation. For Morton & Rao (1977) say that

> The literature on inheritance of intelligence
> has suffered from ... domination of the field
> by psychologists and sociologists with primary
> interests and competence outside genetics,

and Rao, Morton, & Yee (1976, p. 241) have written that

> There can be no dialogue between genetics and the
> social sciences unless ... the latter accepts
> quantitative models and goodness of fit tests.

But the interests of science dictate that neither my gratitude nor my trepidation should stand in the way of my being rude on this occasion.

In a longer paper (Goldberger, 1977) I have undertaken a detailed analysis of both the Birmingham and Honolulu schools' efforts at fitting models to observed kinship correlations for IQ.

The Birmingham school is represented by the articles of Jinks & Eaves (1974) and of Eaves (1975), who modify the classical model of R. A. Fisher. Fisher specified phenotypic assortative mating, permitted non-additive gene effects, ruled out gene-environment correlation, and also ruled out environmental resemblance among persons living together. As a consequence of this last specification, Fisher's model would be rejected out of hand by any set of IQ kinship correlations which includes adoptive families. So the Birmingham school modifies Fisher's model by introducing a common environmental

component which is shared by siblings, and by parents and
children, living together, whether those kin be biological or
adoptive.

But the Birmingham model is logically untenable because
the consequences of the shared environment are not fully
taken into account. It is essentially impossible to construct
a causal model which will produce the Birmingham formulas for
kinship correlations, if only because the conjunction of
phenotypic assortative mating and environmental transmission
from parents to children will generate gene-environment
correlation: Goldberger (1977, pp. 36-37, A1-A15). Few
social scientists would try to publish a set of derived
equations, like the Birmingham formulary, without first
specifying a causal system from which those equations could
be derived. Fewer still would succeed.

I now turn to the Honolulu school.

II. THE HONOLULU VENTURE

The Honolulu school is represented by the series of arti-
cles in the <u>American</u> <u>Journal</u> <u>of</u> <u>Human</u> <u>Genetics</u> -- Morton
(1974), Rao, Morton, & Yee (1974, 1976) -- and by the recent
papers of Morton & Rao (1977) and Rao & Morton (1977). They
build upon the remarkable work of Sewall Wright, and proceed
from an explicit, logically tenable, and internally consistent,
causal model, the heart of which is captured in the path
diagram on p. 229 of Rao, Morton, & Yee (1976). Assortative
mating is on the basis of common environment and genotype
(rather than on the basis of phenotype). Parents transmit
environments as well as genes to their children (who also
share additional common environment). Hence environmental
resemblance among relatives, and gene-environment correlation,
are provided for. Non-additive gene effects, on the other
hand, are ruled out. To assist in the resolution of the determinants of IQ, the model also incorporates a second phenotype,
an index of family environment (e.g. socioeconomic status).
A sharp distinction is permitted between the determination of
IQ in childhood and the determination of IQ in adulthood.

The model has 10 free parameters, which I find convenient to specify as follows:

c = path from common environment to child's phenotype,
h = path from genotype to child's phenotype,
p = path from common environment to adult's phenotype,
q = path from genotype to adult's phenotype,

$\underline{f}$ = path from parent's common environment to child's common environment,

$\underline{x}$ = path from parent's phenotype to child's common environment,

$\underline{u}$ = correlation between environments of spouses,

$\underline{m}$ = correlation between genotypes of spouses,

$\underline{s}$ = correlation of one spouse's genotype with the other spouse's common environment,

$\underline{i}$ = path from common environment to index.

Several derived parameters also appear:

$$\underline{a} = (\underline{s}(\underline{f} + \underline{px}) + \underline{qx}(1 + \underline{m}))/(1 - \underline{f} - \underline{px})$$

= correlation between an individual's genotype and his common environment,

$$\underline{\theta} = (1 - 2 \underline{cha})^{-\frac{1}{2}}$$

= phenotypic standard deviation for adopted children. My notation follows that of Rao, Morton, & Yee (1976) except that I use $\underline{p}$ and $\underline{q}$ in place of their $\underline{cy}$ and $\underline{hz}$.

Various versions of this model have been applied to IQ data by the Honolulu group. Their venture into the IQ debate began modestly enough. Morton (1972) told us that

recent controversy about ethnic differences in behavior is based on two fallacies: first, that a reliable estimate of heritability can be obtained when the environment is not random; secondly, that heritability is relevant to educational strategy.

Morton (1974, pp. 320-321) told us that

each type of relationship introduces another equation and another assumption, generally in the direction of overestimating heritability,

and that

While heritability of IQ in man has usually been calculated as greater than .5, ... it would not be possible to argue strongly against a smaller value.

He went on to say (p. 327) that

one would be quite unjustified in claiming that heritability is relevant to educational strategy.

Within two years, however, Rao, Morton, & Yee (1976, p. 238) had estimated IQ heritability to be $.67 \pm .07$ for children and $.21 \pm .10$ for adults. And this striking difference had led them to conceive the possibility that

adult education of parents could ... have greater effects on academic performance than preschool education of their children.

Nowadays Rao, Morton, & Yee (1977) are telling us that
  the biological and cultural factors involved in
  the inheritance of IQ are resolved,
and Morton & Rao (1977, p. 38) close off their discussion of
"Quantitative inheritance in man" with this announcement:
  The "nature-nurture" controversy was partly an ideological confusion of individuals and populations,
  partly a methodological problem in distinguishing cultural and biological causes of family resemblance. As
  far as that problem has been formulated, it has been
  solved.
  What happened between 1974 and 1976? A rude person might
describe the transition, from skepticism to true belief, as a
comedy of errors.

III. THE HONOLULU MODELS

  The data set analyzed by Rao, Morton, & Yee (1976) was
drawn from the compilation in Jencks (1972) and from Burks
(1928), and is displayed below. For each kinship, $\underline{r}$ and $\underline{n}$
denote the observed correlation and the number of paired
observations on which it is based.

  Table 1. Data Set Analyzed by Rao, Morton, & Yee

	Variables correlated	$\underline{r}$	$\underline{n}$
1.	IQs of identical twins	.89	50
2.	IQs of separated identical twins	.69	19
3.	IQs of siblings	.52	2001
4.	IQs of adopted-adopted siblings	.23	21
5.	IQs of adopted-natural siblings	.26	94
6.	IQ of adopted child and his index	.25	186
7.	IQ of child and his index	.44	101
8.	IQ of parent and child's index	.69	205
9.	IQs of adoptive parent and child	.23	1181
10.	IQs of parent and child	.48	1250
11.	IQs of spouses	.50	887

  To this data set they fit five variants of their basic
model. The most general of those, which I refer to as H1,
sets $\underline{m}$ = $\underline{s}$ = 0, so that spouses' IQs correlate only because

the spouses had similar common environments in their youth. From the elaborate formulary in Rao, Morton, & Yee, we can set out the equations of this model as in the table below, in which the various kinships are labelled by acronyms.

Table 2.   Equations of Model H1

1.	MZTXY	$h^2 + c^2 + 2\,\underline{cha}$
2.	MZAXY	$\theta^2 h^2$
3.	SSTXY	$\tfrac{1}{2}h^2 + c^2 + 2\,\underline{cha}$
4.	FSTXY	$\theta^2 c^2$
5.	FSPXY	$\theta(c^2 + \underline{cha})$
6.	SSAXIX	$\theta \underline{ic}$
7.	SSTXIX	$\underline{i}(\underline{c} + \underline{ha})$
8.	OPTXIY	$\underline{i}\,[\underline{f}(\underline{p}(1 + \underline{u}) + \underline{qa}) + \underline{x}(1 + \underline{p}^2\underline{u})]$
9.	OFPXY	$\theta \underline{c}[\underline{f}(\underline{p}(1 + \underline{u}) + \underline{qa}) + \underline{x}(1 + \underline{p}^2\underline{u})]$
10.	OPTXY	$\underline{c}\,[\underline{f}(\underline{p}(1 + \underline{u}) + \underline{qa}) + \underline{x}(1 + \underline{p}^2\underline{u})] + \tfrac{1}{2}\underline{h}(\underline{pa} + \underline{q})$
11.	FMTXY	$\underline{p}^2\underline{u}$

With $\underline{m} = \underline{s} = 0$, H1 has 8 free parameters, and the formula for the derived parameter $\underline{a}$ reduces to

$$\underline{a} = \underline{qx}/(1 - \underline{f} - \underline{px}).$$

The four other variants of the model, which I refer to as H2 – H5, involve additional restrictions beyond $\underline{m} = \underline{s} = 0$, namely:

H2: $\underline{x} = 0$;   H3: $\underline{x} = 0$, $\underline{q} = \underline{h}$;   H4: $\underline{f} = 0$;

H5: $\underline{x} = 0$, $\underline{f} = 0$.

The estimation procedure is essentially as follows. Let $\underline{\rho}_j = \underline{\rho}_j(\theta)$ denote the expected correlation for the $\underline{j}$-th kinship, where θ denotes the set of $\underline{K}$ free parameters; and let $\underline{r}_j$ denote the observed correlation for the $\underline{j}$-th kinship. The corresponding $\underline{z}$-transforms are

$$\underline{\zeta}_j = \tfrac{1}{2}\log((1 + \underline{\rho}_j)/(1 - \underline{\rho}_j)) = \underline{\zeta}_j(\theta),$$

$$\underline{z}_j = \tfrac{1}{2}\log((1 + \underline{r}_j)/(1 - \underline{r}_j)).$$

For a data set with $\underline{j} = 1, \ldots, \underline{N}$ kinships, choose $\underline{\theta}$ to minimize the weighted least squares criterion

$$\chi^2 = \Sigma_{j=1}^{N} \ \underline{n}_j (\underline{z}_j - \underline{\zeta}_j(\theta))^2 .$$

The value of the criterion when minimized is referred to a chi-square distribution with degrees of freedom equal to $\underline{N} - \underline{K}$. In fact, the Honolulu group works with "bias-corrected" $\underline{z}$-transforms: Rao, Morton, & Yee (1974, pp. 331-332); Rao, MacLean, Morton, & Yee (1975, pp. 519-520); Rao, Morton, Elston, & Yee (1977, p. 150). But I ignore this refinement, which seems to have only negligible impact on the results.

The parameter estimates reported by Rao, Morton, & Yee (1976) for the models H1 - H5 are here displayed in Table 3 along with some auxiliary statistics.

Table 3. Parameter Estimates by Rao, Morton, & Yee

	H1	H2	H3	H4	H5
$\underline{c}$	.306	.423	.496	.266	.424
$\underline{h}$	.819	.835	.757	.789	.835
$\underline{p}$	.711	.916	1.074	.714	.918
$\underline{q}$	.459	.558	.757	.369	1.159
$\underline{f}$	.274	.406	.284	0	0
$\underline{x}$	.243	0	0	.577	0
$\underline{u}$	.985	.595	.434	.980	.595
$\underline{i}$	.858	.752	.642	.812	.752
χ^2	2.71	3.88	9.38	3.60	81.32
d.f.	3	4	5	4	5
$\underline{a}$	.201	0	0	.363	0
$\underline{\theta}$	1.055	1	1	1.086	1

They emphasize the good fits of the models to the data, saying (p. 239) that

> There is remarkable agreement between the observations and a simple model of biological and cultural inheritance ($\chi^2_3 = 2.71$).

For the H1 model, they translate their estimates into decompositions of phenotypic variances, as summarized in Table 4, and emphasize the contrast between the estimates of $\underline{p}$, $\underline{q}$ on the one hand and $\underline{c}$, $\underline{h}$ on the other hand, saying (p. 242),

Adult heritability remains significantly less than
heritability in childhood, presumably because the
leveling effect of the school system is replaced
by varying stimulation in different occupations.
The effect of family environment is significantly
greater for adults than children.

Table 4.   Estimated Variance Components for Model H1

Source	Adult IQ		Child IQ	
Genotype	$q^2 =$	.211	$h^2 =$	.670
Common environment	$p^2 =$	.506	$c^2 =$	.094
Covariance	$2\ pqa =$	.132	$2\ cha =$	.101
Residual		.151		.135
Total		1.000		1.000

IV.   THE HONOLULU ARITHMETIC

If one takes the H1 parameter estimates from Table 3,
inserts them into the equations of Table 2 to get predicted
correlations, and compares those predicted correlations with
the observed correlations in Table 1, one finds a chi-square
value substantially larger than that reported by Rao, Morton,
& Yee. Similarly for models H2 - H5. When I did that exercise in June, I was using a pocket calculator, and hence
recording some intermediate results. I happened to note that
the estimated value of the quantity $i(p + qa)$ remained constant
over the five models, and that its constant value was precisely the observed value of the 8-th correlation. That led me to
conjecture that the authors had accidentally used $i(p + qa)$
as the equation for the 8-th correlation in setting out their
models for estimation. My conjecture proved to be correct,
leading me to conclude that they had fitted five non-models.
Consequently their numerical results, interpretations thereof,
and policy recommendations could be disregarded.
Wondering what would happen if the error was corrected
and the models refitted, I set out to program the models myself. As I was transcribing the 11 equations, I happened to
note that the same long expression in square brackets appeared
in the 8-th, 9-th, and 10-th equations. I gave it a single

symbol to economize on writing. As I was doing so, it dawned
on me that I was writing the H1 model in terms of only 7 free
parameters, rather than the 8 free parameters used in the
Honolulu formulation. The parsimonious reformulation of the
H1 model is displayed in Table 5, with some symbols defined
at the bottom of the table.

Table 5. Reformulated Equations of Model H1

1.	MZTXY	$h^2 + c^2 + 2\ \underline{cha}$
2.	MZAXY	$\theta^2 h^2$
3.	SSTXY	$\frac{1}{2}h^2 + c^2 + 2\ \underline{cha}$
4.	FSTXY	$\theta^2 c^2$
5.	FSPXY	$\theta(c^2 + \underline{cha})$
6.	SSAXIX	θic
7.	SSTXIX	$i(\underline{c} + \underline{ha})$
8.	OPTXIY	$\underline{it}$
9.	OFPXY	θct
10.	OPTXY	$\underline{ct} + \frac{1}{2}\underline{hv}$
11.	FMTXY	$\underline{w}$

$$\underline{a} = \underline{qx}/(1 - \underline{f} - \underline{px})$$
$$\theta = (1 - 2\ \underline{cha})^{-\frac{1}{2}}$$
$$\underline{t} = \underline{f}(\underline{p}(1 + \underline{u}) + \underline{qa}) + \underline{x}(1 + \underline{p}^2\underline{u})$$
$$\underline{v} = \underline{pa} + \underline{q}$$
$$\underline{w} = \underline{p}^2\underline{u}$$

Being a social scientist, I realized that the ability
to rewrite a given model in terms of fewer free parameters has
an immediate consequence: the original set of parameters is
indeterminate, nonestimable, or in social science jargon,
underidentified. For H1, it is a well-defined problem to
choose a set of values for the 7 parameters $\underline{c}$, $\underline{h}$, $\underline{a}$, $\underline{i}$, $\underline{t}$,
$\underline{v}$, $\underline{w}$ to best fit the 11 observations, and the least-squares
principle will produce a unique solution. But it is not a
well-defined problem to choose a set of values for the 8
Honolulu parameters $\underline{c}$, $\underline{h}$, $\underline{p}$, $\underline{q}$, $\underline{f}$, $\underline{x}$, $\underline{u}$, $\underline{i}$ to best fit the

11 observations, and the least-squares procedure will not produce a unique solution, there being an infinity of distinct solutions which fit equally well.

It is easy to verify from Table 5 that, of the 8 Honolulu parameters in H1, only $\underline{c}$, $\underline{h}$, $\underline{i}$ are determinate: $\underline{p}$, $\underline{q}$, $\underline{f}$, $\underline{x}$, $\underline{u}$ cannot be extracted from $\underline{a}$, $\underline{t}$, $\underline{v}$, $\underline{w}$. The paths leading into adult IQ are confounded with the paths of environmental transmission from parents to children. Similar considerations apply to models H2 - H5: in no case is the Honolulu parameter set fully determinate in terms of the present data set. In particular, $\underline{p}$ is never determinate so that the contrast between the decomposition of variances at the adult and child level cannot be sustained. On this count alone, preschool educators may relax; their jobs are not in jeopardy.

What happens when the reparametrized H1 model is fitted? The results, kindly provided to me by the Honolulu group in July, are as follows, in terms of my parametrization :

$$\underline{c} = .286, \qquad \underline{h} = .823, \qquad \underline{a} = .228, \qquad \underline{i} = .903,$$

$$\underline{t} = .762, \qquad \underline{v} = .646, \qquad \underline{w} = .501,$$

with a chi-square value of 3.15 on 4 degrees of freedom. Readers can trace out the combinations of values of $\underline{p}$, $\underline{q}$, $\underline{f}$, $\underline{x}$, $\underline{u}$, which are compatible with these estimates.

There is another problem with the Honolulu modeling of the present data set, which I had pointed out to them several months earlier. In the Newman, Freeman, & Holzinger (1937) study of separated identical twins, which is the sole source of their MZAXY observation, most of the twins had been tested as adults. The logic of the Honolulu causal model indicates that the appropriate equation for such pairs is not $\underline{\theta}^2 \underline{h}^2$, but rather $\underline{\theta}^2 \underline{q}^2$. The Honolulu group realized, as I had not, that making this change would remove the indeterminacy in the H1 model. For, the MZAXY correlation would now isolate $\underline{q}$, and permit the remaining unknowns, $\underline{p}$, $\underline{f}$, $\underline{x}$, $\underline{u}$ to be extracted from $\underline{a}$, $\underline{t}$, $\underline{v}$, $\underline{w}$. In September, Rao, Morton, & Yeé (1977) reported on the fitting of this new model, which I refer to as H1*.

Their parameter estimates for H1* are:

$$\underline{c} = .290, \qquad \underline{h} = .843, \qquad \underline{p} = .707 \qquad \underline{q} = .566$$

$$\underline{f} = .290, \qquad \underline{u} = 1.000, \qquad \underline{x} = .179, \qquad \underline{i} = .969,$$

with a chi-square of 6.45 on 3 degrees of freedom. In terms

of our formulation, these estimates correspond to $\underline{a}$ = .174, $\underline{t}$ = .707, $\underline{v}$ = .688, $\underline{w}$ = .499. With this set of estimates for H1* in hand, Rao, Morton, & Yee (1977) decide that

> the biological and cultural factors involved in the inheritance of IQ are resolved,

while recognizing that $\underline{p}$ and $\underline{u}$ are closely correlated and thus poorly resolved.

Several features of their latest analysis of the 11-observation data set are worth noting:

(1) The burden of resolving the determinants of adulthood IQ rests squarely on the slim shoulders of the MZA observation, based on a sample of size 19. Rao, Morton, & Yee (1976, p. 236) had suggested that "twin research might profitably be left to twins."

(2) The fit has deteriorated so that there is no longer "remarkable agreement between the observations and a simple model". Indeed the chi-square is significant at the 10% level.

(3) With $\underline{u}$ = 1, the common environments of spouses are perfectly correlated: by the time that they walk down the aisle together, the typical bride and groom have shared as much IQ-relevant environmental experience as identical twins who have been raised together since birth.

(4) The estimates are wrong. To verify the last point, it suffices to recognize that the only difference between the H1* model and the corrected-H1 model lies in the 2d equation where $\underline{q}$ replaces $\underline{h}$. Take the corrected H1 estimates provided by the Honolulu group in July, set $\underline{q}$ = $\underline{h}$ = .823, and solve for $\underline{p}$, $\underline{f}$, $\underline{x}$, $\underline{u}$ from $\underline{a}$, $\underline{t}$, $\underline{v}$, $\underline{w}$. Inserted into the H1* formulary, these will produce the same predicted correlations for all kinships as they did when used in the corrected-H1 formulary. Hence they will produce the same chi-square, namely 3.15. This being less than 6.45 establishes that the latest Honolulu estimates are wrong.

Upon refitting the H1* model myself, I find that the best-fitting parameter values are

$$\underline{c} = .285, \quad \underline{h} = .835, \quad \underline{p} = -.782, \quad \underline{q} = .789$$

$$\underline{f} = -.159, \quad \underline{u} = .817, \quad \underline{x} = .375, \quad \underline{i} = .906.$$

These produce a chi-square of 2.61 with 3 degrees of freedom. The fit is excellent, but the signs of $\underline{p}$ and $\underline{f}$ are quite implausible.

It is hard to share the Honolulu group's confidence in their resolution of the biological and cultural factors involved in the inheritance of IQ.

V. THE HONOLULU DATA

Throughout the comedy of errors, the estimates of c and h have remained relatively constant. It is tempting to conclude that the Honolulu venture has at least succeeded in resolving the determinants of <u>childhood</u> IQ. That too would be a mistake.

The structure of the Honolulu models suggests that the estimates of the childhood parameters are heavily dependent on just four observations, the IQ correlations for: identical twins raised together (MZTXY), biological siblings raised together (SSTXY), pairs of adopted children raised together (FSTXY), and pairs of children raised together, one being adopted and the other biological (FSPXY). My conjecture is that that is indeed the case, the remaining equations and observations being irrelevant window-dressing as far as the childhood components of variance are concerned.

For convenience let us confine attention to the cases where $a = 0$ as in H2, H3, H5. The equations for the four key kinships are displayed below along with the observed values used by Rao, Morton, & Yee (1976):

$$\rho_1 = h^2 + c^2, \qquad\qquad r_1 = .89$$

$$\rho_3 = \tfrac{1}{2}h^2 + c^2, \qquad\qquad r_3 = .52$$

$$\rho_4 = c^2, \qquad\qquad r_4 = .23$$

$$\rho_5 = c^2, \qquad\qquad r_5 = .26$$

With this specification, each of the following contrasts provides an estimate of $\tfrac{1}{2}h^2$: $r_1 - r_3$, $r_3 - r_4$, $r_3 - r_5$. With this data set, doubling each contrast in turn gives these estimates of h^2: $2(.89 - .52) = .74$, $2(.52 - .23) = .58$, and $2(.52 - .26) = .52$. When account is taken of their respective sample sizes, these three estimates average out to just about .67, the full model's estimate of h^2. My conjecture is that the same mechanism will essentially operate regardless of the specification of the remainder of the model.

If so, and if our main concern is with the determinants of childhood IQ, it is essential to have a look at the specification, and at the observed values, employed in those contrasts.

First, consider the contrast between r_1 and r_3, that is between MZT and SST. For this contrast to estimate $\frac{1}{2}h^2$ requires that identical twins (who are of the same age and sex) have no more environmental similarity than ordinary siblings (who may differ in age and sex). Evidence against that specification can be found in the very source material on which the Honolulu group drew, namely Jencks (1972, pp. 286, 287, 289): To get their figure for r_3, namely .52, Rao, Morton, & Yee (1974) combined one study of same-sex fraternal twins (r = .63), with the mean of seven studies of ordinary siblings (r = .52). Those underlying figures suggest that identity of age and sex increases environmental similarity. Even the classical twin method applied here would compare the MZT figure, .89, with the DZT figure, .63, producing an h^2 estimate of .52, in place of .74. And that reduction in h^2, be it noted, would occur without any allowance for the possibility that MZTs share more environmental experience than same-sex DZTs. Nor is the MZT figure a fact of nature: Nichols (1970), as reported by Loehlin, Lindzey, & Spuhler (1975, p. 109), found r = .62 in his sample of 36 MZT pairs, so that with a judicious selection of samples, one could contrast the MZT figure of .62 with the DZT figure of .63, and arrive at an estimate of h^2 = −.02.

Second, consider the contrast between r_3 and r_4, that is between SST and FST. To get their figure for r_4, namely .23, the Honolulu group picked one adoptive study and discarded three others given in Jencks (1972, p. 291). Rao, Morton, & Yee (1974, p. 353) did so because the four studies together would be statistically heterogeneous, and would average up to r_4 = .42, a value which is higher than their r_5 = .26, such an ordering between FST and FSP being an anomaly in terms of their general model. With r_4 = .42, be it noted, the contrast between r_3 and r_4 would have estimated h^2 to be .20, in place of .58. Nor are these figures facts of nature. Scarr & Weinberg (1977, Table 6) report

$$r_3 = .42, \qquad r_4 = .39, \qquad r_5 = .30$$

in some 100 families who have adopted black and interracial children. The Texas Adoption Project, according to Scarr (1977, p. 66), has

$$r_3 = .37, \qquad r_4 = .22, \qquad r_5 = .30,$$

as the preliminary results in a sample of some 300 adoptive families. Readers are invited to construct their own estimates of $\underline{h}^2$ from these more recent data sets.

Rao, Morton, & Yee (1976, p. 234) told us that a critical assumption of their analysis is that "foster parents are random". This assumption is demonstrably false. Every adoption study shows that adoptive parents are well above population averages on IQ, education, income, occupational status, indeed on virtually every measurable variable which might be construed as an index of the environment conducive to intellectual development of children. For Burks's (1928) study, which the Honolulu group used, this point was documented at length by Goldberger (1976a,b).

> Rao, Morton, & Yee (1974, p. 357) had told us that
> there are enough problems in human biometrical
> genetics without introducing biased selection,
> which is sufficiently protean to invalidate any
> path analysis, for which we regard random sampling
> as an essential condition.

If they believe that, they should abandon their venture, or at least stop using adoptive family data on IQ, for they will not find adoptive studies in which the general population has been randomly sampled.

Social scientists are familiar with the proposition that selection on one trait has consequences for the means, variances, and correlations of that trait, and of all other traits with which it is correlated. In the present context, there is every reason to believe that environmental variation is limited across adoptive families. If so, the empirical correlations of adopted children with their parents, and with their siblings, will be attenuated. Thus the Honolulu models are misspecified, in precisely the direction which leads to overestimation of heritability.

Social scientists are also acquainted with the proposition that to obtain unbiased estimates of population parameters from nonrepresentative samples, it is necessary to model the selection process itself. In the present context, that task is not an easy one. A start on it might' be made by referring to Karl Pearson (1903). Translated into modern notation, Pearson's analysis tells us that when explicit selection on a single variable in a multinormal distribution takes place, reducing its variance by the ratio $\underline{b}$, then the variance-covariance matrix of the distribution changes from Σ to $\Sigma^* = \Sigma - \underline{b}\,\underline{d}\,\underline{d}'$, where $\underline{d}$ is the column of Σ corresponding to the explicit selection variable. For explicit selection on several variables, reference might be made to Lawley (1943).

VI.   THE HONOLULU APPROACH

There is unlikely to be a serious dialogue between the Honolulu school and social scientists until the former begins to deal seriously with the nonrepresentativeness and heterogeneity which characterize the underlying sources of kinship data on IQ.   In the interim I will take the opportunity to point out some other aspects of the Honolulu approach that came up as, over the past year, I worked through their articles and papers.

A.   Data Sources

To construct their data set, Rao, Morton, & Yee (1974, pp. 352 - 354; 1976, p. 236) made no independent search of the literature but rather relied on Jencks's (1972) compilation.   Consequently, they reproduce Jencks's errors: reversing the sample sizes for the two FMT correlations of Burks, incorrectly adjusting Willoughby's FMT correlation, discarding Outhit's FMT correlation because of a misunderstanding, -- and Jencks's arbitrary guesses at sample sizes. They also introduce some fresh errors -- treating the mean of seven observed sibling correlations as if it were a single observed figure in testing for heterogeneity in the SST category.
Relying on Jencks's compilation, Rao, Morton, & Yee have constructed a data set which draws only on studies conducted before 1940.

B.   Statistical Methods

A methodological theme that runs through the Honolulu articles is that specification errors lead to poor fits. Rao, Morton, & Yee (1974, pp. 336-337, 356) write
> Failure of either assumption tends to give spuriously high estimates of heritability, an error that may in principle be detected by a goodness-of-fit test against other pairs of relatives ...   In sufficiently large samples such discrepancies should be detected by significant deviations from our model.

Rao, Morton, & Yee (1976, pp. 230, 234) write
> A test of goodness of fit should reveal such discrepancies in a well-designed study ...
> The critical assumptions ... are best tested by residual χ^2 in an overdetermined system.

Morton & Rao (1977) write
> If the general hypothesis is acceptable by a
> goodness-of-fit test ... there is little reason
> to distrust distributional or causal assumptions
> which are subsumed by the general hypothesis.

The grounds for their optimism are not apparent. A
general principle is that specification errors lead to biased
estimates but not necessarily to bad fits. Reliance on over-
determinacy is perilous when all, or most, of the misspeci-
fications run in the same direction. (An analogous situation
is familiar to many social scientists: In regression
analysis it is assumed that disturbances are uncorrelated
with the explanatory variables. Violation of that assumption,
as in simultaneous-equation (= reciprocal-causation) models,
makes least-squares estimates biased. But the estimates
themselves contain no hint of the misspecification, because
the calculated residuals are by construction uncorrelated
with the explanatory variables). Another general principle
is that hypothesis tests should not be accepted until their
power against relevant alternatives has been established. I
have seen no evidence that the Honolulu school has investigated the power of their tests for path analysis of continuous
traits.

Morton & Rao (1977) write
> In any case emphasis should be on goodness-of-fit
> tests in a rich body of data rather than on justi-
> fication a priori of any hypothesis about family
> resemblance,

and Rao & Morton (1977) write
> However appealing a model may be, it is a simplifi-
> cation of nature and may always be stigmatized as
> an oversimplification ... To such criticism there
> is only one answer: a statistical test of goodness-
> of-fit, which in samples of adequate size and struc-
> ture can rule out an inadmissible model.

It is instructive to see how these guidelines are employed in
practice.

Rao & Morton (1977) fit an 8-parameter variant of their
model to an expanded IQ data set, consisting of 16 observations. A chi-square of 39.83 results, which on 8 degrees
of freedom is highly significant. Rather than rejecting
the model, they adopt a new criterion of goodness-of-fit.
An F-ratio is invented in which the model chi-square is
deflated by a heterogeneity chi-square, the latter measuring
the variation, across the original studies, of the correlations which were pooled into the 16 observations. An F-ratio
of 1.71 results, and so they adopt that model as "the

parsimonious model for American I.Q.". Noting that the model
seriously misfits MZA, FST, and FSP, they announce:
>These three observed correlations are elevated
>due to assortative placement, and it is a small won-
>der that these correlations are under-predicted by
>our model. Hence these discrepancies do not consti-
>tute evidence against our model.

They go on to say that
>We have shown that genetic analysis of I.Q. data
>is simple, determinate, and consistent over data
>sets.

Rao, Morton, Elston, & Yee (1977) suggest that working
with z-transforms produces estimates and test statistics
with desirable small-sample properties. These claims should
be ignored. As far as I know, it has not been established,
in the multivariate case, that the z-transforms are, in small
samples, multinormally distributed. Furthermore, the
equations of the models are nonlinear in the parameters, so
that only asymptotic theory will be available. (Many social
scientists are familiar with an analogous situation. In
conventional regression analysis with normally distributed
disturbances, least-squares estimates of the regression
coefficients are minimum variance unbiased. But if the
regression function is nonlinear in the parameters, the
least-squares estimates have that property only asymptotically,
their small-sample distributions being unknown).

C. Nuclear Families

>Rao, Morton, & Yee (1976, pp. 238, 242) remark that
>The main defect [of their analysis of the 11 IQ
>observations] is that these data depend on rare
>relationships and fail to make systematic use of
>information available in environmental indices
>and adult sibs in nuclear families. If indices
>of parents and children are determined, uncer-
>tainty about the magnitude of gene-environment
>correlations (s, u), the genetic correlation of
>mates (m), and the causal paths which determine
>family environment can be dispelled ... Further
>resolution is more likely to come from nuclear
>families than from the rare relationships that
>were favored by classical human genetics.

The grounds for such optimism are not apparent. Consider
Table 6, which sets out for nuclear families the equations
of one version of the Honolulu model. In this version, which
corresponds to H2, $m = s = x = 0$, so that $a = 0$ and $\theta = 1$.

There are 7 free parameters, which I take to be c, h, p, q, t, u, i; here $t = fp(1 + u)$. There are 10 correlations with distinct equations; Rao, Morton, & Yee (1976, p. 236) erred in counting 13.

Table 6. A Honolulu Model for Nuclear Families

Variables correlated		Equation
1.	IQs of parents	$p^2 u$
2.	IQ of parent with his index	ip
3.	IQ of parent with spouse's index	ipu
4.	IQs of parent and child	$ct + \frac{1}{2} hq$
5.	IQ of parent with child's index	it
6.	Indexes of parents	$i^2 u$
7.	IQ of child with parent's index	ict/p
8.	Indexes of parent and child	$i^2 t/p$
9.	IQ of child with his index	ic
10.	IQs of siblings	$c^2 + \frac{1}{2} h^2$

This model of 10 equations in 7 parameters makes 3 predictions about the observations; those are in fact the restrictions whose validity is examined by the chi-square test of goodness of fit. From the table, it is easy to see that those 3 restrictions are

$$r_1 r_6 = r_3^2, \qquad r_2 r_6 r_7 = r_3 r_8 r_9, \qquad r_5 r_6 = r_3 r_8 .$$

Observe that the parent-child IQ correlation, r_4, and the sibling IQ correlation, r_{10}, do not enter those restrictions. The model makes no predictions about, and is compatible with any observations on, r_4 and r_{10}. Looking at the same point in another way, we see that those two correlations contain two parameters, h and q, which appear nowhere else in the model. As a consequence, the estimates of c, p, t, u, i will be independent of r_4 and r_{10}; and the estimates of h and q will adjust to perfectly fit r_4 and r_{10}, given the estimates of the other five parameters. Indeed the estimate of h will be independent of r_4.

This sort of preliminary algebraic analysis of the
Honolulu system sheds light on the informational content of
nuclear families with respect to heritability in children and
adults. From this perspective, the Honolulu model looks more
like a theory of the determination of environmental indices
than like a theory of the determination of IQ.

D.   Environmental Indices

A distinctive feature of the Honolulu approach to modeling kinship correlations is the reliance on indices of common
environment. Rao, Morton, & Yee (1974, p. 331) say that
>   indeterminacy was resolved by combining path
>   analysis with the concept of an index and a theory
>   of hypothesis testing.

Rao, Morton, & Yee (1976, p. 236) say that
>   Systematic use of a family environmental index gives
>   a large number of correlations with different ex-
>   pectations.

Morton & Rao (1977) write
>   The concept of an index, defined by regression of
>   phenotype on relevant environmental factors, is
>   extremely flexible and powerful, often making
>   indeterminate data yield a unique solution and
>   greatly reducing standard errors of determined
>   parameters .... Multiple relationships and
>   indices are complementary; and combination of
>   indices with a variety of relationships is the
>   ideal design for separating genetic and cultural
>   inheritance, leaving many residual degrees of
>   freedom for testing the model.

For their IQ models the Honolulu group has indexed common
environment by a single measure of the cultural level of the
home (Rao, Morton, & Yee, 1976), and by father's occupation
scaled into a measure of socioeconomic status (Rao & Morton,
1977). Rao & Morton (1977) tell us that
>   Recent advances in analysis of family resemblance
>   depend critically on indices ... The index of an
>   individual may be created by regressing the pheno-
>   type on relevant observed variables which are not
>   themselves products of the genotype ... Indices
>   could be improved by including parental education
>   as well as occupation, combining these and other
>   socioeconomic indicators by regression with child's
>   phenotype as the dependent variable. Like Burks's
>   culture index this is likely to correlate highly
>   with parental phenotype, but in a way that is

accounted for by the estimate of $\underline{i}$ ... and does not disturb the rest of the analysis.

While social scientists may be happy to learn of the geneticists' interest in socioeconomic variables, they will be puzzled by the role assigned to them. In the Honolulu models for IQ, socioeconomic variables are taken to be mere fallible measures of the unobserved common environment which actually determines IQ. Only one causal path enters into the index (that from common environment), and no causal path emanates from it. Suppose that some of the socioeconomic variables (parental education for example) have a direct effect on the intellectual development of children. Or consider the fact that since socioeconomic status is itself a phenotype, it may well have a genetic component correlated with the genetic component of intelligence. If so, the Honolulu IQ models will be clearly misspecified.

ACKNOWLEDGEMENTS

I am indebted to D. C. Rao and Newton Morton for their care in responding to my many inquiries about their work, to Carol Treanor and S. Mostafa Baladi for computational assistance, and especially to Leon Kamin who provided me with his unpublished analyses of the American IQ samples. My research has been facilitated also by the opportunity to draw on the expertise of Luca Cavalli-Sforza, Dudley Duncan, Marc Feldman, Walter Nance, and Sandra Scarr. Financial support was provided by the Graduate School Research Committee at the University of Wisconsin, the Center for Advanced Study in the Behavioral Sciences, and the National Science Foundation. But none of those persons and institutions should be held responsible for the contents of this paper.

REFERENCES

Burks, B. S. 1928. The relative influence of nature and nurture upon mental development: a comparative study of foster parent – foster child resemblance and true parent – true child resemblance. Twenty-Seventh Yearbook of the National Society for the Study of Education, Part I. Public School Publishing, Bloomington: 219-316.

Eaves, L. J. 1975. Testing models for variation in intelligence. Heredity, 34: 132-136.

Goldberger, A. S. 1976(a). Mysteries of the meritocracy. In The IQ Controversy: Critical Readings (N. J. Block & G. Dworkin, editors). Pantheon, New York: 265-279.

Goldberger, A. S. 1976(b).   Jensen on Burks.   Educational
     Psychologist, 12: 64–78.
Goldberger, A. S. 1977.   Models and methods in the IQ debate,
     Part I. Workshop Paper 7710, Social Systems Research
     Institute, University of Wisconsin, Madison.
Jencks, C. 1972. Inequality: A Reassessment of the Effect of
     Family and Schooling in America.   Basic Books, New York.
Jinks, J. L. & Eaves, L. J. 1974.   IQ and inequality.   Nature,
     248: 287–289.
Lawley, D. 1943.   A note on Karl Pearson's selection formulae.
     Proceedings of the Royal Society of Edinburgh, Section A,
     62: 28–30.
Loehlin, J. C., Lindzey, G., & Spuhler, J. 1975.   Race Differ-
     ences in Intelligence.   W. H. Freeman, San Francisco.
Morton, N. E. 1972.   Human behavioral genetics.   In Genetics,
     Environment, and Behavior (I. Ehrman, G. S. Omenn, & E.
     Caspari, editors).   Academic Press, New York: 247–271.
Morton, N. E. 1974.   Analysis of family resemblance.   I.
     Introduction. American Journal of Human Genetics, 26:
     318–330.
Morton, N. E. & Rao, D. C. 1978.   Quantitative inheritance in
     man.   Yearbook of Physical Anthropology,
     in press.
Newman, H. H., Freeman, F. N., & Holzinger, K. J. 1937.
     Twins: A Study of Heredity and Environment.   University
     of Chicago Press, Chicago.
Nichols, P. L. 1970.   The effects of heredity and environment
     on intelligence test performance in 4 and 7 year white
     and Negro sibling pairs.   Doctoral dissertation,
     University of Minnesota, Minneapolis.
Pearson, K. 1903.   Mathematical contributions to the theory of
     evolution – XI.   On the influence of natural selection
     on the variability and correlation of organs.
     Philosophical Transactions of the Royal Society of
     London, 200: 1–66.
Rao, D. C., Maclean, C. J., Morton, N. E., & Yee, S. 1975.
     Analysis of family resemblance. V. Height and weight in
     Northeastern Brazil.   American Journal of Human Genetics,
     27: 509–520.
Rao, D. C. & Morton, N. E. 1977.   IQ as a paradigm in genetic
     epidemiology.   Population Genetics Laboratory, University
     of Hawaii, Honolulu.
Rao, D. C., Morton, N. E., Elston, R. C., & Yee, S. 1977.
     Causal analysis of academic performance.   Behavior
     Genetics, 7: 147–159.
Rao, D. C., Morton, N. E., & Yee, S. 1974.   Analysis of family
     resemblance. II. A linear model for familial correlation.
     American Journal of Human Genetics, 26: 331–359.

Rao, D. C., Morton, N. E., & Yee, S. 1976. Resolution of cultural and biological inheritance by path analysis. American Journal of Human Genetics, 28: 228-242.

Rao, D. C., Morton, N. E., & Yee, S. 1977. Resolution of cultural and biological inheritance by path analysis: Corrigenda and reply to Dr. Goldberger. Population Genetics Laboratory, University of Hawaii, Honolulu.

Scarr, S. 1977. Genetic effects on human behavior: recent family studies. Yale University, New Haven.

Scarr, S. & Weinberg, R. A. 1977. Intellectual similarities within families of both adopted and biological children. University of Minnesota, Minneapolis.

DISCUSSION

RAO: I would first like to make some specific comments, mostly on his discussion of our latest solution to the 1976 data set (H1* in his notation). We first classified MZA as children rather than as adults in our 1976 paper, which led Dr. Goldberger to suggest that they be classified as adults. When we did this, thus also removing indeterminacy in the H1 model, he charges that "the burden of resolving the determinants of adulthood IQ rests squarely on the slim shoulders of the MZA". It is pertinent to note that, before reclassifying MZA as adults, we fitted all other parameters for various fixed values of u. The remarkable outcome was that, within the acceptable range of values for u as judged by the residual χ^2, the determinants of childhood and adulthood IQ came out close to what we got after reclassifying MZA as adults (e.g., u = 1 gave h = .823, c = .286, y = 2.476 and z = .589). Dr. Goldberger is aware of these results which refute his charge.

The extreme value of u(=1) may reflect post-marital resemblance of the spouses. A smaller value of FMTXY = .33 (see our paper in this volume), obtained on spouses prior to marriage, led to a substantially smaller value of u = .681 for an extended data set of 16 correlations, and other estimates did not change appreciably.

The most serious charge he makes is that our "estimates are wrong". He produced a set of estimates yielding a "chi-square" of 2.61, but concedes that some of his estimates are implausible. More seriously, they are not maximum likelihood estimates (m.l.e.) whereas our's are; m.l.e. of a parameter θ is defined as that value of θ, within the admissible range of θ, which makes the likelihood function as large as possible. For IQ we take the admissible ranges as $0 \leq h, c, u, i \leq 1$ and $y, z \geq 0$; there are additional constraints on these and other parameters due to complete determination equations (Σ_{PC}, Σ_{PA} and Σ_{CC} of our paper in this volume). In claiming our estimates to be wrong Dr. Goldberger disagrees either with the definition of m.l.e. or the admissible ranges of the parameters. In any case he should hesitate to argue in favor of a negative value for p (or y) since he is aware of substantially positive correlations between the IQ and index of adults (OPTXIX in our paper).

His conjecture that kinships other than MZTXY, SSTXY, FSTXY, FSPXY are irrelevant for the resolution of h and c is false; for example, misspecification of the expected correlations for the other kinships as c^2 would inflate the overall estimate of c and deflate that of h. Improper specification of the remainder of the model may often lead to unacceptable fits. In reply to his discussion on adoption studies, I would like to point out that their deletion from the bigger data set did not give different results (see our paper in this volume). It is suggested that we should "deal seriously with the nonrepresentativeness and heterogeneity" of the IQ data. When we did this, by excluding adoptions and other rare relatives to take care of nonrepresentativeness and by introducing an F-test to account for heterogeneity, we are attacked for "inventing" an F-ratio! I may draw Dr. Goldberger's attention to one study I know of on the power of path analysis, presented at the Vth International Congress of Human Genetics (Mexico City, 1976) by Dr. Palovino.

Dr. Goldberger confines his discussion of nuclear families to the special case of m = s = x = 0, and points out that h and z (q) appear just in one correlation each. How does this constitute an argument against the nuclear family approach? Further, by introducing m ($\neq$ 0), and say s = $\sqrt{mu}$, one would see z appearing in four more equations and h appearing in six more equations, and none of the 3 restrictions he gave will hold. The fact is, we have introduced a rather elaborate model for environmental inheritance with many parameters, for the simultaneous resolution of which we need many equations which are introduced through the indices. We have a manuscript on lipoproteins which were analysed under m = s = x = 0. Even so, h, c, y, z and specific maternal effects were successfully resolved in nuclear families. In fact, as I have pointed out while discussing Dr. Li's paper, treatment of assortative mating and cultural inheritance involves arbitrary assumptions for relationships outside nuclear families. These aspects are exactly treated in nuclear families.

Finally, I am curious to know if Dr. Goldberger would like to make a contribution of his own to the IQ debate apart from making a glossary of pitfalls in others' analyses; not that a glossary of pitfalls isn't useful, but I would like to see if he has any new model that leads to results substantially different from ours. Does he propose to apply a new model which meets his objections, or to recommend collection of specifically better data, or both?

MORTON: I would like to testify to the stimulation which Arthur Goldberger has provided through his criticisms. Because of them our paper in these proceedings is much better than the first draft, yet we are no closer to agreement. That would not be surprising if we believed with Marxists that class struggle is reflected in antipathy between proletarian and bougeois science. On the contrary, we argue that to the dispassionate mind the nature-nurture controversy for IQ is settled, unless new data compel a revision. For us the problem is to explain Professor Goldberger.

We readily grant that the IQ data are old and flawed, and critical studies on nuclear families with indices would be welcome. In contrast, the critics of these data are curiously silent about the need for better studies. Instead, they exploit ad hoc arguments. When we illustrated a method to resolve genetic and cultural inheritance by IQ data largely drawn from Burks to obtain homogeneity (Rao et al., 1976), capriciousness was imputed. When we deliberately set out to include all data (Rao and Morton, 1977) using an F test as the standard statistical approach to heterogeneity, Professor Goldberger finds this no more acceptable. If this were an undergraduate debate, we could only admire his spoiling game. Like a certain politician, he responds to an awkward question by "neither yes nor no--quite the contrary."

Ours is a different approach. We look for evidence against our model (by an F test, as appropriate), and find none. We remove the rare relationships like adoptions and identical twins, against which so much rhetoric has been directed, then in a separate analysis we do the same with indices, and find that the results are substantially unchanged. We look at data from other populations, and get the same results. Which of us is using the scientific method?

Since Professor Goldberger does not have or advocate an alternative model or data set, he must use other tactics. One is to find inconsistency between my remarks over a five-year interval in which distribution theory and goodness-of-fit tests for a model of genetic and cultural inheritance were developed. Studies of family resemblance in man are much more appealing as tests of hypotheses than as estimation theory. I have always considered the belief that "heritability is relevant to educational strategy" to be a fallacy (e.g. Morton, 1974), which is why I can pit dispassionate curiosity against his evangelical fervor. Our 1976 remark about educational strategy was not based on the "striking difference" between genetic heritability in children and adults, which has survived all statistical tests, but explicitly on the observation that "the effect of family environment is significantly greater for adults than children." While neither a geneticist nor an economist is expert in educational psychology, the objection of Professor Goldberger to my environmentalism is, in the present context, surprising.

Another tactic is to make statistical quibbles. In the 1976 study we did indeed follow Jencks in pooling several sibling studies. Professor Goldberger calls this a "fresh error", not choosing to note that this illustration in a theoretical paper was disaggregated in our 1977 study, with no effect whatever. His objection to the standard F-ratio has been mentioned. Although he has now introduced z-transforms into the Jöreskog computer program, he is not happy with them because multivariate normality has not been proved. This is irrelevant for independent correlations. Marginal normality of z-transforms was demonstrated by Fisher, whereas neither variance components nor correlations have this desirable property in small samples. In goodness-of-fit tests we are concerned with the distribution of the likelihood ratio, not estimation bias. Maximum likelihood estimation reconciles an overdetermined system, and Professor Goldberger is undoubtedly aware that numerical results do not support his simple-minded argument about Table 6.

It seems unnecessary to list other points of disagreement: they are trivial besides what I believe to be a fundamental but unstated difference. I hold that errors in science are corrected through observational tests, and that pursuit of truth about family resemblance for IQ is interesting and responsible, while repression of such inquiry by any means including sophistry is harmful. I contend that the preposterous claim of American environmentalism, the emptiness of which is palpable to any parent, is an unsound basis for a democratic

society.* If Prof. Goldberger holds to a contrary view, as I
believe he does, he would be more honest to admit that he
objects not so much to our data or methods, as to our conclusion. The discussion would then be concerned with whether
there is any scientific reason to resist significant genetic
heritability in the face of overwhelming evidence. Until he
is prepared to do that, I will borrow one of his tactics.
Just as he challenges us to produce a data set that he cannot
criticise on some ground or other, I defy him to make an
analysis that leads with any semblance of objectivity to
conclusions substantially different from ours.

GOLDBERGER: By offering us an explicit and coherent causal
model, the Honolulu group has facilitated discussion of many
issues in the IQ debate. Their contribution will be dissipated
if their models, methods, and data are held to be exempt from
the usual requirements of scientific discourse.

For the H1* model, the unconstrained likelihood function
is maximized at my parameter values, not theirs. In that
sense, at least, their estimates are wrong. Their parameter
values apparently maximize a constrained likelihood function,
in which certain paths are forced to be non-negative. Imposing
the constraints leads to a substantial increase in the residual
sum of squares (i.e. decrease in the likelihood). That may be
interpreted as evidence against the validity of those constraints in the 11-kinship data set.

When Rao & Morton (1977) fit their current, 8-parameter,
model to an expanded, 16-kinship, data set, the residual sum
of squares is 39.83. Now, their maintained hypothesis has
$\sqrt{n_j}$ $(z_j - \zeta_j)$ asymptotically standard normal. Hence on the
null hypothesis that their model is valid, the residual sum

---

*J. B. Watson, the father of behaviorism, coupled a laud-
able opposition to racism with an indifference to law
and medicine: "Give me a dozen healthy infants, well-formed,
and my own specified world to bring them up in and I'll guarantee to take any one at random and train him to become any
type of specialist I might select--doctor, lawyer, artist,
merchant chief and, yes, even beggarman and thief, regardless
of his talents, penchants, tendencies, abilities, vocations,
and race of his ancestors." [Behaviorism (1925), p.104.] He
made no effort to test this hypothesis, which two generations
of educators have espoused with the enthusiasm of lemmings
for the sea.

of squares is asymptotically chi-square on 8 degrees of
freedom. Reference to a χ_8^2 table shows that they should
decisively reject their model at any sensible significance
level; indeed that is precisely what their own likelihood-ratio
argument would do.

One cannot divide the residual mean square (39.83/8) by a
heterogeneity mean square (142.46/49) and refer the result to
an F-table. I know of no statistical hypothesis on which such
a ratio has the F-distribution, even asymptotically. Of
course, in conventional ANOVA, a heterogeneity (i.e. within-
cell) mean square is used as the denominator of the F-
statistic. But there it serves as an estimate of the underlying sampling variance, a role which is precluded here since
the $\sqrt{n_j}(z_j - \zeta_j)$ have unit variance on the maintained
hypothesis. That the heterogeneity mean square is far in
excess of unity will reinforce, not diminish, the evidence
against the latest variant of the Honolulu model.

Family studies show great promise for refining our
estimates of the regression equations (norms of reaction)
relating socioeconomic achievement measures to their observable
determinants. Work along this line by social scientists
includes Scarr (1977), and the chapters by Leibowitz,
Chamberlain & Griliches, Olneck, and Sewell & Hauser in the
book, Kinometrics: Determinants of Socioeconomic Success
Within and Between Families, Paul Taubman, editor, Amsterdam:
North-Holland, 1977. But I would not encourage family studies
whose objective is to partition phenotypic variance. My
understanding is that heritability estimates are relevant to
predicting the outcomes of selective breeding under constant
environmental conditions, but quite irrelevant to assessing
the potential outcomes of environmental policies. On this
point, I follow an earlier geneticist:

> Each child approaches school with certain
> attitudes and abilities determined by his
> family and neighbors; some of these behavioral
> traits are presumably genetic to an undetermined
> degree. The educational establishment tries to
> optimize the school output and might reasonably
> be expected to diversify goals and content of
> instruction to accommodate individual differences.
> However, the extent to which these differences
> are genetic is completely irrelevant, both to
> educational strategy and the success of that
> strategy. Of course, the genetic determination
> of individual differences remains an interesting
> academic problem, which is insoluble except by
> randomizing the environment... My conclusion is

that measures of heritability when the environment
is not randomized are fraught with uncontrollable
difficulties. Instead of asking the geneticist
to develop a better method of estimation, the
psychologist should perhaps reconsider his reasons
for wanting to estimate heritability when no
selection experiment is envisaged.--N.E. Morton
(1972, pp.262, 255).

HRUBEC: I would hate to see twin research become a casualty of the IQ controversy. It is not always necessary to
make untestable assumptions about environmental sharing
between MZ and DZ twins. In some problems the relevant environmental variables can be identified and data on them can be
obtained. Appropriate methods can be employed for using such
data in genetic analyses. Including information on relevant
environmental variables in twin studies may also take care of
two other points, namely genetic-environmental interactions
and representativeness of the environments of twins compared
to the single born.
     Samples of twins need not always be biased. Twin regis-
tries based on specifiable populations have been established
in Finland, Sweden, Norway, Denmark, and the United States.
That extrapolation from twins to the single born may often be
justified is supported by data from the Health and Nutrition
Examination Surveys of the National Health Survey. These data
show that twins age 6 to 17 years as a group are indistinguishable from the single born with respect to a variety of
developmental traits.
     Models have been developed that partition the various
components of genetic variance in data obtained on twins
together with data on other relatives. Admittedly, these
models are not perfect, more development is needed, and not
all models are applicable to all problems.
     In trying to obtain answers to genetic-epidemiological
questions, twin data represent one of a wide variety of
observational methodologies that can contribute useful information. Monozygotic twins permit one uniquely powerful
research design, sometimes designated as the co-twin control
method. Twin pairs may be available with one member having
experienced a particular treatment or environmental exposure
that is absent in the co-twin. A comparison between members

of such monozygotic pairs excludes all genetic variance, age-related variance, and variance due to all environmental factors shared by pair members. It is usually impossible to control all of these factors in any other way. If uncontrolled, at best such factors introduce noise into the study comparisons so that they reduce the probability of evaluating relationships correctly. At worst they interact with study comparisons and confound them, and thus may lead to erroneous interpretations. In my opinion, it is the co-twin control applications in which twin studies can make the greatest and unique contribution.

RESOLUTION OF MAJOR LOCI FOR QUANTITATIVE TRAITS

R. C. Elston, K. K. Namboodiri and E. B. Kaplan

Department of Biostatistics
University of North Carolina
Chapel Hill, North Carolina 27514

The ultimate goal of genetic analysis is to identify individual genes and how they act. This paper is concerned with how this goal can be achieved by the statistical analysis of quantitative data on related individuals. We define a major locus to be a locus at which there is an allele that has a large effect on a trait, i.e. is megaphenic (1), regardless of the frequency of the allele in the population. Our interest is in determining whether such an allele exists, and what its effect is on the trait being studied; we are not concerned with estimating its frequency in the population.

The power of any statistical analysis to detect an effect increases with the size of that effect relative to other sources of variation in the sample in which it is studied, as well as with the size of the sample itself. Furthermore, for an effect of fixed magnitude and for a given total sample size, the power to detect a difference between two groups increases as the groups become more equally represented in the sample. Thus, to facilitate the detection of a major locus effect, a sample should be chosen in which that locus is as polymorphic as possible. For this purpose it is often useful to select for study families that contain at least one member who has an extreme value of the trait. There are appropriate sampling corrections for analyzing nuclear families that have been so selected (2, 3), but, if the sample consists of one or a few large pedigrees, sampling corrections are not necessary for our purpose. Analyzing such pedigrees as though they are random samples from the population may lead to grossly biased estimates of gene frequency and heritability, but will lead to only trivial biases in determining the mode of inheritance.

It is not known, if a single major locus affects a quantitative trait, how the power of statistical tests to detect that locus depends on the family structure of the sample. We do not know whether one large multigenerational pedigree is more informative for that purpose than the same number of individuals in many nuclear families. But if several major loci affect a trait, then a single large pedigree is more likely to be genetically homogeneous than many nuclear families; and in the latter the mode of inheritance may well be obscured by the genetic heterogeneity from family to family.

In this paper we describe some methods for major gene analysis in pedigree data. The basic method of pedigree analysis (4) is briefly reviewed, and two ways of applying previously described goodness-of-fit tests (5) to pedigree data are described. These goodness-of-fit tests are then applied to a previously published set of pedigree data (6). The data are the serum cholesterol and triglyceride levels on 190 members of a single pedigree; originally data on 195 members were analyzed, but here we have eliminated data on 5 members as a result of finding genetic inconsistencies in the transmission of blood polymorphisms. The pedigree was ascertained via four probands who had either elevated cholesterol levels or a family history of premature death from myocardial infarction.

STATISTICAL METHODS

There are two kinds of persons in a pedigree: persons who have a parent in the pedigree, whom we denote x, and persons who do not have a parent in the pedigree, whom we denote y. We shall use the symbols x and y to denote both the person and the trait measures on that person. The two-allele autosomal locus model assumes that, after age and sex adjustment and transformation (if necessary), each x or y comes from one of three normal distributions, which we call AA, Aa, and aa. The probabilities that y comes from each of these distributions are denoted ψ_{AA}, ψ_{Aa}, and ψ_{aa}, respectively. The probabilities that x comes from each of these distributions depend upon the distributions from which x's parents come and the following three transmission probabilities:

$\tau_{AA\ A}$ = probability that parent from AA transmits A to x

$\tau_{Aa\ A}$ = probability that parent from Aa transmits A to x

$\tau_{aa\ A}$ = probability that parent from aa transmits A to x

If x's two parents transmit A and A, x comes from distribution AA; if A and a, then x comes from distribution Aa; and if a and a, x comes from distribution aa. Thus simple Mendelian transmission corresponds to the null hypothesis: $\tau_{AA\ A} = 1$, $\tau_{Aa\ A} = 1/2$, $\tau_{aa\ A} = 0$. On the other hand, if the distribution from which x comes does not depend on which distributions x's parents come from, the corresponding null hypothesis is $\tau_{AA\ A} = \tau_{Aa\ A} = \tau_{aa\ A} = \tau$. In this case each x comes from distribution AA with probability τ^2, from distribution Aa with probability $2\tau(1-\tau)$, and from distribution aa with probability $(1-\tau)^2$. These probabilities need not be the same as ψ_{AA}, ψ_{Aa}, and ψ_{aa}, respectively, thus allowing for the possibility that measures on individuals born into the pedigree have a different distribution than do measures on individuals marrying into it. In this way the model can accommodate, to a certain extent, the presence of a familial correlation that is environmental in origin. This "environmental" hypothesis is best tested when two of the distributions are identical, since under this model the probabilities that x comes from the different distributions can depend on only one parameter, τ; if there are three distinct distributions, the probabilities must necessarily be binomial proportions.

Under this general model, in which the transmission probabilities can take on arbitrary values between 0 and 1, we can use the likelihood ratio criterion to test many hypotheses; e.g., Mendelian transmission probabilities, equal transmission probabilities, Hardy-Weinberg equilibrium proportions (i.e., $\psi_{Aa} = 2\sqrt{\psi_{AA}\psi_{aa}}$) and dominance (i.e. the distributions AA and Aa are identical or the distributions Aa and aa are identical). In each case, twice the difference between the two maximum log likelihoods, obtained under the unrestricted model and the null hypothesis respectively, is asymptotically distributed as chi-square under the null hypothesis. It has been suggested on the basis of simulation experiments (7) that we can reasonably infer segregation at a major locus in a set of data if pedigree analysis shows that the following criteria are satisfied:

1. There is no significant departure from Mendelian transmission probabilities, and the estimated probabilities are close to 1, 1/2 and 0.

2. There is significant departure from equal transmission probabilities.

3. The multiplicative difference between the two maximum likelihoods obtained under dominant and recessive hypotheses is large; i.e., the hypothesis that AA and Aa are identical has a very different maximum likelihood from that for the hypothesis that Aa and aa are identical. If there is a unique maximum, this criterion is automatically satisfied.

4. The data, when considered as a random sample from some distribution, fit a mixture of two normal distributions significantly better than they do a single normal distribution.

The first two criteria ensure that there is transmission from one generation to the next, but do not guard against the possibility of polygenic inheritance; this is the purpose of the last two criteria. However, it is difficult to specify just how different the likelihoods for the dominant and recessive hypotheses should be; and whether or not two normal distributions fit the data significantly better than a single normal distribution depends on whether the data are transformed or not: data from any continuous distribution, even a bimodal distribution, can be transformed to be normally distributed. For these reasons we decided to investigate the utility of goodness-of-fit tests as further criteria to be met before inferring the presence of a major locus.

Consider any individual in the pedigree, with measurement z. Under the model just described the likelihood of the measurements on all the other persons in the pedigree is the sum of three terms, corresponding to z coming from AA, Aa or aa. These three likelihoods, evaluated under a particular null hypothesis, are proportional to the probabilities, conditional on that hypothesis and the information available in the rest of the pedigree, that z comes from AA, Aa and aa, respectively. Thus under the null hypothesis z can be considered as a random value from a mixture of the three distributions AA, Aa, and aa, the mixing proportions being these conditional probabilities. Alternatively, the mixing proportions can be based on all the information available in the pedigree, the three likelihoods including the measurement of z. In either case, if the cumulative distribution function of this mixture is F, $F(z)$ can be considered as a random observation from the uniform distribution on the unit interval. We determine F, and hence $F(z)$, for each individual, assuming any unknown parameters in F are equal to their maximum likelihood estimates. Then, ignoring the dependencies among them, we test whether the $F(z)$ could in fact be a sample of independently and uniformly distributed random variables. Many test statistics are available for doing this (8) but some lack power and others are sensitive to small sample sizes. On the basis

of empirical results there are four such statistics that have
been recommended (5): three are based, either directly or
indirectly, on Neyman's (9) smooth test, and the fourth is
based on the statistic S' proposed by Lewis (10). In each
case the test statistic is to be compared with a chi-square
with one degree of freedom.

The first statistic tests whether the mean of $F(z)$ is
equal to 1/2. If we have measures on n members of the pedigree, $F_j(z_j)$ corresponding to the jth member, the statistic
is

$$U_1^2 = 12 [\sum_{j=1}^{n} \{F_j(z_j)-1/2\}]^2/n.$$

The second statistic tests whether the variance of $F(z)$ is
equal to 1/12, and is

$$U_2^2 = 180 [\sum_{j=1}^{n} \{F_j(z_j)-1/2\}^2-n/12]^2/n.$$

The third statistic considers the variance of the spacings
between the $F_j(z_j)$. Let $z_{(j)}$ denote the ranked measures, so
that

$$z_{(1)} \overset{<}{_{-}} z_{(2)} \overset{<}{_{-}} \cdots \overset{<}{_{-}} z_{(n)}.$$

Then the n+1 spacings are given by

$$D_j = F_{(j)}(z_{(j)}) - F_{(j-1)}(z_{(j-1)}), \quad j = 1, 2, \ldots, n + 1,$$

where we define $F_{(o)}(z_{(o)}) = 0$ and $F_{(n+1)}(z_{(n+1)}) = 1$. Under
the null hypothesis $1 - (1-D_j)^n$ is uniformly distributed on
the unit interval, and the third statistic is thus

$$U_2'^2 = 180 [\sum_{j=1}^{n+1} \{1/2-(1-D_j)^n\}^2 - (n+1)/12]^2/(n+1).$$

The last statistic utilizes the ranked spacings $D_{(j)}$, defined
so that

$$D_{(1)} \overset{<}{_{-}} D_{(2)} \overset{<}{_{-}} \cdots \overset{<}{_{-}} D_{(n+1)},$$

and is given by

$$L^2 = 144 [2(n+1)-2 \sum_{j=1}^{n+1} j D_{(j)} - \frac{n}{2}]^2/n^2.$$

These same statistics can also be calculated on subsets
of the data, e.g. separately for males and females, to determine if the hypothesized model fits each individual subset;

in this way unsuspected heterogeneities may be revealed. All
the statistics test both the genetic and the environmental
parts of the hypothesized model, and so can help determine
that the complete model fits the data. These statistics can
also be used to test whether the environmental hypothesis, or
even the underlying model with arbitrary transmission probabilities, fits the data. In the case of the environmental
hypothesis with equal transmission probabilities, there are
only two sets of mixing proportions if the measurement on each
individual is excluded to determine them: ψ_{AA}, ψ_{Aa}, and ψ_{aa}
for the y's, and τ^2, $2\tau(1-\tau)$, and $(1-\tau)^2$ for the x's.

RESULTS

     Before fitting the model all measures are adjusted to age
30, using linear regression for males and quadratic regression
for females, and then the measures on females are adjusted to
have the same mean and variance as the measures on males.
Three different transformations are studied for both cholesterol and triglyceride levels: logarithms, the power transformation $z' = (z^p -1)/p$, where p is the maximum likelihood
estimate on the assumption that the 190 values of z' are independently sampled from a normal distribution, and a normalizing transformation--$\Phi^{-1}\{r(z)/191\}$, where Φ is the standardized cumulative normal distribution and $r(z)$ the rank of the
observation z. In each case it is assumed on the basis of
previous analyses (6) that the mean of AA is equal to the mean
of Aa.
     The results of the likelihood ratio criterion and the
four goodness-of-fit tests for cholesterol levels are shown
in Table 1. The likelihood ratio criterion for the Mendelian
hypothesis has three degrees of freedom, that for the environmental hypothesis has two. If we first look at the statistics
based on the likelihood ratio criterion, we see that the
Mendelian hypothesis fits for all three transformations; also,
in each case the environmental model is rejected, indicating
that there is some form of transmission from generation to
generation. It should be noted that these likelihood ratio
tests do not falsely suggest the presence of a major locus
because of skewness of the data <u>per se</u> (7).
     Among the goodness-of-fit tests, the large values of
$U_2'^2$ and L^2 on the normalized scale for the environmental
hypothesis should be ignored as an artifact, since the method
of normalizing causes all the spacings to be equal. Thus
among the first set of four tests, those that do not use the
information on each z to determine its mixing proportions,
only $U_2'^2$ has any discriminating power, and very little at

TABLE 1

Analysis of Cholesterol Levels: Likelihood Ratio (L.R.) and Four Goodness-of-Fit Chi-Square Statistics (i) Excluding Each z to Determine its Mixing Proportions, and (ii) Using All Available Information to Determine the Mixing Proportions.

Transform	Hypothesis	L.R.	(i)				(ii)			
			U_1^2	U_2^2	$U_2'^2$	L^2	U_1^2	U_2^2	$U_2'^2$	L^2
Logarithm	Mendelian	1.0	0.1	0.1	0.3	0.0	0.0	5.5	0.2	0.2
	τ's equal	36.3	0.0	0.7	3.3	0.2	0.0	6.5	4.4	0.2
Normalized	Mendelian	3.4	0.4	0.1	0.0	0.0	0.1	11.5	0.5	0.0
	τ's equal	33.1	0.1	0.3	54.6*	5.6*	5.2	7.6	24.4*	3.2*
p = -1.236	Mendelian	1.1	0.5	0.0	0.7	0.0	0.3	14.1	4.5	1.0
	τ's equal	38.9	0.2	0.0	1.9	0.3	0.0	6.5	4.4	0.3

*Spuriously large values.

that. The second set of goodness-of-fit tests, using all the available information to determine the mixing proportions, have more power. These tests indicate that the major locus model using logarithms fits best: but even here there is significance ($U_2^2 = 5.5$). This lack of fit is reduced somewhat if sex-dependent variances are assumed in the pedigree analysis (for which $U_2^2 = 4.9$) or if the effect of log triglyceride level is eliminated from the log cholesterol level by regressing it out. In the latter case the variable analyzed is 25.16 (log cholesterol) - (log triglyceride), and $U_2^2 = 3.6$; furthermore, the overlap between the two distributions is estimated to be only 1.8% for this variable, the smallest found for any analysis so far performed on these data. But for this variable the lack of fit is similarly reduced under the environmental hypothesis ($U_2^2 = 4.5$).

Table 2 shows the results for triglyceride levels. When logarithms on the normalized scale are used, the likelihood ratio criterion suggests there is segregation at a major locus--not only does the Mendelian hypothesis fit, but there is also significant departure from the environmental hypothesis--and the first set of goodness-of-fit statistics show nothing significant. When the power transformation with p = 0.0697 is used, however, the likelihood ratio criterion marginally accepts both hypothesis, while the first U_2^2 suggests both hypotheses should be rejected. The second U_2^2 goodness-of-fit statistic, however, indicates lack of fit in every case. As was found previously (6), if the effect of log cholesterol is removed from log triglyceride by regressing it out, the likelihood ratio finds both hypotheses quite acceptable. In this case the first set of goodness-of-fit tests shows no significant departure from either hypothesis, but among the second set U_2^2 indicates significant departure from both hypotheses ($U_2^2 = 18.6$ and 9.0 for the Mendelian and environmental hypotheses respectively).

DISCUSSION

We chose to examine the goodness-of-fit tests for these two particular traits because it is now well established by linkage analysis that a major locus for hypercholesterolemia is segregating in this pedigree (11, 12, 13, 14), and because it was hoped that these tests would shed some light on whether or not there is a major locus for hypertriglyceridemia segregating also. It is apparent that only U_2^2 and $U_2'^2$ have any discriminatory power in these situations, and that they are

TABLE 2

Analysis of Triglyceride Levels: Likelihood Ratio (L.R.) and Goodness-of-Fit Chi-Square Statistics (i) Excluding Each z to Determine its Mixing Proportions, and (ii) Using All Available Information to Determine the Mixing Proportions.

Transform	Hypothesis	L.R.	(i)				(ii)			
			U_1^2	U_2^2	$U_2'^2$	L^2	U_1^2	U_2^2	$U_2'^2$	L^2
Logarithm	Mendelian	0.7	0.3	0.1	1.0	0.0	0.2	15.7	0.3	0.0
	τ's equal	11.5	0.0	0.2	0.3	0.0	0.0	13.9	18.2	2.3
Normalized	Mendelian	0.3	0.0	0.0	0.0	0.1	0.0	13.8	0.5	0.5
	τ's equal	23.6	0.0	0.0	67.3*	7.9*	0.0	23.7	41.2*	5.6*
p = 0.0697	Mendelian	6.2	0.1	13.3	1.2	0.4	0.1	28.2	1.5	0.3
	τ's equal	5.5	0.6	6.9	0.1	0.0	0.5	10.5	0.0	0.2

*Spuriously large values

more powerful if they are calculated using the likelihood of the complete pedigree to determine the appropriate mixing proportions for each individual. However, the results of these tests in the analysis of the cholesterol levels suggest they are more useful in determining whether an appropriate transformation has been applied to the data, rather than in discriminating between hypotheses. Since our purpose is not only to detect the existence of segregation at a major locus, but also to resolve as accurately as possible its effect on the phenotype, these goodness-of-fit tests appropriately supplement the likelihood ratio tests.

The results of these tests in the analysis of the triglyceride levels confirm the impression, given by the likelihood ratio tests, that any major locus segregation in this trait may be merely due to its correlation with the cholesterol levels. However, whereas after correction for cholesterol levels the likelihood ratio criterion would indicate acceptance of both hypotheses, U_2^2 would indicate rejection of both hypotheses. This suggests that the model underlying the likelihood ratio tests is inadequate for this trait; and this appears to be confirmed when the second set of goodness-of-fit tests are applied for the underlying model, i.e. when the transmission probabilities are assumed to be equal to their maximum likelihood estimates ($U_2^2 = 9.1$). It is of course possible that some transformation exists for which the model is adequate; but this goodness-of-fit test has detected a lack of fit, for the trait as specified, that is undetected by the likelihood ratio test. The difficulty of finding the appropriate transformation can be avoided by dichotomizing the data, i.e. changing the measure on each individual to an indication only of whether it is above or below a particular threshold. However, the resulting loss in power (15) that can be expected makes a sample size of 190 quite inadequate for this procedure.

It is possible to define analogous goodness-of-fit tests for the polygenic model. For the major locus model, $F_j(z_j)$ is identical to the quotient of two quantities. For the first set of statistics, the dividend is the likelihood of the whole pedigree with $g_u(z_j)$, the density for z_j conditional on genotype u replaced by $G_u(z_j)$, the corresponding cumulative distribution; and the divisior is the likelihood of the whole pedigree with $g_u(z_j)$ replaced by unity. For the second set of statistics, the dividend is obtained by inserting $G_u(z_j)$ next to $g_u(z_j)$, and not instead of $g_u(z_j)$, in the likelihood; and the divisior is simply the likelihood of the whole pedigree. As explained by Elston and Stewart (4), the likelihood of a pedigree under the polygenic model can be expressed in a manner analogous to the likelihood under the major locus model, and so we can define $F_j(z_j)$ in this same way to obtain goodness-of-fit tests for the polygenic model. However, there are computational difficulties that have to be overcome before we can determine the usefulness of these tests.

Another way to resolve the question of whether transmission of a quantitative trait from one generation to the next is monogenic or polygenic is to fit a model containing both types of variation (2, 4) under which we test, separately, the null hypotheses that each is non-existent. We are at present programming the likelihood of a pedigree under such a model, using polynomial approximations to make analytical integration possible; it will be interesting to see whether, using such a model and the likelihood ratio criterion, this single set of data on 190 individuals can unequivocally demonstrate the segregation of a major locus for cholesterol levels. There is such a mixed model program available for nuclear families (15) but, since it does not allow arbitrary transmission probabilities, it is very sensitive to environmentally caused non-normality such as skewness and kurtosis (7, 15).

It should be noted that it is quite possible for a major locus to be segregating and yet find that the environmental hypothesis fits the data well. Equality of the transmission probabilities merely implies that the children's distribution is always the same in the data, regardless of their parents; this will hold true whenever a major locus is segregating if all the parental mating types are the same. If all the matings in a pedigree are Aa x aa, such as might be the case for a rare autosomal dominant segregating in a pedigree from which non-segregating branches (aa x aa) have been eliminated, each child will have one half probability of being Aa and one half probability of being aa. Thus in this situation $\tau^2 + 2\tau(1-\tau) = (1-\tau)^2 = 1/2$, i.e. $\tau = .29$. If, in the case of a rare recessive, all the mating types in the data set are Aa x Aa, each child will have one quarter probability of being aa and three quarters probability of being A-; i.e. $(1-\tau)^2 = 1/4$, or $\tau = 1/2$. If only one mating type occurs in the data it is impossible to distinguish the effect of a major locus from an environmental effect that happens to occur in just that proportion of the children expected under a major locus model.

Finally we should note two things. First, in the absence of any biochemical analysis, the most compelling evidence for the existence of a major locus may come from linkage analysis. We can estimate that over half the human genome is within linkage distance of at least one of the more than thirty polymorphic genetic markers currently known in man (16). Second, whether for segregation analysis or linkage analysis, it is always advantageous to work with traits that differentiate the genotypes as much as possible. We have seen that a

function of both cholesterol and triglyceride levels leads to
a better separation of dominant and recessive phenotypes than
cholesterol levels alone, and in general we can expect multivariate analysis to help resolve major loci. By the same
token that there are traits affected by many loci, we can expect that there are loci affecting many traits; it is therefore not unreasonable to hope that a locus will be better
resolved if we simultaneously study, in a multivariate analysis, more of the traits it affects.

REFERENCES

1. Morton, N. E. (1967). The detection of major genes
    under additive continuous variation. <u>Am. J. Hum.
    Genet.</u> 19:23-34.

2. Morton, N. E. and MacLean, C. J. (1974). Analysis of
    family resemblance. III. Complex segregation of quanti-
    tative traits. <u>Am. J. Hum. Genet.</u> 26:489-503.

3. Elston, R. C. and Yelverton, K. (1975). General models
    for segregation analysis. <u>Am. J. Hum. Genet.</u> 27:31-45.

4. Elston, R. C. and Stewart, J. (1971). A general model
    for the genetic analysis of pedigree data. <u>Hum. Hered.</u>
    21:523-603.

5. Elston, R. C. and Stewart, J. (1973). The analysis
    of quantitative traits for simple genetic models
    from parental, F_1 and backcross data. <u>Genetics</u> 73:
    695-711.

6. Elston, R. C., Namboodiri, K. K., Glueck, C. J.,
    Fallat, R., Tsang, R. and Leuba, V. (1975). Study
    of the genetic transmission of hypercholesterolemia
    and hypertriglyceridemia in a 195 member kindred.
    <u>Ann. Hum. Genet.</u> 39:67-87.

7. Go, R. C. P., Elston, R. C. and Kaplan, E. B. (1978).
    Efficiency and robustness of pedigree segregation
    analysis, <u>Am. J. Hum. Genet.</u> 30:28-37.

8. Pyke, R. (1965). Spacings, <u>J. Roy. Statist. Soc. B.</u>
    27:395-449.

9. Neyman, J. A. (1937). Smooth test for goodness of
    fit. <u>Skand. Aktuar.</u> 20:150-199.

10. Lewis, P. A. W. (1965). Some results on tests for Poisson processes. <u>Biometrika</u> 52:67-77.

11. Elston, R. C., Namboodiri, K. K., Go, R. C. P., Siervogel, R. M., and Glueck, C. J. (1976). Probable linkage between familial hypercholesterolemia and third complement component (C3). Baltimore Conference (1975): Third International Workshop on Human Gene Mapping. Birth Defects: Original Article Series, XII, 7, 1976, 294-297, The National Foundation, New York.

12. Ott, J., Schrott, H. G., Goldstein, J. L., Hazzard, W. R., Allen, F. H., Jr., Falk, C. T., and Motulsky, A. G. (1974). Linkage studies in a large kindred with familial hypercholesterolemia. <u>Am. J. Hum. Genet.</u> 26:598-603.

13. Berg, K. and Heilberg, A. (1976). Linkage studies on familial hyperlipoproteinemia with xanthomatosis: normal lipoprotein markers and the C3 polymorphism. Baltimore Conference (1975): Third International Workshop on Human Gene Mapping. Birth Defects: Original Article Series, XII, 7, 1976, 266-270, The National Foundation, New York.

14. Berg, K. and Heiberg, A. (1977). Confirmation of linkage between familial hypercholesterolemia with xanthomatosis and the C3 polymorphism. IVth International Workshop on Human Gene Mapping, Winnipeg, Manitoba, Aug. 14-18.

15. MacLean, C. J., Morton, N. E. and Lew, R. (1975). Analysis of family resemblance. IV. Operational characteristics of segregation analysis. <u>Am. J. Hum. Genet.</u> 27:365-384.

16. Elston, R. C. and Lange, K. (1975). The prior probability of autosomal linkage. <u>Ann. Hum. Genet.</u> 38:341-350.

DISCUSSION

OTT: I would like to congratulate Dr. Elston on his presentation of the various statistical tests that can be

used for the detection of major genes in pedigree data. I
have two comments to make, the first referring to a question
of robustness of these tests and the second presenting one of
my own approaches.

1. The procedures mentioned by Dr. Elston are intended
to test whether one can reject the null hypothesis (H_0) that
there is no major gene contributing to Z_j, the measurement
on the j-th individual. Most of these procedures are designed
for independent individuals which is thus part of the description of H_0. The alternative hypothesis (H_1) one would like to
accept with a certain statistical power is that of the
presence of a 'major gene. The problem arises that these
procedures could also be powerful with respect to a deviation
from H_0 other than that specified by H_1. One such deviation
might be that in the presence of polygenic effects, the
members of a pedigree are not statistically independent. In
a different context, this problem has been addressed by Sing
and Rothman (Ann. Hum. Genet. 39:141, 1976) where non-
independence of the data alone was indeed shown to make a
test significant although the effects the test was designed
to detect were completely absent. For the chi-square test of
homogeneity in a two-by-two table, Cohen (J. Amer. Statist.
Ass. 71:665, 1976) studied the effects of clustered sampling,
i.e., sib-pairs were sampled rather than independent
individuals. It was again shown that chi-square is inflated
by the presence of a correlation between the two members of a
sib-pair. It would be interesting to know whether the tests
presented by Dr. Elston share this behavior, i.e., that they
have some tendency to show a significance even in the absence
of a major gene so that investigators using these tests will
have to exercise some caution in their interpretation.

2. The design of several of our Seattle studies is that
of ascertaining a random sample of individuals and studying
the families of those individuals (index cases) whose observed
measurements lie above a certain cut-off point, i.e., who
show an elevated value. The rationale behind this design is
that a major gene raising the measurements (e.g., lipid levels)
that is rare in the population will be enriched in the index
cases and thus also in their relatives. There are several
statistical problems with this data design, e.g., the family
members are not independent while the probands are, and the
mean of the measurements in each family clearly depends,
among other things, on the value of the index case. To test
the hypothesis (H_0) of no major gene, I have developed the
following likelihood ratio test. In the absence of a major
gene but allowing for environmental and polygenic effects

(correlation between relatives), the observations in the families of index cases follow a conditional multivariate normal distribution given the index case's observation while the values of all randomly ascertained individuals just follow a univariate normal distribution. For mathematical ease, attention is restricted to siblings of index cases. The test now focuses on a comparison between the variance among the random individuals and the within-sibship variance which is expected to be greatly increased by the presence of a major gene. A simple F-test is inefficient because (i) siblings are not independent and (ii) under the null hypothesis of only environmental and polygenic effects, the variance in these selected sibships is smaller than that among the random individuals. To make the test insensitive to skewness, a power transformation (with estimation of the exponent) is incorporated similar to that used by Morton et al. (Am. J. Hum. Genet. 29:52, 1977). The test was applied to cholesterol and triglyceride values (adjusted for age and sex) of 991 randomly ascertained individuals (age 30-59) in the Seattle area (Boman et al., in preparation). For each of the two lipids separately, n siblings of those index cases with a lipid value above their 90th percentile were used (n = 97 for cholesterol, n = 131 for triglyceride). The lipid value of the index case was the only selection criterion for the sibships, i.e., no presorting of the data was attempted. The within-sibship variance of the cholesterol values turned out to be slightly smaller than expected under polygenic inheritance, i.e., with this test, no major gene for cholesterol could be found in this data. This does not preclude the presence of a major gene too rare to be detected by this test (I have not yet investigated the power of this test). However, for the triglyceride values, the within-sibship variance was 1.3 times higher than expected under polygenic inheritance (one-sided p-value = .014) which can safely be interpreted as evidence for the presence of a major gene in these data. An appropriate transformation (approximately logarithmic) of the lipid levels was performed automatically by the test.

ELSTON: Dr. Ott's concern about the robustness of the goodness of fit tests we have presented is not to be taken lightly; we certainly do need to know more about the properties of these tests. It is interesting to note that the first set of tests, in which each individual's value is not used to determine the mixing proportions, showed virtually no power. The average of all these statistics in Tables I and II, excluding those for $U_2'^2$ and L^2 on the normalized scale,

is less than unity; this is less than the expected value of
chi-square on the (impossible) assumption that every
hypothesis tested is true. This is thus a situation in which
nonindependence of the observations appears to lead to a
deflated chi-square. The second set of tests, in which there
is greater correlation among the transformed data points
F(z), do show more power; in this case our only evidence for
robustness is in the results they give when used on the
cholesterol values, for which we know that there is segregation at a major locus.

MORTON: I agree with most of your remarks, but a few seem
to be of the type that Galton stigmatized as "general
impressions are never to be trusted". You assume that ascertainment bias is negligible in large pedigrees, but this has
never been tested: since the form as well as the content of
the pedigree is affected by ascertainment, I doubt your
assumption. It would be correct to say that ascertainment
correction has not yet been developed for pedigrees. Note
that either incomplete ascertainment or nonindependence of
relatives invalidates the tests of phenotypic distributions.
    Transmission frequencies provide a supplementary test of
hypotheses, but their utility is limited by the fact that
only two special cases have any known interpretation: (1) if
the τ's are equal, there is no specific evidence for genetic
determination either polygenic or megaphenic, although as
Elston suggests the power to detect genetic factors by transmission frequencies may be low; (2) if the τ's have the
Mendelian frequencies 1, 1/2, and 0, this is consistent with
some genetic determination. However, we cannot interpret any
other values of the τ's, except to conclude that the model is
invalid for some reason, which may depend on the form of the
distribution, ascertainment bias, etiological heterogeneity,
or other unspecified alternatives.
    We have shown that skewness increases the type I error in
nuclear families. Since this is a special case of pedigrees,
the simulation of Go et al. (1978) which purports to show that
skewness is not a disturbing factor must be regarded with
suspicion. We prefer to remove skewness by a power transform
unless the data are reduced to a dichotomy or trichotomy.
    As we use nuclear families, parents determine phenotypic
distributions: Elston finds this their principal value in
pedigree analysis. Iselius (1978) has demonstrated that
partitioning pedigrees into nuclear families does not appreciably affect power or bias estimates if displacement is large,
as for hypercholesterolemia; pedigree analysis has low power
and reliability to test for genes with small displacement.

The precision of ascertainment correction in nuclear families and their more complete specification of family environment, polygenes, and a major locus must be weighed against the claim of pedigree analysis to provide some undetermined increase in power. Some of the most promising studies at the present time compare different models and methods of analysis on the same data. It will be interesting to see whether different approaches lead to substantially different conclusions.

REFERENCES

1. Go, R.C.P., Elston, R.C., and Kaplan, E.B., Am. J. Hum. Genet. 30, 28-37 (1978).
2. Iselius, J., Clin. Genet. (in press, 1978).

ELSTON: The statement that ascertainment biases in determining the mode of inheritance are trivial in large pedigrees has been tested for hypercholesterolemia in the pedigree we discuss; as many as four probands led to the discovery of the pedigree, but the only discernible bias, when analyzed as though it were randomly drawn from the population, was in the estimate of gene frequency. This testing is analogous to Iselius' demonstration that partitioning pedigrees into nuclear families (and, presumably, without rigorous correction for ascertainment bias) does not appreciably affect power or bias estimates.

Transmission probabilities certainly have their limitations, but they also have there advantages. Skewness has been shown to increase the probability of accepting the hypothesis of a major gene under a model in which the only way skewness can be allowed for is by the presence of a major gene. Having transmission probabilities in the model allows for environmentally caused skewness; this is both clear theoretically and has been demonstrated by simulation. It does not, however, allow for polygenic inheritance or sibling environmental correlation which, when they both occur in certain intensities together with skewness, can lead to spurious results.

SING: I would like for you to clarify a couple of points. First, is the test you are describing based on Tau's invariant with respect to the displacement between AA, Aa, and aa? Secondly, you point out that you used the evidence for admixture of distributions as an a priori criterion for conducting your analysis. Then you transformed to normalize the data before fitting the Tau's. This seems to me to represent a contradiction. Isn't information on the Tau's being lost by removal of the skew?

ELSTON: The tests are asymptotically valid, i.e. if the null
hypothesis is true it is rejected with a probability equal to
the presumed significance level, whatever the displacement.
The power of the tests, on the other hand, depends very much
on the displacement relative to the environmental variation
(as well as on other factors, such as pedigree structure); if
there is no displacement, i.e. the means of the three distributions are equal, the tests will be completely powerless.
Transforming the data prior to analysis might be expected to
alter the displacement among the distributions that best fit
the model, and hence also the power of the tests.   We therefore studied two normalizing transformations, and found they
had virtually no effect on the likelihood ratio tests in the
case of cholesterol.   Thus from this example we <u>tentatively</u>
conclude that the likelihood ratio tests are not much affected
by normalizing transformations if there is a major gene
segregating in the data.   But it must be remembered that the
likelihood ratio test we have presented for the Mendelian null
hypothesis is not very powerful against a polygenic alternative.

PEDIGREE ANALYSIS OF THE LINKAGE BETWEEN

HLA AND HEMOCHROMATOSIS

K. Kravitz,[1] M. Skolnick,[1] C. Edwards,[2] G. Cartwright,[2]
B. Amos,[3] D. Carmelli,[1] and B. Baty[1]

[1]Department of Medical Biophysics and Computing, University of
Utah, LDS Hospital, Salt Lake City, Utah 84143

[2]Department of Internal Medicine, University of Utah Medical
Center, Salt Lake City, Utah 84132

[3]Department of Microbiology and Immunology, Duke University
Medical Center, Durham, North Carolina 27710

Hemochromatosis is a disorder in which the absorption of
iron is increased. While it is generally agreed that hemochromatosis has a genetic etiology, the exact mode of inheritance has generated a good deal of debate. Recently an association between hemochromatosis and the HLA A3, B7, and B14
alleles (most notably the 3,7 and 3,14 haplotypes) has been
reported (1). This association led to an investigation of
linkage between the HLA loci and the locus of a major gene
for hemochromatosis. The quantitative trait used was transferrin saturation, the single best indicator of the disease
safely measurable on a large set of pedigree members. The
complete set of phenotypic measures on the pedigree is described elsewhere (2). This paper describes the analytic
methods used to resolve a major locus for a quantitative
trait (3) and to demonstrate linkage.

PEDIGREE ANALYSIS

The mode of inheritance of hemochromatosis and possible
linkage between a postulated hemochromatosis locus and histocompatibility antigen loci was investigated by comparing
likelihoods of various models. Likelihoods were calculated
(4, 5) using a program for linkage analysis between a discrete marker locus and a locus with continuous phenotypic
expression (6, 7).

MATERIALS

Analysis was performed on three subsets of a large Mormon pioneer family. Transferrin saturation values and HLA haplotypes were known for 27 individuals in a core pedigree, consisting of six clinical cases and near relatives. Models were also tested on two extensions of the pedigree, both of which contained the core pedigree. The first extension consisted of 84 pedigree members with percent transferrin saturations and HLA haplotypes. The second extension included 159 individuals with transferrin saturation values and an additional 38 dead or unsampled individuals who were used to show relationships between the pedigree members. One hundred seven of the individuals of this second extended pedigree were HLA typed.

MODELS

The underlying model for the inheritance of elevated transferrin saturation used is a single locus with two alleles. The phenotypic expression of each genotype is given by a Normal distribution. The assumptions of the model are the same as those described by Elston et al. (3). Dominant, recessive, and intermediate models were investigated (Table 1). Normal values were taken from Cartwright (8), and abnormal values were estimated from the distribution in the pedigree (Figure 1). The values for the final intermediate model were derived from pedigree members of known genotype after linkage with HLA was established. The HLA A, B, and C loci and B cell types were considered as a single locus as they are tightly linked and segregate together in this pedigree. Three haplotypes were defined: HLA 3,7 HLA 29,12 (which showed co-segregation with some of the abnormal values in this pedigree) and all others pooled. The haplotype frequencies in Caucasians for the HLA 3,7 and HLA 29,12 were taken from Thomson et al. (9) as 0.055 and 0.0065 respectively. Use of a fourth allele did not affect the LOD scores.

TABLE 1.

Mean and Standard Deviations of Phenotype Distributions

Model	Homozygous Normal		Heterozygous		Homozygous Abnormal	
	$\overline{X}$	σ	$\overline{X}$	σ	$\overline{X}$	σ
Dominant	35.0	7.5	85.0	15.0	85.0	15.0
Recessive	35.0	7.5	35.0	7.5	85.0	15.0
Intermediate (Initial)	35.0	7.5	45.0	10.0	85.0	7.5
Intermediate (Final)	33.8	6.8	40.4	11.9	87.3	8.0

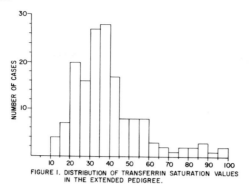

FIGURE I. DISTRIBUTION OF TRANSFERRIN SATURATION VALUES IN THE EXTENDED PEDIGREE.

RESULTS

The likelihoods of the dominant and recessive models on the first extended pedigree were compared without the HLA haplotype data. The likelihood for the dominant model (1.4×10^{-125}) was very close to that for the recessive (1.5×10^{-124}). This led to the consideration of the initial intermediate model which gave a higher likelihood (5.5×10^{-120}).

When the HLA data were included, the intermediate model showed a higher LOD score (Table 2) and a much higher likelihood than both the dominant and recessive models. The mean of the heterozygote distribution was then varied between 85% and 35% to find the value which maximized the likelihood. This was done without the HLA phenotypes in the extended pedigree. The likelihood maximized at a mean of about 40 (Figure 2).

TABLE 2. LIKELIHOODS FOR Three Genetic Models and LOD Scores for Linkage with HLA, Using Three Pedigree Sizes.

Model	Pedigree	Likelihood	LOD for HLA Linkage
Dominant	Core	1.7×10^{-72}	-7.5
	Extension 1	4.7×10^{-176}	-12.2
	Extension 2	4.5×10^{-306}	-15.9
Recessive	Core	1.7×10^{-67}	2.6
	Extension 1	4.8×10^{-162}	0.8
	Extension 2	6.3×10^{-286}	-0.2
Intermediate (Initial)	Core	1.6×10^{-64}	3.7
	Extension 1	3.8×10^{-155}	3.1
	Extension 2	5.8×10^{-267}	5.1
Intermediate (Final)	Core	7.2×10^{-63}	3.2
	Extension 1	7.6×10^{-150}	4.4
	Extension 2	2.6×10^{-253}	5.6

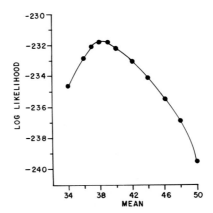

FIGURE 2. LOG LIKEHOOD PLOTTED AS A
FUNCTION OF THE MEAN OF THE
HETEROZYGOTE DISTRIBUTION.

To reconfirm the above estimates, each person of known
phenotype in the 84 member pedigree was assigned a genotype
on the basis of their HLA types, and the presence or absence
of abnormality attributable to each haplotype (2). The means
and standard deviations calculated for each genotypic group
are shown in Table 1 for the final intermediate model. These
values showed close agreement with the maximum likelihood
obtained from the pedigree analysis, and were then used as
the parameters in the linkage analysis, yielding a LOD score
of 5.6 in the extended pedigree with a recombination fraction
close to zero. As the pedigree size increased, the LOD for
linkage dropped dramatically for the dominant and recessive
models with the LOD score of 2.6 for the recessive decreasing
to 0.2 in the largest pedigree. The LOD for the initial
intermediate model fluctuated, where the LOD for the final
intermediate model increased steadily, even though there were
no clinically overt manifestations in the extension to the
core pedigree.

The major gene hypothesis was further examined for the
initial and final intermediate models by varying the segregation parameter, and noting the point at which the likelihood
maximized on the extended pedigree. This analysis was carried
out twice for each model on the whole pedigree, first excluding the HLA haplotype information, and then including it. In
the initial model, without the HLA data, the likelihood maximized at a segregation parameter close to 0.6. Similar results
were obtained when the HLA data were included. In the final
model without the HLA data, the likelihood increased as the
segregation parameter increased past 0.9. When HLA was included in the final model, results consistent with a major gene
hypothesis were again obtained: The likelihood maximized at
a segregation parameter about 0.6.

DISCUSSION

This study strongly suggests that a hemochromatosis gene locus is closely linked to the HLA loci. The mode of inheritance of hemochromatosis appears to be primarily recessive, with heterozygotes showing only mild abnormalities. It should be pointed out that multi-locus recessive models could give similar likelihoods and that the lack of greatly increased consanguinity reported (10) could favor the existence of the two genes necessary for the disease at different loci. The analysis does tell us that two copies of chromosome 6, each carrying an abnormal gene, are necessary for the full expression of the disease.

One reason for the low penetrance in heterozygotes is that females generally show a lesser degree of gene expression due to menstrual bleeding and pregnancy. This study used a single penetrance function for both males and females, and so the estimate of the penetrance was lower than would be expected for males alone. An analysis using separate male and female penetrance distributions and a multivariate index for the phenotype is currently underway. The fact that only 4 out of 21 female heterozygotes were abnormal clearly lowered the mean of the heterozygote distribution, causing considerable overlap with the normal homozygote distribution. This overlap in the final intermediate model probably caused the likelihood to maximize at a segregation parameter approaching 1.0. However when HLA data were considered, the likelihood maximized near 0.6. Furthermore the initial intermediate model, in which there was greater separation between normal and heterozygote distributions, showed major gene segregation both with and without the HLA data. The maximum likelihood occurred when the segregation parameter was above 0.5. The explanation of this finding is that we have studied a family noted for having a cluster of clinical cases in one sibship, implying an ascertainment bias. However, the estimate of linkage and the parameters for the genotypes of the intermediate model should be unbiased as there was no bias for HLA types. It should also be stressed that in most cases in this pedigree the gene was expressed in individuals who do not drink alcoholic beverages. In places where considerable alcohol is consumed, the heterozygote would show a much greater degree of abnormality. Thus the heterozygote distribution might be closer to the affected distribution, making the disease look more dominant.

The analysis showed that increasing the pedigree size, even without additional clinical cases, provided information necessary for the proper resolution of the genetic model.

REFERENCES

1. Cannings, C., Thompson, E.A. and Skolnick, M.H., Adv. Appl. Prob., in press.

2. Edwards, C., Kravitz, K., Skolnick, M., Amos, D.B., Carroll, M., Bray, P., Johnson, A. and Cartwright, G., submitted for publication.

3. Elston, R.C., Namboodiri, K.K. and Kaplan, E.B., these proceedings.

4. Elston, R.C. and Stewart, J., Hum. Hered. 21, 523-542 (1971).

5. Kravitz, K., Technical Report No. 9, Department of Medical Biophysics and Computing, University of Utah (1977).

6. Simon, M., Bourel, M., Fauchet, R. and Genetet, B., Gut 17, 332-334 (1976).

7. Thompson, E.A., Technical Report No. 5, Department of Medical Biophysics and Computing, University of Utah (1977).

8. Cartwright, G., "Diagnostic Laboratory Hematology," 4th Ed., Grune and Stratton, New York, 1968.

9. Thomson, G., Bodmer, W.F. and Bodmer, J., in "Population Genetics and Ecology" (S. Karlin and E. Nevo, Eds.), Academic Press, Inc., 1976.

10. Simon, M., Alexandre, J., Bourel, M., Le Marec, B., and Scordia, C., Clin. Genet. 11, 327-341 (1977).

ACKNOWLEDGEMENT

Supported by NIH grants AM-04489, CA-16573, GM-10367, GM-07464, RR-05428, and FR-00064.

LINKAGE AND THE POWER OF A PEDIGREE STRUCTURE

E.A. Thompson,* K. Kravitz, J. Hill, and M.H. Skolnick

Department of Medical Biophysics and Computing
University of Utah, LDS Hospital,
Salt Lake City, Utah   84143

*also King's College, Cambridge, England

When considering questions of modes of inheritance, the efficiency of different pedigree structures to discriminate between alternative models is a fundamental aspect of study design. The importance of three generation pedigrees as opposed to nuclear families for linkage studies is well known (1). The efficiency of multi-generational families over nuclear families to estimate parameters of the monogenic model has been studied (2). The purpose of this paper is to quantify the concept of discriminating power of different pedigree structures for linkage studies which, in the absence of any biochemical analysis, is the most compelling evidence for the existence of a major locus (3). With this knowledge in hand, it may be possible to increase the efficiency of performing marker studies by sequential sampling of large pedigrees (4).

THEORY

There are several possible criteria which may be used to assess the utility of an experimental design. In one simulation study (2) the standard errors of parameter estimates obtained for a specified genetic model on different pedigree structures were compared. A measure of the intrinsic information content of an experiment with regard to its power to distinguish between two hypotheses of interest is provided by the expected log-likelihood difference (5, 6). The expected log-likelihood function has been used as a criterion of the efficiency of different genetic marker systems to distinguish alternative hypotheses of genealogical relationships and to infer unknown pedigree structures (7). Here the problem is reversed; we consider the power of different pedigree structures to demonstrate linkage between a marker system and a disease locus.

The probability of a set of phenotypes (p) observed on a pedigree, as a function of the recombination fraction (r) between the two loci, is the likelihood function for r ,

given allele frequencies at both loci. This likelihood is
denoted by Lp(r) . The hypothesis that the loci are un-
linked thus has likelihood Lp(0.5) , and for the given
observed phenotypes the log-likelihood difference between
any specific hypothesized r-value of interest, r* , and the
alternative of no linkage is $\log_{10}(Lp(r*) / Lp(0.5))$. (As
is usual in linkage studies we use logs to base 10 in calculating LOD scores (8).)

In computing expected LOD scores all possible phenotype
combinations on the pedigree must be considered. The expectations we compute are conditioned on the phenotypes of some
members of the pedigree. These "propositi" are individuals
whose marker and disease phenotypes are assumed known, and
expectations are taken over the probability distribution
over the set of all phenotype combinations for other members
of the pedigree. The set is denoted by ρ . Since the likelihood function is simply the probability of any specific
phenotype combination, the probability conditioned on the
types of the propositi may be written

$$Lp(r) \ / \ \sum_{p \varepsilon \rho} Lp(r)$$

where r is the (unknown) true value of the recombination
fraction. Thus the required expectation is

$$I(r*;r) \ = \ \frac{\sum_{p \varepsilon \rho} Lp(r) \ \log_{10}(Lp(r*) \ / \ Lp(0.5))}{\sum_{p \varepsilon \rho} Lp(r)}$$

By standard likelihood theory (6), this expected log-likelihood function is maximized with respect to the hypothesized
r* when this is equal to the true value r ;

$$\max_{r*} \ I(r*;r) \ = \ I(r;r)$$

$$= \ \frac{\sum_{p \varepsilon \rho} Lp(r) \ \log_{10}(Lp(r) \ / \ Lp(0.5))}{\sum_{p \varepsilon \rho} Lp(r)}$$

METHODS

The computation of Lp(r) follows the standard pedigree
analysis formulation (9) using a different algorithm (10, 11,
12). The method for summation over phenotype combinations ρ

is based on an algorithm which generates all compatible combinations of genotypes (13) or phenotypes (14).

Unfortunately, even for the simplest case of a 2-phenotype disease locus and a 2-allele codominant marker locus, there are 6 phenotypes and hence up to 6^n phenotype combinations where n is the number of individuals in the pedigree in addition to the propositi. This inevitably leads to the summation being based on only a random sample from the set of all possible elements of ρ . Even with sampling, the largest pedigree attempted so far on the Data General Eclipse is of 10 members.

The pedigrees examined fall into three categories:
(1) A parental couple with n children for n ranging from 1 to 8 with one parent affected.
(2) A set of 4-person pedigrees illustrating a wide variety of potential study designs (Table 1).
(3) A set of pedigrees consisting of two connected copies of smaller pedigrees, in order to illustrate the increased information due to larger pedigrees (Table 2).

TABLE 1. THE EXPECTED LOD SCORES FOR 12 FOUR-PERSON PEDIGREES. THE PROPOSITUS (SHADED) IS FIRST ASSUMED TO BE A HETEROZYGOTE, THEN A HOMOZYGOTE.

Pedigree	Phenotype of Propositus Affected MN	Affected M
1	.273	$< 10^{-5}$
2	.216	$< 10^{-5}$
3	.187	.039
4	.182	$< 10^{-3}$
5	.123	.184
6	.110	.171
7	.099	.102
8	.072	.106
9	.063	.019
10	.053	.108
11	.041	.062
12	.029	.079

TABLE 2.   THE EXPECTED LOD OF TWO INDEPENDENT PEDIGREES (COLUMN A) COMPARED WITH ONE LARGER PEDIGREE WHICH IS APPROXIMATELY TWICE THE SIZE OF THE FIRST AND SIMILAR IN STRUCTURE (COLUMN B); AND THE PERCENT INCREASE IN INFORMATION CONTENT OF B RELATIVE TO A. PROPOSITI (SHADED) ARE AFFECTED AND HETEROZYGOUS (TYPE MN).

Pedigree Number	r	A Pedigree	$2 \times E(LOD)$	B Pedigree	$E(LOD)$	% Increase in Information
1	.3		0.47×10^{-2}		3.25×10^{-2}	591%
	.0001		.224		.518	131%
2	.3		1.39×10^{-2}		3.78×10^{-2}	172%
	.0001		.546		.844	55%
3	.3		1.88×10^{-2}		4.46×10^{-2}	137%
	.0001		.765		1.09	42%
4	.3		4.08×10^{-2}		8.01×10^{-2}	96%
	.0001		.432		.674	56%

For this first study we have considered a simple dominant disease with complete penetrance and allele frequency 0.01, and the allele frequency at the codominant marker locus (referred to as MN) was 0.5 for each allele. The two recombination fractions represent tight ($r = 0.0001$) and loose linkage ($r = 0.3$).

RESULTS

The first set of pedigrees considered illustrates the increase in information content with increasing family size. Beginning with two parents, one of whom is the propositus, offspring are added one at a time, and for each sibship size $I(r;r)$ is computed. The propositus in each case is affected and heterozygous, type MN. In Figure 1, $I(r;r)$ is graphed as a function of the number of offspring. $I(r;r)$ for one offspring is zero. It initially increases rapidly with increased family size. The increase in information with each additional sib decreases.

Of all the 10 member pedigrees examined so far, a couple with eight children is the optimal structure. When both parents have known phenotype, the maximal $I(r;r)$ is provided by an affected individual who is heterozygous for the marker locus married to an unaffected individual who is homozygous for the marker locus. This combination is four times better than any other and emphasizes the advantage in studying the parents before studying the offspring. Figure 1 also illustrates the ease of demonstrating tight linkage compared to loose linkage.

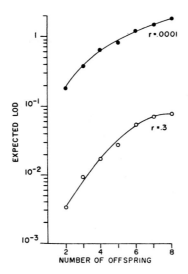

FIGURE I. THE EXPECTED LOD SCORE FOR
TWO VALUES OF r AS A FUNCTION
OF SIBSHIP SIZE.

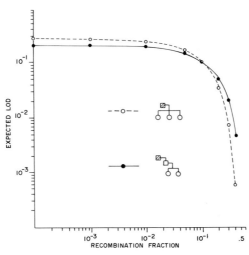

FIGURE 2. THE EXPECTED LOD SCORE AS A FUNCTION OF
RECOMBINATION FRACTION FOR TWO FOUR MEMBER
PEDIGREES.

The results for the 4-member pedigrees are given in Table 1 which shows that whenever the propositus is a parent, the pedigrees with a heterozygous propositus have a much higher expected LOD score than the same pedigrees with a homozygous propositus. In the pedigrees in which the propositus is an offspring, the opposite is true. There is also a tenfold difference in the information content of the pedigrees explored where the propositus is a heterozygote, and a 10,000 fold difference in information content between pedigree structures when the propositus is homozygous for the marker locus. Analysis of several selected 4-member pedigrees for a range of recombination fractions shows that even for the most informative pedigrees the information content drops sharply for r greater than 0.1 (Figure 2).

Table 2 illustrates the importance of having one large pedigree as opposed to two independent small ones. In each case tested, the combined pedigree is more powerful than the sum of its two parts. Even though the two most informative 4-member pedigrees were chosen, a greater than 50% increase in power was obtained from the combined pedigrees. This increase is due to the phase information implicit in the relationship between the propositi.

CONCLUSION

To establish linkage, the phase of the marker locus with respect to the disease locus must be established. This can be done by studying large sibships and/or by having sibships related in a pedigree structure. Since affected individuals provide more information as parents if heterozygous at the marker locus and as children if homozygous, the marker genotype of the propositus will determine which part of the pedigree should be studied further.

The large differences in the information content of different pedigree structures show the importance of evaluating potential information both before and sequentially during the course of a linkage study. Ideally, analysis of data would proceed in parallel with the marker data collection process, so that expected LOD scores can be used to decide which family members should be studied next.

REFERENCES

1. Edwards, J.H., <u>Brit. Med. Bull.</u> 25, 58-64 (1969).
2. Go, R.C.P., Elston, R.C. and Kaplan, E.B., <u>Am. J. Hum. Genet.</u>, in press.
3. Elston, R.C., these proceedings.
4. Cannings, C. and Thompson, E.A., <u>Clin. Genet.</u> (1978).
5. Fisher, R.A., <u>Proc. Camb. Phil. Soc.</u> 22, 700-725 (1925).
6. Edwards, A.W.F., "Likelihood", Cambridge University Press (1972).
7. Thompson, E.A., <u>SSI</u> 15, 477-526 (1976).
8. Morton, N.E., in "Methodology in Human Genetics" (W.J. Burdette, Ed.), pp. 17-52. Holden-Day, San Francisco, 1962.
9. Elston, R.C. and Stewart, J., <u>Hum. Hered.</u> 21, 523-542 (1971).
10. Cannings, C., Thompson, E.A. and Skolnick, M.H., <u>Adv. Appl. Prob.</u>, in press (1977).
11. Thompson, E.A., Technical Report No. 5, Department of Medical Biophysics and Computing, University of Utah (1977a).
12. Thompson, E.A., Technical Report No. 6, Department of Medical Biophysics and Computing, University of Utah (1977b).
13. Cannings, C., Skolnick, M.H., de Nevers, K. and Sridharan, R., <u>Comp. and Biomed. Res.</u> 1, 393-407 (1976).
14. Kravitz, K. and Hill, J., Technical Report No. 10, Department of Medical Biophysics and Computing, University of Utah (1977).

ACKNOWLEDGEMENT

Supported by NIH grants CA-16573 and GM-07464

GENETIC EPIDEMIOLOGY

RECURRENCE RISKS AS AN OUTCOME OF SEGREGATION ANALYSIS

J. M. Lalouel

Population Genetics Laboratory
University of Hawaii
Honolulu, Hawaii 96822

I. INTRODUCTION

Increasing recognition of the importance of genetic factors in common disorders will surely affect medical practice, research, and education in many respects (1), up to the very concept of disease; "disease is an abstraction, the reality is the inability of one person's homeostasis, conditioned by his genotype and a lifetime of special experiences, to maintain equilibrium" (1).

For the genetic 'counselor', this trend means a growing involvement with disorders of complex inheritance, for which an efficient approach to calculation of recurrence risks is needed. Such calculation is conditional on determination of a likely model of inheritance, and it is presented here as an outcome of segregation analysis. Rather than systematically assuming a multifactorial model of inheritance, a more analytic approach, in search of major gene effects, should prevail as, besides risk calculation, it may permit identification, if only in probability, of individuals under high genetic risk, which may be relevant for therapeutic decision or prevention.

II. SIMPLE AND COMPLEX MODES OF INHERITANCE

Most disorders in man present, to a varying degree, familial aggregation. The Mendelian model of single factor inheritance has proven itself valid to explain the patterns of familial transmission of an impressive number of generally rare disorders.

A. Mendelian Disorders

In the simplest situations, this has been arrived at by direct observation or statistical analysis of familial data, retaining that Mendelian hypothesis best supported by the observed segregation within mating types. When dealing with a collection of familial data, it was realized that the mode

255

of ascertainment of probands had to be taken into account
(2,3).

When observed segregation ratios deviated from expected
Mendelian ratios, it became necessary to rely on more
elaborate methods, with greater emphasis on tests of genetic
hypotheses under more general models than on estimation of
segregation frequencies. This was done by Morton (4,5) by
extension of existing formulae (6,7,8) based on the Likelihood Principle. The analysis allows one to distinguish between
mutations, phenocopies and incomplete penetrance; heterogeneity of genetic entities, if not revealed by prior analyses,
may be resolved by separation of mating types. The work of
Morton and Chung on muscular dystrophy (9,10) has clearly
demonstrated the power of this approach.

For such disorders, the inference provided by segregation
analysis about the genetic mechanism responsible for their
occurrence was often reinforced by the demonstration of a
single biochemical defect, leading in some instances to very
efficient curative methods. Recurrence risk in a given
family could easily be calculated, and this initiated the
practice of genetic counseling.

B. The Genetic Basis of Common Disorders

With regard to more common disorders, familial aggregation presents a number of often recalled features (e.g. 11)
that cannot be readily explained by simple Mendelian models.
Reported associations between incidence of affection and
various genetic as well as environmental factors (e.g. 12,
in connection with congenital malformations) revealed the
necessity of considering the effect of both the genetic
constitution and the environment in the development of
affection.

Two conceptually quite different models have been
proposed to describe the patterns of familial aggregation of
common diseases, the generalized single locus model and the
multifactorial model. Both have been frequently enough
presented in the literature to allow us to assume them known.
More relevant here are the theoretical considerations that
have led to their introduction in relation to the study of
common disorders.

The generalized single locus model is simply an extension
of single factor Mendelian models with incomplete penetrance,
specified as a probability of affection for each genotype.
Hence actual occurrence of affection, given the genotype of
an individual, is only a function of random environmental
factors. A conceptual liability scale can be constructed,

affection occurring when liability exceeds a threshold. However, there is, built in this model, some degree of prejudice in considering penetrance not to be influenced by other genetic factors (not to mention common environment).

In connection with a dichotomy normal versus affected, the multifactorial model of inheritance, first advanced by Pearson (13,14), and considered again by various authors during the last decades (15,16,17,18,19,20), postulates that the cumulative effect of numerous weak, independent factors, genetic or environmental, determines liability to affection, which occurs when liability exceeds a threshold. This is sometimes referred to as quasi-continuous variation, and how the concept of a threshold in relation to affection can be envisioned, whether developmental, biochemical, mechanical, or imposed by the observer for semantic economy, was clearly presented by Edwards (17).

C. Recurrence Risks in Complex Inheritance

Discrimination between both models has been attempted with little success for a variety of common disorders, using familial data reduced to pairs of relatives of varying degrees (e.g. 21,22,23,24). Assuming that some conditions on the estimability of parameters are met (25,22), it was shown (26, 27) that the power of such methods to discriminate between these models could be expected to be weak. Moreover, as we shall indicate later, reduction of familial data to pairs of relatives is usually done without consideration for ascertainment and variation of risk among families under the multifactorial model.

It would therefore seem that genetic counselors can choose arbitrarily one particular model, compute relevant parameters by some ad hoc method, and calculate risks for various family histories, or ignoring other familial information, quote non-specific empirical figures. However, this is in striking contrast to the rigorous approach that prevails in simple modes of inheritance. The calculation of recurrence risks in complex inheritance should be made as specific as possible by careful delineation of the disorder under study, use of familial information, and adoption of a model whose validity and parameters have been established by rigorous analysis of appropriate data collected according to a well-defined sampling procedure.

III.   SEGREGATION ANALYSIS UNDER THE MIXED MODEL

     The observational distinction between 'hereditary
disorders' and common disorders, where the genetic composition as well as the environment must obviously exert some
influence, should not be maintained when the determination of
the relative influence of both factors is considered as a
problem in statistical inference. As Edwards (18, figure 1
and p.59) made clear, the ineluctable character of simple
Mendelian disorders may be due to an alteration of a unique,
essential, metabolic pathway. When alternative pathways
exist, or when a disorder results from some alteration in a
complex metabolic network, observation is far removed from
the specific alteration, and it is easily conceived that
occurrence of affection will depend on both the genetic constitution and the environment.
     Similarly, the dichotomy normal versus affected should
be avoided whenever possible, particularly when it is merely
an arbitrary classification of a continuous variable. The
resolution of etiological heterogeneity and the identification
of genetic correlates of illness will greatly increase the
specificity and power of genetic analyses, allowing more
efficient counseling, prevention, or therapeutic decisions.
This reconsideration of the concept of disease in medical
practice, the need for which Childs (1) argued most clearly,
is in accordance with the Hippocratic doctrine of diathesis,
as Edwards (17) pointedly reminded us.

A.   The Mixed Model of Inheritance

     If the assumption of constant penetrance is unescapable
in the genetic analysis of rare disorders, it should not be
kept when dealing with common disorders, as suggested by the
preceding discussion. Moreover, a general model of inheritance should combine a single gene concept with multifactorial
inheritance, rather than assuming a priori that penetrance is
solely a function of random environment, as in the generalized
single locus model. A general model would then include simple
modes of inheritance as well as multifactorial inheritance,
with a continuum of models between these extremes, as
advocated by Edwards (17).
     The mixed model of inheritance (28,29) has the appro-
priate generality. It postulates an underlying scale of
liability to which a major locus, a polygenic component, and
environment contribute independently. A quantitative trait
x may be measured, such that

$$x = g + c + e \qquad\qquad [1]$$

with corresponding variances

$$V = G + C + E \qquad\qquad [2]$$

where g is the effect due to the major locus, c is the breeding value due to an indefinitely large number of additive genetic factors, and e is the environmental contribution. The trait x is related to affection through the general liability

$$w = x + k \qquad\qquad [3]$$

k being an environmental effect, normally distributed, with mean zero and variance W. "In principle w cannot be measured (unless W = 0), but rather a threshold, Z, yields affection when w > Z. Therefore liability determines a risk function which we shall call

$$Q(a) \equiv (2\pi)^{-1/2} \int_{a}^{\infty} e^{-h^2/2} \, dh \qquad\qquad [4]$$

where $a = (Z - x)/\sqrt{W}$. This subsumes affection like diabetes, which could be defined on the trait of glucose intolerance, with Z specifying the value of glucose intolerance above which an individual is classified as diabetic. In this case $W = 0$ and $Q(a) = 1$ if $x > Z$; $Q(a) = 0$ if $x < Z$. Also included is affection like myocardial infarction, which cannot be defined on serum cholesterol but is associated with hypercholesterolemia. Then $\sqrt{V/(V + W)}$ is the correlation between cholesterol (x) and phenotypic liability to infarction (w) (29)". Clearly, reference to these disorders is only illustrative, as they are likely to be etiologically heterogeneous.

When the trait x is not measured, but rather information is available on a dichotomy normal/affected or a trichotomy normal/intermediate/affected, affection is then defined by a threshold (or two thresholds for a trichotomy), the threshold being determined by prevalence of affection, assumed known from other evidence. Although definition of a threshold in relation to incidence of affection may in some instances be appropriate, the word incidence actually often stands for prevalence in the literature dealing with quasi-continuity, as indeed made explicit by Falconer (20).

The major locus is assumed biallelic, producing three genotypes. The distance between the homozygous means on the liability scale is called displacement, t. The relative position of the heterozygous class is called the degree of

dominance, d. By convention, if the heterozygote mean is
near the lower homozygote, the locus is called recessive, if
near the higher one it is called dominant, and if in the
middle, it is called additive. The relative sizes of the
genotypic classes are determined by the gene frequency, q,
as panmixia is assumed. The polygenic and environmental
factors are assumed independent and normally distributed.
The proportions of the total variance V due to the polygenic
effect is denoted H, hence $H = C/V$.

The environmental contribution may be further partitioned into two components, environment common to sibs and random
residual, accounting for proportions of the total variance B
and R respectively. Variation in prevalence with sex and age
can be treated by a shift of the liability scale when only
affection status is available, or by covariance adjustment
when a quantitative trait x is measured, although implicit
assumptions associated with these operations should be
validated.

B. Segregation Analysis of Nuclear Families

Just as in simple modes of inheritance, the calculation
of specific recurrence risks will require that the most likely
hypothesis has been determined, and its parameters estimated,
from an earlier analysis of familial data that are representative of a reference population. This cannot be achieved by
the mere compilation of case reports from the literature, but
requires a survey with a carefully designed sampling scheme,
sampling which will be taken into account in the analysis by
estimating the probability of ascertainment of probands (4).

In this context, Morton (28) has advocated the use of
nuclear families, writing the likelihood of the children
conditional on parental phenotypes (29). It is a compromise
between power, feasibility of the survey with adequate
sampling correction, homogeneity of diagnostic procedures
(30), representativeness, and economy of unsupported assumptions. To allow for an effect of environment common to sibs
reduces the chance of confounding this effect with dominance
due to segregation of a major gene (31). Separation of mating
types allows one to test for paternal or maternal effects
and etiological heterogeneity. Writing the likelihood of
sibships conditional on parental phenotypes makes it possible
to sample families through parental phenotypes, which may
facilitate the study of disorders with low recurrence rates
or with early onset, particularly the congenital malformations, and may prove less sensitive to biases due to selection. Internal consistency of the parts of the model or

various sources of heterogeneity are to be tested by likelihood ratio tests, possibly involving partition of the data according to ethnic group or clinical criteria. Provided these precautions have been taken, calculation of recurrence risks will be based on the parameters of that hypothesis best supported by the data in accordance with the rigorous Likelihood Principle. In such an approach, particular models such as the generalized single locus model or the multifactorial model are simply particular hypotheses concerning the nullity of some parameters of the mixed model, that can be tested against the full, unrestricted model.

IV. OTHER APPROACHES

In marked contrast, analyses of pairs of relatives neglect ascertainment and do not provide for separation and tests of heterogeneity among mating types. Besides decreasing power, the reduction of familial data to pairs of relatives by methods such as Weinberg's proband method is not adequate as soon as there is not a constant probability of segregation, and heritability estimates will be biased by not accounting for intra-class correlations and correlations between correlations. The consideration of more distant degrees of relationship, expected to improve the power of discrimination between competing hypotheses, will certainly increase biases in relation with recollection or temporal variation in diagnostic procedures as well as environmental conditions. The choice between two competing hypotheses in different parameter spaces by chi-squares of goodness of fit seems also questionable.

As for the analysis of pedigrees (32,33,58), it should theoretically provide more power in discriminating major gene effects by its use of more extensive familial information, on the condition that a number of disturbing effects such as environmental correlations or temporal trends can be controlled, and that handling of ascertainment can provide valid inference on a well defined reference population. In the present state of development of this approach, the mixed model is not operational, and we are under the impression that, while pedigree analysis may prove valuable in the detection of rare major genes, possibly as a complement to segregation analysis of nuclear families, the latter better allows, at the present, sampling in a well-defined reference population, tests of hypotheses, and estimation of parameters which can be used for calculation of recurrence risks.

V.   CALCULATION OF RECURRENCE RISKS

Given familial information on a certain disorder, the
risk to which a specified member of the family is exposed can
be calculated, provided that a genetic hypothesis and estimates of its parameters have been supported by a careful
analysis of an appropriate reference population. The recurrence risk for this individual is the expectation of the
frequency of occurrence of this disorder in a large number of
identical families with same history belonging to the same
population; it is therefore a probability defined as a property of a conceptual chance set-up. In complex inheritance,
risk varies among families with the same history, a point to
which we shall return. We shall now present methods of computation of phenotype and genotype probabilities conditional
on familial information with some examples, whereas an ensuing
discussion will explore the potential usefulness of these
calculations in research as well as medical practice.

A.   Calculations in Simple Modes of Inheritance

In simple modes of inheritance, the statistical hypothesis to which segregation analysis has lent best support
and the parameters that have maximized its likelihood, together with parameters estimated in a reference population,
such as mutation rate or gene frequency, will be used for
calculation of recurrence risks or probability of being of a
given genotype. Because it involves discrete probability
distributions, hand calculations are easy, if sometimes cum-
bersome, and can be greatly facilitated by adoption of a
probabilistic formulation allowing rapid calculations (34,35,
36,37). However, calculations may still be rather involved,
so that a general computer program, PEDIG (38,39), following
the same probabilistic formulation, has proven of great help
in counseling situations.
In complex inheritance however, phenotype-genotype corre-
spondences involve continuous distributions and calculation
of specific recurrence risks requires the use of a computer.

B.   Methods and Computer Programs for the Multifactorial Model

For multifactorial inheritance, Smith (40) developed a
computer program, RISKMF, which allows calculation of specific
recurrence risks using pedigree information, involving approximation of a normal distribution by a polychotomy and using

information on relatives more distant than first-degree
through the approximation of pedigree reduction; an extension
to this program, RISKCT, allows consideration of a quantitative trait correlated with liability (41). Another approximation to this problem was given by Mendell and Elston (42)
for a restricted number of relatives. More exact calculations
involve changes of variables by which multiple integrals can
be reduced to single integrals involving univariate normal
density and cumulative distribution functions in some simple
situations (43); extensions to arbitrary pedigrees (44) still
involve stringent restrictions on acceptable pedigrees.

     For the generalized single locus model, no particular
procedure was offered to calculate recurrence risks. However,
the computer program PEDIG could still be used, specifying
phenotype distributions conditional on a given genotype.

C.   Methods and Computer Programs for the Mixed Model

     For the mixed model, the computer program RISK was devel-
oped by MacLean (unpublished) for nuclear families, while we
wrote the program OCCUR for calculation of recurrence risks
in pedigrees.

1.   Probabilistic Formulation

     In the convenient notation of Heuch and Li (39), PH indi-
cates a phenotype, G a genotype, and I information on a collection of individuals, while subscripts 1,2 and C specify a
triple father, mother, and child, and subscript D refers to
other descendants of these parents. In the following, we
give a formulation in terms of discrete probabilities, as the
continuous polygenic distribution is to be approximated by a
polychotomy; this still applies when PH is a quantitative
measurement for, where probabilities are replaced by probability densities multiplied by their corresponding differential
elements, the latter cancel as they enter both numerator and
denominator in all formulations.

     For nuclear families, the computer program RISK (MacLean,
unpublished) computes recurrence risks, under the mixed model,
for a child C as (45, appendix)

$$P(PH_C^* | PH_1, PH_2, I_D)$$

$$= \frac{\Sigma_{G_1, G_2} P(PH_C^* | G_1, G_2) P(I_D | G_1, G_2) P(G_1, G_2 | PH_1, PH_2)}{\Sigma_{G_1, G_2} P(I_D | G_1, G_2) P(G_1, G_2 | PH_1, PH_2)} \qquad [5]$$

the asterisk denoting affection. Although quite appropriate
for nuclear families, this formulation cannot be generalized
to pedigrees. The extension we propose here was made possible
by neglecting environment common to sibs, introducing the
fundamental assumption that:

$$P(PH|G,I) = P(PH|G) \qquad\qquad [6]$$

and by considering only pedigrees without loops.

Computation of the phenotype probability distribution
for some individual C in a pedigree requires specification
of his conditional genotype probabilities $P(G_C|PH_1, PH_2, I_1,$
$I_2, I_D, I')$, given phenotype information on his parents PH_1
and PH_2, on pedigree members linked to him through his
parents (cognates as well as affinals), I_1 and I_2, on
descendants of his parents I_D with C excluded, and on other
individuals linked to the parents through these descendants
as affinals, I'.

With $I \equiv (PH_1, PH_2, I_1, I_2, I_D, I')$, the conditional
probabilities $P(G_C|I)$ can be expressed in terms of the
transition probabilities $P(G_C|G_1, G_2)$:

$$P(G_C|I) = \Sigma_{G_1,G_2} P(G_C|G_1, G_2) P(G_1,G_2|I),$$

and we have

$$P(G_1,G_2|I) = \frac{P(PH_1,PH_2,I_D|G_1,G_2,I')P(G_1|I_1)P(G_2|I_2)}{P(PH_1,PH_2,I_D|I_1,I_2,I')},$$

where calculation of the denominator is replaced by norming
and

$$P(PH_1,PH_2,I_D|G_1,G_2,I') = P(PH_1|G_1)P(PH_2|G_2)P(I_D|G_1,G_2,I').$$

This is the formulation of Heuch and Li (39), and we followed
their procedure to obtain $P(G_C|I)$. The probabilities
$P(G_1|I_1)$, $P(G_2|I_2)$ and $P(I_D|G_1,G_2,I')$ are calculated by an
appropriate recursive algorithm (39). This brief outline
is all that is necessary to introduce the numerical functions
that have to be defined under the mixed model.

2. Calculations Under the Mixed Model

Calculations under the mixed model, following this approach, are made possible by use of the independence between major locus and polygenic component, and by a discrete approximation of the continuous polygenic genotype distribution. As in Smith (40) and Morton and MacLean (29), a standardized normal distribution is partitioned into n intervals, the (n-2) interior intervals being of equal length with densities concentrated at their mid-point, while the two exterior intervals are bounded by ± 4 standard-deviations, using Hastings formula (46) for numerical calculations. Heritability of the polygenic component is incorporated by scaling.

Four numerical functions must be specified to compute the prior genotype distribution for individuals without ancestors $P(G)$, the transition probabilities $P(G_c|G_1,G_2)$, the phenotype distribution of an individual given his genotype $P(PH|G)$, and the phenotype distribution of an individual given the parental genotypes $P(PH_c|G_1,G_2)$. Let g_i denote the effect of the i-th major gene genotype and c_j that of the j-th polygenic genotypic class. Then $P(g_i)$ and $P(g_i|g_{1k},g_{2\ell})$ are given in Morton and MacLean (29, tables 1 and 3); $P(c_j)$ is obtained according to the discrete approximation, presented above, to a normal distribution of mean zero and variance C due to the polygenic effect; the prior distribution $P(G)$, (which is a vector with event $G_{i \cdot j} \equiv (g_i,c_j)$), is obtained by calculating $P(g_i,c_j) = P(g_i)P(c_j)$, for all i,j. The transition probabilities $P(c_j|c_{1k},c_{2\ell})$ are obtained by calculation of the area under a normal distribution of mean $(c_{1k} + c_{2\ell})/2$ and variance C/2 in the j-th interval, using Hastings' formula, and probabilities $P(G_c|G_1,G_2)$ are obtained as products of appropriate terms for major gene and polygenic effects.

Conditional phenotype distributions $P(PH|G)$ and $P(PH_c|G_1,G_2)$ are computed as given in table I, using again a discrete approximation and Hastings' formula. In actual calculations, $P(PH_c|G_1,G_2)$ is obtained as

$$P(PH_c|G_1,G_2) = \Sigma_{G_c} P(PH_c|G_c)P(G_c|G_1,G_2)$$

for married individuals and as

$$P(PH_C|G_1,G_2) = \Sigma_i P(g_{Ci}|g_{1j},g_{2k}) P(PH_C|g_{Ci},c_{1\ell},c_{2m})$$

for single individuals, thus reducing computing time and errors of approximation.

Whenever a quantitative trait x may be measured for some pedigree members, we assume that either x or affection status is available; if both were available, it is assumed that knowledge of x is more informative that knowledge of affection status, as in Morton and MacLean (29), which is reasonable whenever x is a relatively good indicator of phenotypic lia-bility w, that is whenever $\sqrt{V/(V+W)}$ is substantial.

If a measurement x_C is available for the individual C at risk, the risk for C to be affected is independent of pedigree information. When affection is defined on x itself, (W=0), then the risk figure is 0 or 1 according to whether $x_C \leq Z$ or $x_C > Z$; when x is a correlate of phenotypic liability to affection w, then the risk for C to be affected is given by $Q((Z-x)/\sqrt{W})$, where Q is defined as in table I.

Although emphasis has been put on calculation of $P(PH_C|I)$, another altogether interesting output is the deter-mination of $P(G_C|I)$ and $P(G_C|I,PH_C)$, for all G_C; the former is the genotype probability distribution, for the individual C at risk, conditional on pedigree information, whereas the latter is the genotype probability distribution for C condi-tional on pedigree information and information on C itself, if any. Examples will follow which, it is hoped, stress the potential usefulness of such calculations in relation with counseling as well as prevention or therapeutic decision.

3. Accuracy of the Discrete Approximation

In order to determine how many genotypic classes, n, are necessary to provide a reasonable approximation to the continuous polygenic distribution, risk for an individual in a given pedigree was computed for various values of n and various parametric values covering the likely range of applications (table II). It can be seen in this table that taking n=18 will generally guarantee sufficient accuracy in practice, particularly when one considers the magnitude of the standard-errors associated to the estimates of the para-meters of the model. Another check is provided by comparing risk figures computed with our program with the exact calcu-lations of Curnow (43) in simple situations where information is available on 2 first-degree relatives (table III). In the current version of our program, written for a 32K CDC3100, n is taken as 18 for the mixed model.

TABLE I Calculation of Conditional Probabilities
of Having Phenotype PH

PH	$P(PH \mid g_i, c_j)$
Unknown	1
Quantitative value x*	$f\left(\dfrac{x - g_i - c_j}{\sqrt{E}}\right)$
Affected	$Q\left(\dfrac{Z - g_i - c_j}{\sqrt{E + W}}\right)$
Normal	$1 - Q\left(\dfrac{Z - g_i - c_j}{\sqrt{E + W}}\right)$

PH_C	$P(PH_C \mid g_{Ci}, c_{1\ell}, c_{2m})$
Unknown	1
Quantitative value x*	$f\left(\dfrac{x - g_{Ci} - \bar{c}_{\ell m}}{\sqrt{C/2 + E}}\right)$
Affected	$Q\left(\dfrac{Z - g_{Ci} - \bar{c}_{\ell m}}{\sqrt{C/2 + E + W}}\right)$
Normal	$1 - Q\left(\dfrac{Z - g_{Ci} - \bar{c}_{\ell m}}{\sqrt{C/2 + E + W}}\right)$

Z: threshold; $\bar{c}_{\ell m} = (c_{1\ell} + c_{2m})/2$; C: variance
due to the polygenic effect; E: variance due to
random environment; W: liability noise. f stands
for the normal density function, Q stands for the
normal cumulative distribution function.

*For quantitative trait given, probability obtains
after multiplication of the density here given by
its differential element.

TABLE II   The Effect of Varying the Number of Classes, n, of
the Polychotomy on Recurrence Risk Calculations.   The Multifactorial Model is Assumed, and Two Different Population
Prevalences, .001 and .01, are considered.

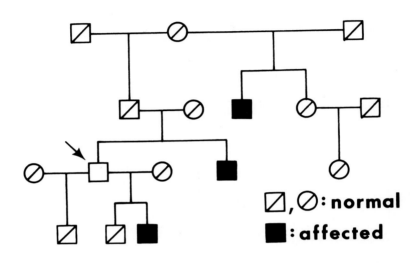

	n	.001	.01
	10	.17576	.21845
	14	.16976	.21398
	18	.16857	.21378
H = .80	22	.16804	.21367
	26	.16775	.21362
	30	.16759	.21358
	40	.16737	.21353
	10	.05582	.11160
	14	.05494	.11110
	18	.05467	.11091
H = .50	22	.05455	.11082
	26	.05448	.11077
	30	.05444	.11074
	40	.05439	.11070

TABLE III   The Risk of Affection for the Next Child in a
Few Simple Situations, Comparing Curnow's (43) Results
(C) With Ours (0).   The Multifactorial Model is Assumed,
With H = .8 and I = .005.   FA: father;   MO: mother;
CH: child.   1: affected;   0: normal;   -: unknown.

FA	1	1	0	1	1
MO	1	0	0	-	-
CH	-	-	-	1	0

(C)	.3770	.0610	.0044	.1630	.0555
(0)	.3776	.0609	.0044	.1632	.0558

We also compared our calculations with those of Bonaiti-
Pellié and Smith (47) and Spence, Westlake, Lange and Gold
(48) under the multifactorial model. Retaining arbitrarily
line 19 of table II of the former authors, it can be seen in
table IV that there is rather good agreement between our calculations and theirs which involve pedigree reduction. Moreover, for their example of figure 1 (47, pp. 375-376), we
obtain a risk of .188 where they give .186. Although accurate
enough for the examples considered, their calculations might
turn out more approximate in more complex situations, partic-
larly when information on a quantitative trait is available
for a number of second or more distant relatives.

As for the calculations of Spence, Westlake, Lange and
Gold (48), it is not clear, in their table III, whether non-
affected individuals are to be considered normal or unknown;
for some representative situations reported in table V, good
agreement obtains when non-affected individuals are assumed
to be normal, and consideration of a polychotomy with 30
classes instead of 18 led to changes affecting the calculations by a term at most equal to .0005.

4. The Question of Confidence Limits for Recurrence Risks

The risk calculation, while a probability, is nevertheless an estimate and as such can be considered to have
estimation error about it, coming from two sources: errors
of estimates of the parameters of the model, and error due
to the fact that the risk applies to an inference class of
similar family histories that are not homogeneous with respect
to genetic parameters. While Smith (40) offered a possible
estimate of variance of risk to account for the latter
source, MacLean (unpublished, see also 45) suggested the use
of a tolerance measure. Defined for nuclear families, the
x% tolerance of a family is the probability that a family
has a risk greater than x%, by analogy with the common
statistical concept, and is therefore a monotonically
decreasing function of risk over the range (0,1).

We do not see, however, how confidence limits could be
used in practical counseling situations, where one is concerned with the future outcome of a single trial and no mean
cost can be attached to alternative decisions.

VI. SOME NUMERICAL EXAMPLES

A first example (table VI) shows how the specificity of

TABLE IV A Comparison Between Some of Bonaiti-Pellié and
        Smith (47) Calculations (S) With Ours (0).

Pedigree:

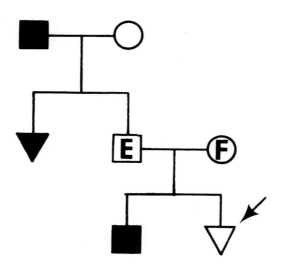

Model: Multifactorial model, H = .84
         Sex specific liabilities:
               Prevalence among males: .0013
               Prevalence among females: .0007

Recurrence risks:

Event E	Event F	(S)	(0)
normal	normal	.063	.063
affected	normal	.123	.133
normal	affected	.275	.281
affected	affected	.472	.507

TABLE V   A Comparison Between Some of Spence et al. (48)
Calculations (S) With Ours (0)

Pedigree:

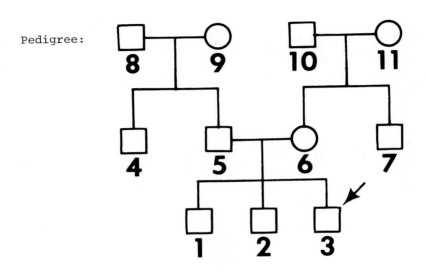

Model: Multifactorial model, H = .80
Sex specific liabilities as in table IV.

Recurrence risks:

Affected individuals	(S)	(0)*	(0)**
1, 5, 8	.12	.113	.132
1, 5, 10	.20	.186	.232
5, 7	.09	.092	.126
1, 5, 7	.19	.184	.232
1, 5, 4	.11	.112	.132
1, 4	.05	.049	.071

*Assuming others 'normal'.
**Assuming others 'unknown'.

TABLE VI The Specificity of Risk Calculations According to Whether or not Sex and Birth-order Specific Liabilities are Considered

Pedigree:

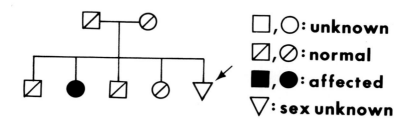

| □,○: unknown |
| ⊠,⊘: normal |
| ■,●: affected |
| ▽: sex unknown |

Model: Multifactorial model, H = 0.79
Incidence at birth according to sex and birth-order:

Sex	Overall	Birth-order			
		1	2	3	4+
Male	.00478	.0064	.0046	.0041	.0020
Female	.00118	.0019	.0008	.0007	.0007

Recurrence risks:

	Sex of individual at risk	
	Male	Female
One liability class	.032	.032
Sex specific liabilities	.056	.018
Sex and birth-order specific liabilities	.030	.013

a recurrence risk can be increased by taking into account sex
or birth-order effect. The disorder is pyloric stenosis, and
the model is the multifactorial model with H = .79, best
supported by a recent segregation analysis of British data
(45). Even in such a simple situation, it can be seen that
the risk calculation varies between .013 and .056, for
the same family history, with consideration of sex and birth
order specific liabilities.

The example of table VII is intended to show on one
hand how the recurrence risk varies according to the model
specified, and on the other hand the difference there is in
considering one individual unknown or normal in a pedigree.
The parameters of the three models considered were the
maximum likelihood estimates in segregation analysis of
pyloric stenosis in mating types with normal mothers (45),
where the mixed model and the multifactorial model yielded
similar likelihoods, whereas the generalized single locus
model (H = 0) led to a $X_1^2 = 5$ versus the unrestricted model.

It can be seen that, although normal individuals do not, a
priori, contribute much information in the recurrence risk
calculation for a rare disorder and in the absence of a
quantitative trait (40), this does not apply when his genotypic liability, conditional on his ancestors, expose him to
an elevated risk. This is particularly so under the mixed
model, as it may affect appreciably the conditional probabilities of major gene transmission in the pedigree.

The example of table VIII shows how informative a
quantitative trait may be in risk calculations, even when
this measurement is close to the average value expected a
priori in a normal individual. That the power of discrimination between competing hypotheses could be very much
increased by consideration of a quantitative trait was well
demonstrated (31); a similar increase in the specificity of
a recurrence risk calculation can consequently be expected.

This examination is pursued further in table IX, where
tentative estimates of the parameters of the mixed model in
relation with cholesterolemia are given, and an hypothetical
relation between cholesterolemia, x, and phenotypic liability
to infarction, w, according to [3], is assumed, with a linear
correlation of .70; prevalence of affection is assumed to be
.003. For the hypothetical pedigree presented, it is shown
how phenotype and genotypes probabilities vary according to
whether information is available only on the nuclear family
of the individual at risk or on the whole pedigree. Assuming
the individual at risk unknown, the probabilities for either
of his parents to be carrier, conditional on pedigree, were
found to be .74 for his father and .10 for his mother. In
a similar situation in practice, one may be led to measure

TABLE VII The Effect of Considering an Individual 'normal'
as 'unknown' on Recurrence Calculations Under Various Models.
Sex and Birth-order Specific Liabilities as in table VI.

Pedigree:

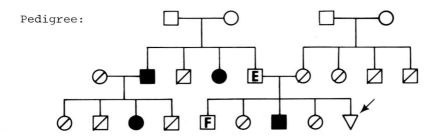

Models:

Model	Parameters					
	V	U	D	T	Q	H
1	1	0	1	1.7	.001	.785
2	1	0	1	2.0	.004	0
3	1	0	-	-	-	.79

Recurrence risks:

Events*	Model	Sex of individual at risk	
		Male	Female
E_1, F_2	1	.108	.061
	2	.069	.032
	3	.060	.028
E_2, F_2	1	.070	.036
	2	.068	.031
	3	.045	.020
E_2, F_1	1	.079	.041
	2	.068	.032
	3	.051	.023

*Events: E_1: 'unknown'; E_2: 'normal'. F_1:
'unknown'; F_2: 'normal'.

TABLE VIII   The Specificity of Recurrence Risk Calculations
in Relation With Consideration of a Quantitative Trait.

Pedigree: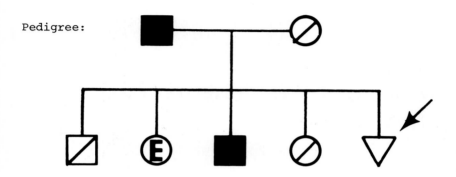

Model: Multifactorial model, H = .79, W = 0
         Sex and birth-order specific liabilities as in
            table VI.

Recurrence risks:

		Sex of individual at risk	
	Event	Male	Female
E_1:	normal	.071	.034
E_2:	unknown	.075	.035
E_3:	x = 0.0	.030	.012

TABLE IX   Illustration of the Information Contributed by
Nuclear Family and More Distant Relatives as Well as Quantitative Measurements in the Calculation of Phenotype and Genotype
Probabilities.   A: affection;   C: carrier of major gene;   F:
nuclear family;   I: all pedigree.

Pedigree:

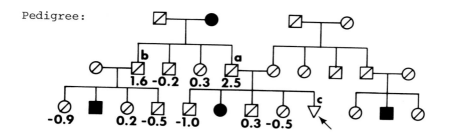

Model:

V	U	D	T	Q	B	H	W	Prevalence
1	0	.5	4.8	.002	0	.5	1.0	.003

Some useful results under this model:

	1	2	3
Major genotypes	1	2	3
Genotypic values	4.79	2.39	-.0096
Frequencies in population	.00000	.00399	.99600
P (Affection/Genotype)	.72666	.13476	.00247
P (Genotype/Affection)	.00097	.17932	.81971

Recurrence risks and genotype probabilities:

Information	$P(A\|F)$	$P(C\|F)$	$P(C\|F,A)$	$P(A\|I)$	$P(C\|I)$	$P(C\|I,A)$
Affection status only	.017	.063	.612	.092	.410	.947
Quantitative traits, and:						
x_C unknown	.029	.217	.898	.066	.468	.980

	$P(A\|x_C)$	$P(C\|F)$	$P(C\|F,x_C)$	$P(A\|x_C)$	$P(C\|I)$	$P(C\|I,x_C)$
$x_C = 2.0$	.026	.217	.583	.026	.468	.866
$x_C = -0.1$	.000	.217	.009	.000	.468	.019

cholesterol levels on the father's relatives. Arbitrary
values have therefore been assigned here which would be
compatible with individual a being heterozygous, individual b
having a value intermediate between heterozygote and normal
homozygote means, and others measurements being compatible
with normal genotype at the major locus. This example,
although a hypothetical one, reveals a number of interesting
features: $P(A|I)$, the risk conditional on pedigree informa-
tion, decreases when quantitative values are taken into
account, whereas $P(C|I)$, the probability of being carrier,
increases, suggesting a reduced polygenic contribution to the
risk; conditional on pedigree and affection, the individual
at risk, if affected, would very likely be carrier, which
might be of interest for therapeutic decision; however,
conditional on pedigree and a quantitative value of - 0.1,
the individual at risk is very likely to be homozygous normal.
Genotype probabilities, conditional on an individual's
measurement and his pedigree information, may be a valuable
guide for prevention or therapeutic decision, as we shall
suggest again in the discussion.

VII. DISCUSSION

Most common disorders are nosologic entities, generally
defined in the absence of familial studies; this certainly
has generated diseases categories of great etiologic heterogeneity. It follows that the first step in elucidating the
genetic basis of common disorders will consist in resolving
these broad categories into more homogeneous, or specific,
etiologic entities. Smith (49) suggested statistical analysis
of pairs of relatives in order to test for the existence of
genetic correlations between disease forms, under the multifactorial model. It may however prove more fruitful to
search for megaphenic effects due to the segregation
of a major gene (50), by studying biological correlates of
affection in a random sample, in a series of affected probands, in a sample of probands and their relatives or in a
large kindred (51); segregation analysis may prove particularly useful at this stage, as it permits selection of
families through extremely deviant parents, study of the
conditional likelihood of their offspring, and various heterogeneity tests; linkage of a quantitative trait with a marker
(52) is another possible approach.
A number of difficulties arise in connection with the
study of a quantitative variable in families, particularly in

distinguishing between environment common to sibs and dominance effects, or between skewness and the effect of a major
gene (31). Path analysis of pairs of relatives (29,53) or
of nuclear families (54) may complement segregation analysis
in assessing environmental effects, and correction for
skewness in a mixture of normal distributions may be done by
transformation (55).

Variation of incidence with age is another important
difficulty, which cannot be entirely resolved by consideration
of age-specific prevalences. The various ways in which age
might have an effect on total liability were considered by
Falconer (20), who also provided some tests of particular
hypotheses concerning this effect under the multifactorial
model. Mean and/or variance of total liability may vary
with age, and these variations may be accounted for by genetic
and/or environmental effects. The situation is still more
complex when one considers a quantitative trait x related to
phenotypic liability to affection, w. The various theories
of aging (e.g. 56,57), either pathogenetic or etiologic, as
well as the restricted number of studies relating to genetic
effects on aging (56), do not allow a general treatment of the
relationship between age effects and incidence of affection.
Careful analyses of the variations of mean and variance of x
as well as of the variance W with age should be done for any
given disorder before a model is constructed to account for
these effects.

Although it will necessarily involve simplifying
assumptions, a model explicitly accounting for an age effect
may prove useful in counseling, prevention, and therapeutic
decision, as the following, hypothetical, example intends to
show (table X). Consider an affection related to a quantitative trait x, according to the mixed model; assume that
genetic liability, $g + c$, is independent of age, and that
variation of prevalence with age is accounted for by a change
of mean of x and/or of w, the variances V and W being independent of age. Then e represents environmental effects
that are independent of time, together with individual
temporal fluctuation and measurement error; x_a, at age a, is
normally distributed with mean μ_a and variance V; after age
correction, it satisfies equation [1]. Parameters of the
mixed model are estimated by segregation analysis of the age-
corrected quantitative trait, and W is estimated from data on
sibships where both affection status and quantitative trait
are available (29, eq. 20 and 21). Age-group specific
prevalences define various thresholds on the distribution of
phenotypic liability w. For a specific family history, one
can calculate the genotype distribution of an individual.

TABLE X   Ulterior Risk of Affection Conditional on Current
    Information.   () and a, b refer to Liability Classes,
                    A: 'affection'.

Pedigree:

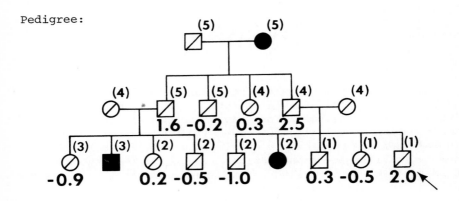

Model: as in table IX, but 5 liability classes are defined,
         in relation with age-group specific prevalences, as:

(1)	(2)	(3)	(4)	(5)
.0010	.0020	.0035	.0050	.0060

Risk calculations:

x_a	a	b	$P(A_a|x_a)$	$P(C|x_a)$	$P(A_b|x_a)$	$P(C|I)$	$P(C|I,x_a)$	$P(A_b|I,x_a)$
2.0	1	3	.007	.028	.017	.453	.875	.090
2.0	1	5	.007	.028	.028	.453	.875	.129
-0.1	1	3	.0000	.0002	.0014	.453	.022	.0019
-0.1	1	5	.0000	.0002	.0027	.453	.022	.0036

conditional on his current quantitative value, after age correction, and pedigree information, $P(G|I,x_a)$. We see that pedigree information, together with the genetic model, may allow detection of high risk individuals, if only in probability. With the present assumption, the ulterior risk of affection at an age b > a, event denoted A_b, conditional on current information, is approximately (neglecting temporal correlation of random environmental effects):

$$P(A_b|I,x_a) = \Sigma_G P(A_b|G)P(G|I,x_a), \qquad [7]$$

in view of the present assumption and [6], $P(A_b|G)$ being calculated as indicated in table I. It can be seen in table X how ulterior risk of affection varies with simultaneous consideration of pedigree information, I, as well as current age-corrected quantitative value, x_a. A model allowing for a change of variance components W_a, and possibly also V_a, with age a may be more realistic; the possibility of considering such trends, by age-group or in a continuous manner, is related to the availability of data from which such inference could be made.

Consideration of the probability distribution $P(G|I,x_a)$ may prove useful for therapeutic decision. The prospects for prevention may be appreciated by recalculating $P(G|I,x_a)$ when the reduction of variance associated with manipulation of environmental factors (random, common to sibs, or common to parent and offspring) has been estimated by path analysis; this stresses the importance there is in studying environmental correlates of affection. $P(G|I,x_a)$ may also be used to select high risk individuals for further biochemical studies.

An interesting feature of models assuming a constant genetic liability, at least for a given life-period, is that age of onset is related to genetic liability; another is that, if W_a increase with age a, early measurement of a quantitative trait better allows recognition of high risk cases, therefore more specific forecasting and more effective prevention.

Currently, our program OCCUR does not allow for inbreeding or environment common to sibs. Were the latter substantial, the program RISK, restricted to nuclear families, should be used. Various extensions to this program can easily be made, for example to allow for age-group specific variance components E_a and W_a, sex-linked major gene, or linkage of major gene to one or several markers.

The specificity of risk calculations will depend on the availability of appropriate data and their rigorous analysis. For a number of disorders, published data were reduced to pairs of relatives, and use of the multifactorial model for risk calculation is inescapable; however, whenever the original data consists of nuclear families obtained through well-defined sampling, they should hopefully be submitted to segregation analysis, for tests of heterogeneity, tests of hypotheses, and more efficient estimation.

VIII. REFERENCES

1. Childs, B., Am. J. Hum. Genet. 29, 1-13 (1977).
2. Weinberg, W., Arch. Rass. Ges. Biol. 9, 165-174 (1921).
3. Weinberg, W., Z. Ind. Abst. Vererb. Lehre 48, 179-228 (1927).
4. Morton, N.E., Science 127, 79-80 (1958).
5. Morton, N.E., Am. J. Hum. Genet. 11, 1-16 (1959).
6. Haldane, J.B.S., Ann. Eugen. 8, 255-262 (1938).
7. Haldane, J.B.S., Ann. Eugen. 14, 339-341 (1949).
8. Finney, D.J., Ann. Eugen. 14, 319-328 (1949).
9. Chung, C.S., Morton, N.E., Am. J. Hum. Genet. 11, 339-359 (1959).
10. Morton, N.E., Chung, C.S., Am. J. Hum. Genet. 11, 360-379 (1959).
11. Curnow, R.N., Smith, C., J. Roy. Statist. Soc. A 138, 131-168 (1975).
12. Carter, C.O., Brit. Med. Bull. 32, 21-26 (1976).
13. Pearson, K., Phil. Trans. Roy. Soc. A 195, 79-150 (1900).
14. Pearson, K., Biometrika 3, 131-190 (1904).
15. Grüneberg, H., Proc. Roy. Soc. B. 138, 437-451 (1951).
16. Penrose, L.S., Acta Genet. 4, 257-265 (1953).
17. Edwards, J.H., Acta Genet. 10, 63-70 (1960).
18. Edwards, J.H., Brit. Med. Bull. 25, 58-63 (1969).
19. Falconer, D.S., Ann. Hum. Genet. 29, 51-76 (1965).
20. Falconer, D.S., Ann. Hum. Genet. 31, 1-20 (1967).
21. Elston, R.C., Campbell, M.A., Behav. Genet. 1, 3-10 (1970).
22. Reich, T., James, S.W., Morris, C.A., Ann. Hum. Genet. 36, 163-184 (1972).
23. Kidd, K.K., Cavalli-Sforza, L.L., Soc. Biology 20, 254-265 (1973).
24. Kidd, K.K., Spence, M.A., J. Med. Genet. 13, 290-294 (1976).

25. James, J.W., Ann. Hum. Genet. 35, 47-50 (1971).
26. Smith, C., Clin. Genet. 2, 303-314 (1971).
27. Krüger, J., Humangenetik 17, 181-252 (1973).
28. Morton, N.E., Am. J. Hum. Genet. 26, 318-330 (1974).
29. Morton, N.E., MacLean, C.J., Am. J. Hum. Genet. 26, 489-503 (1974).
30. Edwards, J.H., Am. J. Medicine 34, 627-638 (1963).
31. MacLean, C.J., Morton, N.E., Lew, R., Am. J. Hum. Genet. 27, 365-384 (1975).
32. Elston, R.C., Stewart, J., Hum. Hered. 21, 523-542 (1971).
33. Elston, R.C., Yelverton, K.C., Am. J. Hum. Genet. 27, 31-45 (1975).
34. Murphy, E.A., Mutalik, G.S., Hum. Hered. 19, 126-151 (1969).
35. Murphy, E.A., Ann. Hum. Genet. 34, 73-78 (1970).
36. Chase, G.A., Murphy, E.A., Bolling, D.R., Clin. Genet. 2, 141-148 (1971).
37. Murphy, E.A., Chase, G.A., "Principles of Genetic Counseling", Year Book Medical Publishers, Chicago (1975).
38. Heuch, I., Li, F.H.F., Clin. Genet. 3, 501-504 (1972).
39. Heuch, I., Li, F.H.F., "Instructions for use of the Computer Program PEDIG", Oslo and Ann Arbor (1973).
40. Smith, C., Am. J. Hum. Genet. 23, 578-588 (1971).
41. Smith, C., Mendell, N.R., Ann. Hum. Genet. 37, 275-286 (1974).
42. Mendell, N.R., Elston, R.C., Biometrics 30, 41-57 (1974).
43. Curnow, R.N., Biometrics 28, 931-946 (1972).
44. Lange, K., Westlake, J., Spence, M.A., Ann. Hum. Genet. 39, 485-491 (1976).
45. Lalouel, J.M., Morton, N.E., MacLean, C.J., Jackson, J., J. Med. Genet., in press (1977).
46. Hastings, C., "Approximations for Digital Computers", Princeton Univ. Press, Princeton (1975).
47. Bonaiti-Pellié, C., Smith, C., J. Med. Genet. 11, 374-377 (1974).
48. Spence, M.A., Westlake, J., Lange, K., Gold, D.P., Hum. Hered. 26, 327-336 (1976).
49. Smith, C., Ann. Hum. Genet. 39, 281-291 (1976).
50. Morton, N.E., Am. J. Hum. Genet. 19, 23-34 (1967).
51. Elston, R.C., Namboodiri, K.K., Glueck, C.J., Fallat, R., Tsang, R., Leuba, V., Ann. Hum. Genet. 39, 67-87 (1975).
52. Haseman, J.K., Elston, R.C., Behav. Genet. 2, 3-19 (1972).
53. Rao, D.C., Morton, N.E., Am. J. Hum. Genet. 26, 767-772 (1974).
54. Rao, D.C. et al., in preparation.

55. MacLean, C.J., Morton, N.E., Elston, R.C., Yee, S.
     Biometrics 32, 695-699 (1976).
56. Walford, R.L., "The Immunologic Theory of Aging",
     Munksgaard, Copenhagen (1969).
57. Spiegel, P.M., in "Developmental Physiology and Aging",
     P.S. Timiras (ed.), MacMillan, New York, pp.564-580
     (1972).
58. Cannings, C., Thompson, E.A., Skolnick, M.H., Adv. Appl.
     Prob., in press (1977).

DISCUSSION

MORTON: A few years ago there was a flurry of interest in
training paramedics for genetic counseling centers.   In
principle such personnel could learn to use computer programs
that exchange data on a unique pedigree for a specific risk.
However, they could not conduct original studies nor apply
segregation analysis to determine risk parameters.   Since
specification of risk is definitive of genetic counseling, no
serious center can dispense with a professional genetic
epidemiologist.   The deplorable level that now prevails was
illustrated by John Edwards' simple test on risks for sex-
linked lethals. Most of the members of the European Society
of Human Genetics did not attempt the test; of those who did,
the majority made gross errors.   This was a particularly easy
situation, since assumptions were explicitly stated; in
practice, uncertainty about fitness and mutation rates raises
more complicated problems.   Beyond these straightforward
Mendelian cases, in the area of complex inheritance, the
specification of risk is still more difficult.   One wonders
how many medical geneticists could give reasonably accurate
predictions. Will quality control and licensure of medical
geneticists assure modest competence in the risk prevision
which operationally defines genetic counseling?

COMMON DISEASES

The concept of host factors in disease is as old as medicine, but systematic study began only when public health measures had reduced the impact of infectious disease on industrial societies. During the last decade considerable progress has been made in the genetic epidemiology of common diseases, despite problems raised by cultural inheritance and etiologic heterogeneity. At least for chromosomal aberrations and other causes of spontaneous abortion, monitoring of potential mutagens and teratogens has become so feasible as to be mandatory.

GERMINAL AND SOMATIC MUTATION IN CANCER

Alfred G. Knudson, Jr.

The Institute for Cancer Research
Fox Chase Cancer Center
Philadelphia, PA 19111

Any hypothesis that invokes two or more mutations can account for three categories of epidemiologic observation on the origin of cancer: (a) the
potent influence of age, (b) the importance of environmental factors, and (c) the importance of heredity in
some instances. It can also account for the long
latent period between exposure to a carcinogen and
the development of a cancer, as well as the chromosomal
abnormalities so often seen in cancer cells. From
mathematical models fitted to age-specific incidence
data on normal and genetically predisposed individuals
it is concluded that two mutations are essential for
tumors of children and some tumors of adults, while
three are required for most tumors of adults. Two
mutations may be critical for oncogenesis by rendering a cell homozygously abnormal at one of a set of
tissue-specific genes that regulate proliferation. A
third "mutation" may consist of a crucial step in
clonal evolution of chromosomal changes that are
required for expression of malignancy in many tumors
of the adult. The somatic mutation rates deduced
from the two-mutation model are compatible with rates
observed for human cells in vitro.

I. THE INCIDENCE OF CANCER: AGE, ENVIRONMENT, AND HEREDITY

The single most evident factor influencing the incidence
of cancer is age. Most cancers occur in late adulthood and

their incidences steadily increase with age. Epidemiologists
have long been intrigued with the observation that the age-
specific incidences for many cancers are virtually a simple
power function of time. This is especially true for the
gastrointestinal cancers. Some adult cancers, including breast
cancer, deviate from this pattern in that the increase in
incidence changes at advanced ages. However, the principal
deviation occurs in the first decade of life, where there is
a peak in incidence of a set of cancers peculiar to early
life, including Wilms' tumor of the kidney, neuroblastoma,
and retinoblastoma. These general patterns of incidence for
the cancers of adults and children are universal and must
therefore receive primary consideration in any hypothesis
on the origin of cancer.

Epidemiologists have also demonstrated that environment
is a major factor in determining the incidence of cancer. The
single most outstanding example is that of lung cancer, the
incidence of which has risen in many countries in this century
as a consequence of cigarette smoking. On the basis of both
population and family studies it has been concluded that
environment is more important than heredity for most cancers.
This conclusion has been based largely upon geographic differences in the incidence of specific tumor types. Thus in
Japan, relative to the United States, the incidence of carcinoma of the stomach is high and of the colon and breast, low.
Support for the role of environmental factors in this difference comes from the observation that the offspring of Japanese
migrants to the United States, notably here to Hawaii, experience cancers at rates more nearly like those observed in
the United States (1). The nature of the environmental factor
in such instances is unknown, although dietary agents have
been suspected. It should be noted that geographic differences
are not necessarily environmental in origin; for example,
Ewing's sarcoma is less common in Africa than in the United
States, but it is also rare among blacks in the United States
(2). The relative importance of environment has also been
shown from numerous family studies, including studies on twins.

Yet there is no doubt that in some instances heredity
plays a major role in carcinogenesis. "Cancer families" have
been known since the last century. In one of the earliest examples hereditary cancer occurred in the colon and was
associated with adenomatous polyps in the same organ. This
condition, polyposis of the colon, is clearly dominantly inherited, and, unless the colon is removed, there is virtual
certainty that carcinoma will ultimately develop at a mean
age of about 40 years. Since many cases die before the end
of the reproductive period, natural selection acts against the

responsible gene and the incidence of the disease is presumably
determined by mutational equilibrium. This kind of equilibrium
accounts for the fact that, although many such examples of
dominantly inherited predisposition to cancer are known, none
is common.

Some hereditary conditions predispose to cancer because
of a peculiar susceptibility to environmental agents. Probably the best known, and best studied, example is xeroderma
pigmentosum, a recessively inherited condition that predisposes to skin cancer. The development of this cancer is
limited to areas of the body exposed to sunlight. Genetic
predisposition to environmental carcinogens could be widespread without being detected easily. The possibility that
such may be the case with lung cancer will be discussed later.
In fact it is even possible that a major fraction of cancers
might be due to the combined action of environmental agents
and genes that by themselves produce little phenotypic effect.

The incidences of some tumors seem to show neither environmental nor genetic influence. They are distributed with
virtually constant incidence throughout the world. Wilms'
tumor of the kidney is an example (3). Nonhereditary
variation seems to play little or no role in the
causation of such a cancer, although it should be noted that
this does not eliminate the universal environmental factor
such as cosmic rays. These cancers may arise as a result of
"spontaneous" or "background" processes not associated with
either genetic or environmental variation.

With respect to causation, human cancers may be divided
therefore into four classes, according to the presence or
absence of identifiable hereditary (H) or environmental (E)
factors; i.e., they may be H - E+, H + E-, H + E+, or
H - E- (4). Any hypothesis on the incidence of cancer must
consider these classes as well as the influence of age.

II.   MUTATION AND CANCER

A.   Environmental Agents and Somatic Mutation

In 1914 Boveri first articulated the concept that cancer
might be due to mutation in somatic cells (5). He based his
idea on reports of abnormal mitoses in cancer cells and noted
that cancer was associated with stimulation of proliferation,
with aging, with exposure to certain environmental agents, par-

ticularly X-rays, and with certain hereditary conditions, notably xeroderma pigmentosum. Boveri concluded that genetic change in one cell of a dividing cell line can give rise to cancer.

Attempts to verify this hypothesis have been partially successful. One necessary, although not sufficient condition, viz., that cancers should have a single cell origin, is fulfilled for most malignant tumors. Unlike the tissues from which they arise, tumors in females heterozygous at the X-linked glucose-6-phosphate dehydrogenase locus are not mosaic for these markers (6).

While it is true that chromosomal abnormalities are found in most tumors, it is also true that they are not usually specific and that they continue to evolve, suggesting that they are secondary rather than primary. In addition some cancers, especially some acute leukemias, seem to have no chromosomal aberrations, even when examined with refined banding techniques (7). However, other tumors are so regularly associated with specific chromosomal abnormality that the latter may well account for neoplastic transformation. Examples are the Philadelphia chromosome of chronic myelocytic leukemia and a chromosome 14 abnormality in various lymphoid neoplasms, including Burkitt's lymphoma (8). Of course the absence of chromosomal abnormality in some cancers does not rule out genetic change, since many mutations are not apparent microscopically.

Some of the strongest evidence that cancer may result from somatic mutation comes from the demonstration that environmental carcinogens, including ultraviolet and X-rays and many chemicals, are mutagenic as well. Two recessively inherited conditions of man, xeroderma pigmentosum and ataxia telangiectasia, have been particularly useful in this respect. In both instances a predisposition to cancer is associated with defective repair of DNA damage produced by radiation, in the former case ultraviolet, the latter, ionizing (9, 10). These disorders demonstrate that cancer can be induced by environmental agents via alteration in DNA, i.e., mutation. Considerable support for the idea that chemical carcinogens also act via mutagenesis comes from the observation that in their active carcinogenic forms most of them are mutagenic as well (11).

Viral carcinogenesis also entails somatic mutation in the broadest sense, in that part or all of the genomes of DNA tumor viruses, or DNA transcripts of the genomes of RNA tumor viruses, are integrated into host cell DNA (12). In animals viral transcripts may even be integrated into the DNA of germ cells and transmitted to subsequent generations as dominant genes (13). Although we do not have any unequivocal viral tumors in man, one tumor, Burkitt's lymphoma, is highly suspect. It is interesting that individual Burkitt tumors reveal a single cell origin by the test of X-mosaicism, although separate tumors in the same individual may show different active X-chromosomes (14).

The tumors produced by environmental agents do not seem to be different from "spontaneous" tumors or from hereditary tumors, suggesting either that phenotypic expression of tumor is limited regardless of cause or mechanism or that a common mechanism operates regardless of cause. A mutational hypothesis states that hereditary cancers, environmental cancers, and spontaneous cancers are all caused by mutation. Spontaneous cancers would be produced at a rate determined by "background" mutation, while environmental mutagens would increase these rates and therefore the incidence of a particular cancer. We have noted that two hereditary conditions, xeroderma pigmentosum and ataxia telangiectasia, cause a still further increase in rates of mutation in response to selected mutagen-carcinogens. We now ask whether this is a general or special phenomenon for predisposing genetic states.

B. Genetic States Predisposing to Cancer

Since cancers are so often chromosomally aberrant, it is perhaps not surprising that several conditions characterized by generalized, prezygotic, chromosomal abnormalities are associated with an increased risk of cancer. The best known trisomic state for which this is true is Down's syndrome. The mechanism by which this occurs is not known but clonal evolution of abnormal karyotypes has been reported in the blood cells in this disease and presumably could lead to leukemia, the principal neoplasm that affects these children (15). There are other examples of predisposition to karyotypic instability and cancer associated with a genetic abnormality. Thus in one family with inherited translocation involving chromosomes 7 and 20, a child with acute myeloid leukemia had not only this translocation but trisomy 8 in leukemic cells, T lymphocytes, and skin fibroblasts (16). The trisomy 8 was probably the immediately predisposing factor in the leukemia since it has been observed repeatedly in just the leukemic cells of patients with acute myeloid leukemia (17).

There is one specific chromosomal abnormality, an interstitial deletion of the long arm of chromosome 13, that occurs prezygotically and predisposes with very high probability to a specific tumor, retinoblastoma. The incidence of bilateral tumors and of the ages of appearance of these tumors is similar to those features in the much more common hereditary form of retinoblastoma in which there is no deletion in somatic cells generally (18). It is a reasonable hypothesis that a gene preventing retinoblastoma is located in this part of chromosome 13 and that it can be eliminated by deletion or altered by mutation. It is also interesting that some retinoblastoma tumors have a deleted chromosome 13 even though other cells are normal, suggesting that the same genetic change can be involved in both hereditary and non-hereditary cases (19).

Two conditions that predispose to cancer, xeroderma pigmentosum (XP) and ataxia telangiectasia (AT), have already been regarded as doing so via defective repair of DNA damage. Another condition that may operate in this fashion is Fanconi's anemia (FA). Chromosomal abnormalities develop in somatic cells in all three of these conditions. In XP there are excessive numbers of pseudodiploid clones containing reciprocal translocations; in AT chromosomal breaks and rearrangements are common and one particular type of translocation involving chromosome 14 seems to be related to the predisposition for lymphoreticular neoplasms; and in FA chromosome breaks and interchanges, especially between nonhomologous chromosomes, occur excessively (20, 21, 22). Persons heterozygous for AT and FA may also be predisposed to cancer, a possibility that could assume considerable quantitative importance since these heterozygotes comprise approximately one per cent of the population (23).

An intriguing kind of predisposition to cancer is one that depends upon host activation of chemical carcinogens. It is clear from carcinogenesis studies in animals and mutagenesis studies in bacteria that some chemicals are inactive in their native states but are activated by enzymes present in animal tissues (11). It has been suggested that lung cancer is much more likely to occur in smokers who are genetically endowed with high inducibility of the activating enzyme aryl hydrocarbon hydroxylase (AHH) (24). Although serious doubt has recently been cast on this conclusion, it still remains a possibility that genetic polymorphisms of this type exist (25).

Other conditions which predispose to certain cancers, especially lymphoreticular neoplasms, are rare immunodeficiency diseases. One of these, Duncan's disease, is particularly interesting because it implicates a virus in the origin of one kind of cancer. This disease has been associated with progressive and fatal lymphocytic proliferation following infectious mononucleosis (26). The Epstein-Barr virus produced a disorder distinct from, but related to, infectious mononucleosis and Burkitt's lymphoma in these subjects.

Immunological markers have been associated with many diseases, including cancer. Great effort has been spent searching for associations between specific HLA types and specific cancers. The most convincing association is that between the antigen Sin 2 and nasopharyngeal carcinoma in Chinese (27). This association could be physiologically unrelated or related, the former reflecting linkage disequilibrium, the latter, some unusual immunological response to the Epstein-Barr virus which has been implicated in the origin of this cancer.

A long-standing immunological curiosity is the observation that individuals with blood group A are more susceptible to cancer of the stomach than are those with O or B (28). Now there may be an explanation for this observation. Hakomori et al. (29) have discovered that gastric tumors and normal gastric mucosa may contain a Forssman (F) antigen closely related to A. Tumors arising from F^- mucosa (most individuals) were surprisingly F^+, and vice versa. It is therefore possible that oncogenesis in stomach cancer involves emergence of an A-like antigen that O and B individuals recognize as foreign and may reject.

The most striking relationship between heredity and cancer, however, is shown by the "cancer families" alluded to earlier. Polyposis of the colon is just one example. Another striking example is provided by families like that first reported by Warthin (30) and later elaborated upon by Lynch and Krush (31). These families show dominant transmission of a gene highly penetrant for cancer of the colon and endometrium. Many such dominantly transmitted tumors are known. Experience with one of these, retinoblastoma, suggests that, as treatment of childhood cancer improves, other tumors in this age group will prove to be heritable; in fact, evidence has already been presented in support of the heritability of some cases of neuroblastoma (32) and Wilms' tumor of the kidney (33). For retinoblastoma it is estimated that about 40 per cent of cases result from acquisition of a dominant retinoblastoma gene, most often by new germinal mutation. The probability that such gene carriers will develop tumor is approximately 95 per cent and it has been estimated that the mean number of tumors per gene carrier is three (34). The overall incidence of retinoblastoma is approximately five per 100,000 children, so

the incidence of tumor in children who do not carry this gene
is three per 100,000; the gene increases risk of tumor approximately 100,000 times (35).

C.   The Relationship of Germinal and Somatic Mutations

     For XP and AT the relationship between the germinal muta-
tion that causes the hereditary conditions and the presumed
somatic mutations that lead to cancer seems clear; under certain conditions of environmental exposure the somatic mutation
rates will be greatly increased and so also the probability
of cancer. If it is shown that genetic polymorphisms exist
for activation of mutagenic carcinogens, they too would be ex-
plainable in terms of a somatic mutation model. In other instances, such as Down's syndrome, the mechanism is not
understood but there is evidence to suggest karyotypic instability that in effect increases somatic "mutation". On
the other hand, the 13 deletion syndrome and the dominantly
inherited cancer genes do not seem to predispose to cancer by
increasing mutation rate.

     The dominant gene for a tumor such as retinoblastoma is
very specific for a particular tissue, and the prospect that a
person carrying the gene will not develop a tumor is very
small. Yet at the cellular level oncogenesis is a rare event;
only 3 or 4 cells among millions will on average be transformed to tumor cells. This phenomenon suggests that another
event must occur, and its frequency further suggests that the
event may be a mutation. A first event can be conceived as a
germinal mutation that makes all of the target cells in a
specific tissue susceptible to transformation by a second,
somatic mutation (34).

     Approximately 60 per cent of retinoblastoma cases are non-
hereditary. How does this form relate to the hereditary form?
The model developed for the hereditary form may be applied
here too, except that the first event is conceived as a
somatic mutation (34). Both forms would therefore entail a
sequence of two mutations. Any cell that sustains both would
be transformed into a tumor cell.

     Such a model would help to explain the well known latency
observed for environmental carcinogenesis. Many years usually
intervene between exposure and development of cancer. If a
single mutation were involved there should be no latent
period, except for the time required to render a tumor
clinically apparent. But such a long latency is also known

for readily observable skin tumors arising in skin previously
irradiated. Presumably an environmental mutagen can produce a
first mutation in a cell line, and "spontaneous" mutation can
produce a second mutation much later. On the other hand,
irradiation of a person carrying a germinal mutation might
lead to tumor after a relatively brief period. Such seems to
be the case when patients with the dominantly inherited
nevoid basal cell carcinoma syndrome receive craniospinal
irradiation for medulloblastoma. Strong (36) has reported
that basal cell carcinomas may appear in the irradiated skin
within months instead of years.

   If we assume that two mutations in a normal cell can
transform it into a tumor cell, what might be the relationship
between the mutations? Three possibilities can be considered;
(a) the second mutation might occur in or near the site of the
first mutation, further changing the gene; (b) it might occur
at the same gene site in the homologous chromosome, rendering
the cell homozygously mutant at that site; or (c) it might
occur at an entirely different site. The first of these seems
unlikely in view of the fact that retinoblastoma can occur
when the first mutation is a very large deletion of the long
arm of chromosome 13; there seems to be no remaining locus at
which a second mutation could occur (18).

   The second possibility is important because different
tumors would be different single (recessive) gene disorders.
In an individual who inherits such a gene from both parents,
every cell would presumably become a tumor cell. Such matings
have not been recorded in man or other vertebrates, but it is
interesting that in the fruit fly homozygosity for a lethal
larval gene transforms all neuroblasts in the brain (37).
Another mechanism that could produce homozygosity would be
somatic recombination in a heterozygous cell. In fact this
could be the "second mutation". Any agent or gene that is
known to increase the rate of somatic recombination should
increase the incidence of tumor in heterozygous cells,
whether the latter are in carriers of cancer genes or in
normal individuals in whom one somatic cancer mutation has
occurred. Bloom's syndrome in man may well produce its high
incidence of diverse cancers in this manner. In this syndrome
there is a great increase in both sister chromatid exchanges
and homologous chromosome exchanges (38). Heterozygous cells
in which the latter has occurred would segregate some
homozygous daughter cells.

III. MUTATION MODELS FOR THE INCIDENCE OF CANCER

A. Cancers of Adulthood

As noted in the beginning of this presentation the incidences of adult cancers increase steadily with age. For cancers of colon and stomach the incidence (I) may be related
mathematically to age (t) by the expression

$$I = kt^{r-1}$$

The meaning of this relationship, and particularly the meaning
of r has aroused great interest. Nordling first suggested
that r might represent the number of mutations a cell must
accumulate before it is transformed into a tumor cell (39).
It is assumed that target cell number is constant and that new
mutations accumulate in proportion to the product of mutation
rate and time, t. Thus if r = 1, the age-specific incidence
of a tumor would be constant, if r = 2 it would rise linearly
with time, and so on. For many tumors the value of r is in
the range of 6-7 (40). Such a number is obviously much
greater than the number of events suggested in the previous
section. It also calls for rates of somatic mutation that
would be considerably higher than have been estimated for
mammalian cells.

Some cancers do not show this simple relationship. Thus
for cancer of the lung the value of r is greater than 8. However, for non-smokers, among whom this tumor is rare, the
value of r is between 5 and 6 (40). Since smoking greatly increases the probability that cancer will occur, it is reasonable to suppose that somatic mutation rates increase after
smoking is begun. If the age specific incidence is therefore
plotted against years of smoking, the value of r is approximately the same as for non-smokers. Similarly, for cancer of
the prostate the value of r is much higher, even as high as
11 or 12 in some populations (40). If it is assumed that some
factor is introduced after birth and significantly increases
mutation rates, the estimate of r will be lower. Thus sub-
traction of 20-30 years from actual ages places the value of r
into the range 6-8 (40).

For other cancers, notably of breast, endometrium, and
ovary, the values of r change; in each of these cases it decreases at advanced age. In addition there is a marked decrease in r for breast cancer around the time of menopause.
It is generally thought that these decreases might be the result of endocrine changes that limit tumor cell survival and

growth or that reduce the number of target cells available for transformation.

As a result of their consideration of these various perturbations, Armitage and Doll (41) concluded that the basic premise of Nordling was correct and that the observed age-specific incidences for cancer in the adult were best explained by multiple mutations. Subsequently these same authors (42) expressed concern for lack of direct evidence supporting so many steps as 6 or 7 and for the magnitude of somatic mutation rates that would probably be required. They therefore proposed a two-mutation model in which a first mutation would produce a cell with a selective growth advantage over normal cells such that it would grow exponentially. But this model was criticized by Ashley (43) for its deviation from observation at advanced age and suggested that a three-mutation model previously introduced by Fisher (44) would fit observation more satisfactorily. Fisher's proposal was that a growth advantage might apply to cells confined to the basement compartment of epithelium such that they would increase radially with time and their number would increase in proportion to the square of time. Thus cells with one mutation would be produced linearly with time and their total number would increase with the third power of time. If a second mutation were to operate similarly then cells with two mutations would increase with the sixth power of time. A third, and final, mutation would cause an accumulation of cancer cells with the seventh power of time. If this notion were correct, $r = 7$, and the age-specific incidence of a three-mutation tumor should increase with the sixth power $(r - 1)$ of time, a two-mutation tumor with the third power of time. This relationship is expressed by the equation $r - 1 = 3(n - 1)$, where $\underline{n}$ is the number of mutations. Ashley observed that for several human cancers, including leukemia, lymphoma, connective tissue sarcomas, and brain tumors, the age-specific incidences vary with the second to fourth power of time.

Although Fisher's hypothesis fits well to observation there is no direct way to test it. An indirect test was undertaken by Ashley (45), who applied Burch's idea (46) that the number of somatic events should be reduced by one when one of them is inherited, as with the dominantly inherited cancers. Ashley suggested that for carcinoma of the colon arising in patients with polyposis of the colon the value of $\underline{r}$ should be reduced by one if Nordling's original idea were correct, or reduced by three if Fisher's idea were correct. Ashley estimated the reduction to be two. However, Ashley's curve was not a true tumor incidence curve since it only measured the manner in which gene carriers were affected by one tumor,

i.e., penetrance for cancer. The curve becomes a power
function when tumor number is calculated, using a Poisson
distribution to relate penetrance (P) to tumor number. Since
all persons with the gene developed tumor with time, $P(\infty) = 1$,
and $P(t)$, the quantity Ashley measured, is related to the mean
number of tumors by the equation

$$P(t) = P(\infty)\left[1 - e^{-m(t)}\right].$$

A plot of the values of m(t) gives a power function in which r
is 2-3 less than its value for carcinoma of the colon in the
general population (47).

The number of events (mutations) responsible for the development of most tumors of adulthood may therefore be
three. This would fit well to observation in the case of
carcinoma arising in subjects with polyposis of the colon. A
first, inherited, mutation may cause some loss of regulatory
control of DNA synthesis. A second mutation would then lead
to formation of an adenomatous polyp and a third one to
carcinoma. The crucial step in oncogenesis would be the
second one, while the one responsible for malignancy would be
the third. A comparison of benign tumors and the malignant
tumors arising from them might define the nature of the
third step at least. The most obvious possibility derives
from the observation that karyotypes of benign tumors are
nearly normal, or even normal, while those of malignant tumors
of the kind that show a value for r of seven or so are invariably very abnormal. The simplest hypothesis, then, is
that the third step represents clonal evolution of karyotype.

Clonal evolution obviously does not occur in one step,
but it may seem to entail one step in that the tumor will continue to appear benign until a clone develops that has a
growth advantage. Once the tumor is malignant further clonal
evolution will only accentuate its malignant character. One
could imagine that years might transpire for the transition
from benign to malignant, while acceleration of malignancy
would occur in a very short time. Therefore the appearance of
malignancy would seem to involve one threshold event in the
evolution of abnormal karyotypes.

As noted previously, some tumors of adulthood show age-
specific incidences that rise with approximately the third
power of time. These would be compatible with Fisher's model
for a two-mutation tumor. Here two events would seem to be
sufficient for malignancy, or the third event may occur so
regularly and be so intimately connected to the second that it

is not separable. It is interesting that the acute leukemias are in this group and are also known in many instances to demonstrate minimal, or even no, abnormality in karyotype. Conceivably the release from growth control provided by two mutations leads to benign tumors in some tissues and to malignant tumors in others. This possibility is especially appealing for the tumors of children.

B.   Cancers of Childhood

The possibility that tumors of childhood may arise as a result of two mutations has already been presented. Such a model can account for the existence of hereditary and nonhereditary forms of the same tumor by the same process. The peak incidence in early life is explained by the disappearance, through differentiation, of the normal embryonic cells that are the targets for the expression of the two mutations. For hereditary cases only one of these mutations occurs in somatic cells and it therefore becomes possible to relate the age-specific incidence of tumor to number of cells, number of cell divisions, and rates of somatic mutation per cell division (48).

For this model affected individuals are divided into two classes, one hereditary (H) and one nonhereditary (N). Since the risk of tumor is very high in the former, multiple tumors can occur. When the target organ is paired, tumors may be bilateral (B) or unilateral (U). Cases are collected according to age (t) at diagnosis of first tumor and according to eventual bilaterality or unilaterality. The fractions of cases still not diagnosed at time t are designated $N(t)$ for nonhereditary cases, $HU(t)$ for hereditary unilaterals, and $HB(t)$ for hereditary bilaterals. These fractions can then be related by a Poisson distribution to mean numbers of tumors at time t, $m(t)$ for hereditary cases and $q(t)$ for nonhereditary ones. The following relationships are readily derived (49):

$$HU(t) = \frac{e^{-m(t)/2} - e^{-m(\infty)/2}}{1 - e^{-m(\infty)/2}}$$

$$HB(t) = \left[HU(t) \right]^2$$

The term $m(\infty)$ is the mean number of tumors that ultimately develop. The equation for nonhereditary tumors may be further simplified, since $q(\infty) < 10^{-4}$ for tumors occurring in children who do not carry a predisposing gene:

$$N(t) = \frac{e^{-q(t)} - e^{-q(\infty)}}{1 - e^{-q(\infty)}} = 1 - \frac{q(t)}{q(\infty)}$$

These means, m and q, can be related to numbers of embryonic cells, numbers of cell divisions in these cell lines, and somatic mutation rate per cell division. A stem cell (S) becomes an intermediate mutant cell (I) after a first mutation that may be either germinal or somatic. A second, somatic mutation, occurring at a rate μ, converts the latter cell to a cancer cell (C). The number of tumor cells, $m(t)$ or $m(\infty)$, is then a product of μ and the total number of cell divisions that have occurred, $a(t)$ or $a(\infty)$:

$$m(t) = \mu \cdot a(t)$$

$$m(\infty) = \mu \cdot a(\infty)$$

A new function, $f(t)$, can be defined as $a(t)/a(\infty)$, and signifies the fraction of all cell divisions that have occurred by t. Hence

$$m(t) = m(\infty) \cdot f(t).$$

$HU(t)$ and $HB(t)$ therefore become functions of $m(\infty)$ and $f(t)$.

| The derivation of an expression for $N(t)$ is much more complex because it entails formulation of the number of intermediate mutant cells present at any time, $I(t)$. However it can be shown (48) that $N(t)$ bears the following relationship to $f(t)$, $a(\infty)$ and a new entity, the initial number of tissue-specific target cells present, $b(0)$:

$$N(t) = 1 - f(t) - \frac{f(t) \ln f(t)}{\ln a(\infty)/b(0) - 1}$$

In cases where there are data for $N(t)$, $HU(t)$, and $HB(t)$, and where estimates of $a(\infty)$ and $b(0)$ can be made, values of $f(t)$ can be computed. From a set of data on retinoblastoma published by Bonaïti-Pellie et al. (50) values of $f(t)$ were computed which then permitted calculation of theoretical values for $N(t)$, $HU(t)$, and $HB(t)$. From Table I it is seen that the fit of observation to theory is very good.

TABLE I   Predicted and Observed Distributions
of Retinoblastoma Cases (48)

Age (months)	HB(t) 236 cases pred.	HB(t) 236 cases obs.	HU(t) 22 cases pred.	HU(t) 22 cases obs.	N(t) 346 cases pred.	N(t) 346 cases obs.
0	1.00	1.00	1.00	1.00	1.00	1.00
10	0.53	0.54	0.73	0.73	0.86	0.85
20	0.22	0.26	0.47	0.46	0.67	0.66
30	0.05	0.06	0.23	0.18	0.41	0.41
40	0.01	0.03	0.11	0.09	0.22	0.22
50	0.00	0.02	0.06	0.00	0.13	0.13
≥ 60	0.00	0.01	0.04	0.00	0.09	0.09

C.   Mutations and the Incidence of Cancer

In the model for childhood cancer formulations were also made for the two somatic mutation rates, μ for the conversion of I cells to C cells, and ν for the conversion of S cells to I cells. If the mutation rates are assumed to be equal, as would be the case if the mutations occur in homologous genes, a rate of approximately 5×10^{-7} mutations per locus per cell division is found for retinoblastoma (48). This rate is similar to a recently recorded rate of 8×10^{-7} for one of the HLA loci (51).

For each childhood tumor the probability that the second, cancer producing, mutation will occur is related to a somatic mutation rate. As a result some mean number of tumors will be produced per unit of population of intermediate cells. The total incidence of tumor in a population of children is therefore directly related to the generation of intermediate cells. For nonhereditary cases these cells are produced in proportion to a first somatic mutation rate ν and for hereditary cases, to a germinal mutation rate, μ_g, so the total incidence of tumor is dependent upon these two rates: incidence = $k_1 \mu_g + k_2 \nu$ (35). The incidence of tumor will not fall below that determined by spontaneous mutation rates but may increase in the presence of environmental mutagens or in the event of increased survival value of hereditary cases.

IV.   REFERENCES

1. Haenszel, W., and Kurihara, M., <u>J. Natl. Cancer Inst.</u> 40, 43 (1968).
2. Fraumeni, J.F., and Glass, A.G., <u>Lancet</u> 1, 366 (1970).
3. Editorial, <u>Lancet</u> 2, 651 (1973).
4. Knudson, A.G., Cancer 39, 1882 (1977).
5. Boveri, T., "Zur Frage der Entstehung maligner Tumoren," p. 64. Gustav Fischer, Jena, 1914.
6. Fialkow, P.J., <u>Adv. Cancer Res.</u> 15, 191 (1972).
7. Mitelman, F., and Brandt, L., <u>Scand. J. Haematol.</u> 13, 321 (1974).
8. Manolov, G., and Manolova, Y., <u>Nature</u> 237, 33 (1972).
9. Cleaver, J.E., <u>Nature</u> 218, 652 (1968).
10. Paterson, M.C., Smith, B.P., Lohman, P.H.M., Anderson, A.K., and Fishman, L., <u>Nature</u> 260, 444 (1976).
11. Ames, B.B., Sims, P., and Grover, P.L., <u>Science</u> 176, 47 (1972).
12. Temin, T., <u>Science</u> 192, 1075 (1976).
13. Jaenisch, R., <u>Proc. Natl. Acad. Sci. USA</u> 73, 1260 (1976).
14. Fialkow, P.J., Klein, G., and Clifford, P., <u>Lancet</u> 2, 629 (1972).
15. Lejeune, J., Berger, R., Haines, M., Lafourcade, J., Vialatte, J., Satge, P., and Turpin, R., <u>C.R. Acad. Sci.</u> (Paris) 256, 1195 (1963).
16. Riccardi, V.M., Humbert, J., and Peakman, D., <u>Am. J. Hum. Genet.</u> 27, 76A (1975).
17. Ford, J.H., Pittman, S.M., Singh, S., Wass, E.J., Vincent, P.D., and Gunz, F.W., <u>J. Natl. Cancer Inst.</u> 55, 271 (1975).
18. Knudson, A.G., Meadows, A.T., Nichols, W.W., and Hill, R., <u>New Engl. J. Med.</u> 295, 1120 (1976).
19. Hashem, N., and Khalifa, S., <u>Hum. Hered.</u> 25, 35 (1975).
20. German, J., Gilleran, T., LaRock, J., and Regan, J.D., <u>Am. J. Hum. Genet.</u> 22, 10A (1970).
21. McCaw, B.K., Hecht, F., Harnden, D.G., and Teplitz, R.L., <u>Proc. Natl. Acad. Sci. USA</u> 72, 2071 (1975).
22. Schroeder, T.M., and German, J., <u>Humangenetik</u> 25, 299 (1974).
23. Swift, M., in "Cancer and Genetics" (D. Bergsma, Ed.), Birth Defects Original Article Series, Vol. 12, No. 1, p. 133, The National Foundation - March of Dimes. Alan R. Liss, New York, 1976.
24. Kellermann, G., Shaw, C.R., and Luyten-Kellermann, M., <u>New Engl. J. Med.</u> 289, 934 (1973).

25. Paigen, B., Gurtoo, H.L., Minowada, J., Houten, L., Vincent, R., Paigen, K., Parker, N.B., Ward, E., and Hayner, N.T., New Engl. J. Med. 297, 346 (1977).

26. Purtilo, D.T., Cassell, C.K., Yang, J.P.S., Harper, R., Stephenson, S.R., Landing, B.H., and Vawter, G.F., Lancet 1, 935 (1975).

27. Simons, M.J., Wee, G.B., Day, N.E., Morris, P.J., Shanmugaratnam, K., and de The', G.B., Int. J. Cancer 13, 122 (1974).

28. Aird, I., Bentall, H.H., and Roberts, J.A.F., Brit. Med. J. 1, 799 (1953).

29. Hakomori, S., Wang, S.M., and Young, W.W., Proc. Natl. Acad. Sci. USA 74, 3023 (1977).

30. Warthin, A.S., Arch. Int. Med. 12, 546 (1913).

31. Lynch, H.T., and Krush, A.J., Cancer 27, 1505 (1971).

32. Knudson, A.G., and Strong, L.C., Amer. J. Hum. Genet. 24, 514 (1972).

33. Knudson, A.G., and Strong, L.C., J. Natl. Cancer Inst. 48, 313 (1972).

34. Knudson, A.G., Proc. Natl. Acad. Sci. USA 68, 820 (1971).

35. Knudson, A.G., Pediat. Res. 10, 513 (1976).

36. Strong, L.C., in "Genetics of Human Cancer" (J.J. Mulvihill, R.W. Miller, and J.F. Fraumeni, Eds.), p. 401. Raven Press, New York, 1977.

37. Gateff, E., and Schneiderman, H.A., Wilhelm Roux' Archiv 176, 23 (1974).

38. Chaganti, R.S.K., Schonberg, S., and German, J., Proc. Natl. Acad. Sci. USA 71, 4508 (1974).

39. Nordling, C.E., Brit. J. Cancer 7, 68 (1953).

40. Doll, R., J. Roy. Stat. Soc. Ser. A. 134, 133 (1971).

41. Armitage, P., and Doll, R., Brit. J. Cancer 8, 1 (1954).

42. Armitage, P., and Doll, R., Brit. J. Cancer 11, 161 (1957).

43. Ashley, D.J.B., Brit. J. Cancer 23, 313 (1969).

44. Fisher, J.C., Nature 181, 651 (1958).

45. Ashley, D.J.B., J. Med. Genet. 6, 376 (1969).

46. Burch, P.R.J. Nature 195, 241 (1962).

47. Knudson, A.G., in "Genetics of Human Cancer" (J.J. Mulvihill, R.W. Miller, and J.F. Fraumeni, Eds.), p. 391. Raven Press, New York, 1977.

48. Hethcote, H.W., and Knudson, A.G., Proc. Natl. Acad. Sci. USA, in press.

49. Knudson, A.G., Hethcote, H.W., and Brown, B.W., Proc. Natl. Acad. Sci. USA 72, 5116 (1975).

50. Bonaïti-Pellie, C., Briard-Guillemot, M.L., Feingold, J., and Frezal, J., J. Natl. Cancer Inst. 57, 269 (1976).

51. Pious, D., and Soderland, C., Science 197, 769 (1977).

LIKELIHOOD ANALYSIS OF BREAST CANCER PREDISPOSITION

IN A MORMON PEDIGREE

J. Hill, D. Carmelli, E. Gardner, and M. Skolnick

Department of Medical Biophysics and Computing
University of Utah, LDS Hospital,
Salt Lake City, Utah 84143

Heritability studies of breast cancer to date have yielded inconclusive results about the contribution of genetic factors to the manifestation of the disorder. A 47-fold increase in risk to sisters of women with pre-menopausal and/or bilateral breast cancer has been demon-strated by incorporating a heterogeneous model which discriminates between pre- and postmenopausal cases (1). In contrast, previous investigators who used a homogeneous model found only a 2-3 fold risk increase to first degree relatives of probands. It was further noted that males seem to transmit the trait equally well as females but with a reduced tendency to express it. The purpose of this paper is to further clarify these observations of increased risk to relatives of breast cancer victims by proposing a model of inheritance of a predisposition to breast cancer through a major dominant gene with age-dependent penetrance. The penetrance was constructed from the "multi-hit" model of carcinogenesis as a function of age, sex, and genotype.

I.   MATERIALS

The following analysis was performed on data collected by Dr. Eldon Gardner for Kindred 107. This kindred was first investigated in 1947, reinvestigated in 1958 and fully surveyed again in 1976 (2), by which time there were 44 cases of breast cancer or benign tumor and 42 cases of cancer or tumor at other sites of a total of 1446 related individuals. Most of those first reported to have had benign tumors had developed breast cancer by 1976 despite some surgical interventions. Ages of onset of benign breast tumors and cancers were tabulated, and most were found to be pre-menopausal. Inspection of the age-incidence data, reproduced in Figure 1, suggested an age, sex, and genotype dependent penetrance. The discontinuity between the under-50 and over-50 age groups was interpreted as the admixture in the kindred of the two subgroups suggested by epidemio-logical studies, the early-onset high-risk group expressing a genetic predisposition while the late-onset low-risk group expresses nongenetic or sporadic forms of cancer.

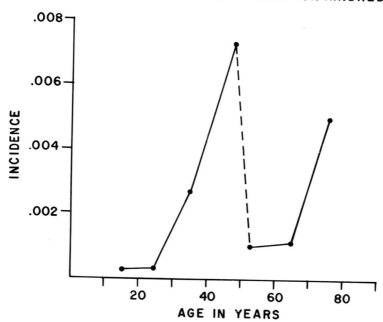

Figure 1.

II. METHODS

From this age-incidence data, two penetrance functions were constructed, one for each of the two subgroups observed, and incorporated into the genetic model fitted to the pedigree. These functions were constructed after the somatic mutation model (3) which in its simplest form supposes that a stem cell becomes cancerous when each of n specified loci have mutated. If the probabilities of occurrence of each of the n events are considered to be small, the Poisson probability that all n events will have occurred by time T in years is approximately

$$P(T) = A \cdot T^n$$

where A is the product of the probabilities of each of the n events.

Or

$$Log_{10}P(T) = nLog_{10}T + nLog_{10}A$$

This last equation yields the familiar linear relation of a log-log plot of incidence versus age for cancers in general and provides the physiologic interpretation of slope as the number of events or "hits" involved in the expression of cancer. This model of cancer also provides a simple accounting of the interaction of genetics and environment, as some of the events may be inherited and the remainder acquired from the environment. In the case of the genetically predisposed subgroup, one would expect to see a penetrance function with decreased slope and increased y-axis intercept (the $nLog_{10}A$ term) due to inheritance of one or more of the events.

The two penetrance functions described above and the Mendelian dominant mode of inheritance were incorporated into a pedigree likelihood analysis method developed and programmed for computer application (4, 5) and executed on a Data General Eclipse mini-system. The two parameters of the genetic penetrance, A and n, were allowed to approach successively their maximal values, while the parameters of the nongenetic penetrance were extracted from the late-onset age-incidence data by a least-squares technique and held constant throughout a grid-search of the genetic penetrance parameters. Comparison of the nongenetic penetrance extracted from Kindred 107 with that extracted from the Utah population incidence, which is significantly lower than the national incidence, demonstrated a close concurrence. This reinforced the initial interpretation of the age-incidence data as representing two kinds of cancer, the late-onset subgroup being primarily composed of nonpredisposed sporadics (see Figure 2). Line A in this figure represents the maximized penetrance function fitted to the phenotypic data by a grid-search of the likelihood surface defined by the two parameters, A and n, of the genetic penetrance. Notice that the slope is reduced to 1.3 while the y-axis intercept is increased.

For both subgroups the penetrance functions for males were initially constructed with the same slopes but with A (the y-axis intercept) set at 1/100th the value extracted for females, based on the Utah incidence statistics for male breast cancer. Note however that there are two documented cases of male breast cancer of some 33 total cases, which is rather larger than 1%. A parameterization of this scale factor for predisposed males yielded a maximal likelihood value of 0.37 times the female penetrance, but had only a slight effect on the likelihood.

Thus the model tested distinguished two types of breast cancer individuals and assigned a penetrance function for each, those who carried the dominant cancer gene and had on the order of a thousand times greater risk of expressing the

disorder at a given age (see Figure 2), and those who were
genetically normal and expressed breast cancer at the Utah
population incidence.

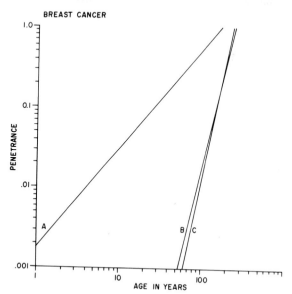

PENETRANCE AS A FUNCTION OF AGE. LINE A IS THE MAXIMIZED
GENETIC PENETRANCE. B IS TAKEN FROM THE UTAH POPULATION
STATISTICS, AND C WAS EXTRACTED FROM THE LATE-ONSET GROUP
FROM KINDRED 107. SLOPES ARE 1.3,4.97 AND 5.07 RESP.

Figure 2

The likelihood calculated using this genetic model which
allowed for both genetic and nongenetic forms of cancer was
compared to the likelihood of a completely nongenetic or
sporadic model which retained the multi-hit penetrance function but assumed the penetrance to be independent of genotype.
This was done by using a single penetrance extracted from the
Utah incidence data for all three genotypes. A LOD score was
then obtained by calculating the Log_{10} of the ratio of the
likelihood generated by the genetic model to the likelihood
generated by the sporadic model. That model which yields the
highest LOD score is taken to be the one that fits the pedigree data the best.

III. RESULTS

LOD scores of 21.5 for breast cancer and 36.1 for all
cancers were calculated for Kindred 107 using the maximized
penetrance found by grid searches of the two penetrance parameters and an assumed gene frequency of .001. (The likelihood is the probability of observing the pedigree given the

genetic model, gene frequency, and segregation.) The likelihood function was found to be robust and fairly insensitive
to the assumed population frequency, entering the calculations through the original ancestors, whose phenotypes are
unknown, and through founder spouses. The likelihood maximized at a gene freuency of 0.25 which is quite unrealistic
and most probably is an artifact introduced by the many
instances of skipped generations in the pedigree. Skipped
generations have been found to introduce artifacts into many
of the likelihood cross sections, making interpretation of
population gene frequency and segregation bias impractical.
A simple dominant model with complete (0 or 1) penetrance
was also fitted to Kindred 107 for an estimate of the effect
of the time-dependent penetrance and yielded a LOD score of
6.0. A recessive model was also tested but yielded a negative LOD.

Other interesting results were uncovered during the
search for maximizing parameters. The amount of scatter, or
noise, in the phenotypic data provided a wide range of nearly
equal likelihoods. Although the penetrance does have a
single peak, the variance about this peak is large which
precludes the possibility of making an accurate estimate of
the number of inherited events or hits (see Figure 3). No
significance can be ascribed at this point to the numerical
difference between the slopes of the genetic and nongenetic
penetrances beyond the apparent inheritance of one or more
events.

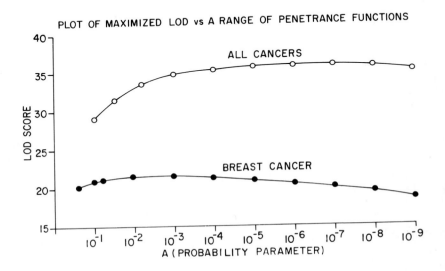

Figure 3

The LOD score is surprisingly insensitive to the parameters of the nongenetic penetrance function, which references the incidence among genetic "normals." This is no doubt due to the fact that 96% of the members of Kindred 107 are phenotypically classified as unaffected, and the majority of these will be given a high probability by the peeling program of not having carried the gene predisposing for breast cancer.

Pedigree analysis offers a method of analyzing co-segregation of different cancer sites which may indicate whether a single gene is responsible for the enhanced incidence at other sites, most notably in the urogenital system. Unfortunately, attempts to maximize segregation against penetrance were unsuccessful, probably due to the effect of the skipped generations in the kindred. The peeling algorithm can compensate for skipped generations in a likelihood grid-search by biasing segregation towards high values and reducing penetrance; since the pedigree likelihood is the product of penetrance and segregation, they can be inversely modified without significantly affecting the overall likelihood, thus preventing a clear peak for optimal segregation. Another attempt to test for co-segregation will be made by breaking down the pedigree into nuclear families and applying traditional segregation analysis.

IV. SUMMARY

The initial numerical analysis of Kindred 107, using a genetic model of predisposition to cancer inherited as a dominant gene with selective penetrance constructed from the somatic cell mutation theory has yielded a high probability that there is a major gene for breast cancer segregating in the kindred. This likelihood is 10^{22} times greater than the likelihood that the observed distribution of breast cancers might have occurred sporadically and 1036 times greater for all cancers in the kindred from a single gene. There is, however, more scatter or less tendency to cluster with all cancers considered together than with breast cancer alone. Traditional segregation analysis on the nuclear families may clarify the issue of co-segregation of sites and lead to a nonsite-specific model of inheritance of a predisposition to cancer with differentially specific penetrances by site. More pedigrees are being ascertained in an attempt to find a similar pattern of inheritance. We suggest that the reason a single major gene effect has not been clearly demonstrated in previous risk analyses of relatives of probands is the dilution of the effect by the more frequent cancers of the second type, the nongenetic or sporadic cancers, and by failure to include age-dependent penetrance. Thus pedigree analysis provides an elegant method of modeling both types of cancer on a single pedigree and distinguishing the genetic

component through maximum likelihood analysis. The use of
large multi-generation pedigrees incorporates the horizontal
information of traditional segregation analysis along with
the vertical information which provides insight into the mode
of inheritance. Similar and more detailed applications of
this approach to informative pedigrees may provide
insights into the genetics of cancer.

V.   REFERENCES

1.   Anderson, D.E., Cancer 34, 1090-1097 (1974).
2.   Gardner, E.J., Hill, J., Skolnick, M. and Carmelli, D.,
     in preparation.
3.   Knudson, A.G., these proceedings.
4.   Cannings, C., Thompson, E.A. and Skolnick, M., Adv. Appl.
     Prob., in press (1978).
5.   Thompson, E.A., Technical Report No. 5, Department of
     Medical Biophysics and Computing, University of Utah
     (1977).

ACKNOWLEDGEMENT

Supported by NIH grants CA-16573 and GM-07464

GENETIC EPIDEMIOLOGY

ETIOLOGICAL DIVERSITY IN THE PSYCHOSES

Steven Matthysse

Mailman Research Center
McLean Hospital, Belmont, Mass. 02178

Geneticists contemplating the problem of schizophrenia usually conclude that real progress will be made only after biochemical correlates are identified. Biochemists, on the other hand, tend to become discouraged because time and again biochemical studies report "no significant difference" between schizophrenics and controls. Fortunately, a way out of this dilemma is becoming increasingly apparent. We have to recognize the likelihood that schizophrenia – even when conservatively defined – can result from a number of different causes, and adapt our research strategies accordingly. The current methods virtually guarantee that "no significant difference" will be found between schizophrenics and controls, if the disorder is etiologically heterogeneous, since they are based on random samples of patients. We may have to accustom ourselves to asking less of our hypotheses, and not discarding them quite so readily.

As an example, let us consider the "dopamine hypothesis" of schizophrenia. There is substantial evidence in favor of this hypothesis, althought it is all indirect. Drugs of the phenothiazine or butyrophenone type, which are used to treat schizophrenia, are known to be dopamine blockers – i. e. they bind to the postsynaptic dopamine receptor and prevent the binding of the naturally occurring neurotransmitter (1). These drugs do not bring about a complete cure, but they are able to decrease the intensity of the patient's psychotic preoccupations and thought disorder, improve his ability to concentrate, and make his behavior less bizarre. Their effect on the number of schizophrenic patients who have to be permanently hospitalized has been truly revolutionary (Fig.1). The correlation between clinical potency and affinity for binding to the dopamine receptor is remarkably good (Fig.2).

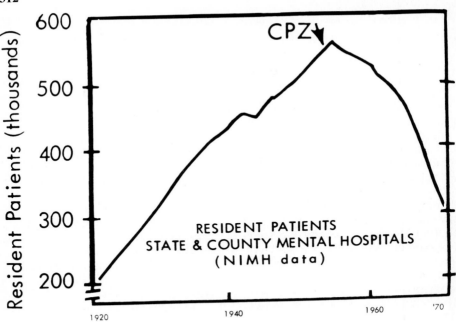
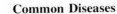

Fig. 1.   Effect of the introduction of antipsychotic drugs on the number of hospitalized patients.   From Davis (2).

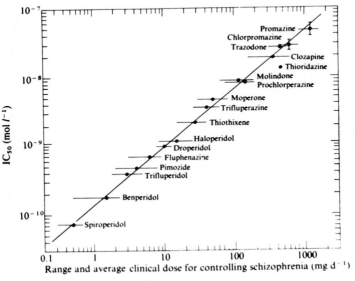

The IC₅₀ values (ordinate) are the concentrations of the antipsychotic drugs which reduce the stereospecific component of ³H-haloperidol binding by 50%. The abscissa indicates the average values (and ranges) of doses used for schizophrenia.

Fig. 2.   Correlation between clinical potency and affinity for the dopamine receptor.   From Seeman (3).

A number of drugs of the phenothiazine type exist which are not used in the treatment of psychosis (Fig. 3), and none of these structural analogues is an effective dopamine blocker - with one exception, thiethylperazine. This drug passes all the tests for a dopamine antagonist, but it has not generally been regarded as useful in schizophrenia. However, a recent study shows that this drug, too, is an effective anti-psychotic in appropriate doses (5), so this exception turns out to prove the rule.

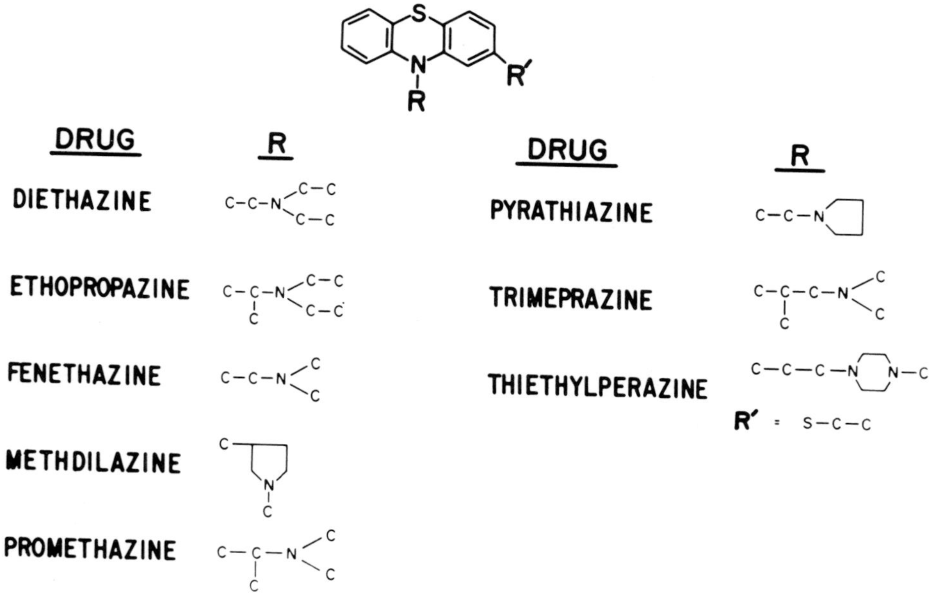

DRUG	R	DRUG	R
DIETHAZINE	C-C-N< C-C / C-C	PYRATHIAZINE	C-C-N◁
ETHOPROPAZINE	C-C-N< C-C / C-C (C)	TRIMEPRAZINE	C-C-C-N< C / C (C)
FENETHAZINE	C-C-N< C / C	THIETHYLPERAZINE	C-C-C-N◯N-C
METHDILAZINE	(pyrrolidine-N-C)		R' = S-C-C
PROMETHAZINE	C-C-N< C / C (C)		

Fig. 3. Phenothiazines not used in the treatment of psychosis (4).

With this favorable background, it is disappointing that all of the attempts to prove an excess of dopaminergic trans-mission in the brain of schizophrenic patients have found "no significant difference". There is no significant elevation of cerebrospinal fluid homovanillic acid (the chief metabol-ite of dopamine); no significant decrease in serum prolactin (prolactin is under inhibitory control by dopamine, so if there is too much dopamine there should be too little prol-actin); no significant decrease in brain dopamine-beta-hydroxylase or monoamine oxidase (decreases in these enzymes could elevate brain dopamine) (1).

However, in every one of these studies there are a number of patients whose biochemical measurements are precisely what the theory would have predicted (Figs. 4-7). This does not prove that the hypothesis is correct--they could merely represent sampling fluctuations--but it does emphasize the need for methods capable of distinguishing between random variability and underlying heterogeneity.

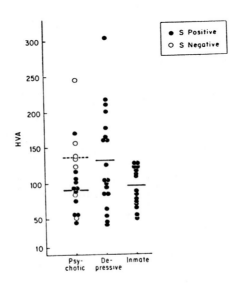

Fig. 4. Cerebrospinal fluid homovanillic acid in patients and controls. From Bowers (6). Bowers notes that patients without "first rank symptoms" according to the criteria of Schneider tended to have higher HVA values.

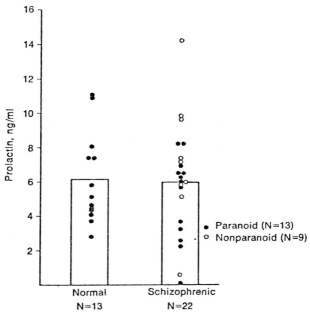

Fig. 5. Serum prolactin levels in patients and controls. From Meltzer (7). Note extremely low values in two patients. Meltzer comments "Two of the patients did have very low initial prolactin levels....However, such low levels have been reported in some normals, so it seems unlikely that the low levels in these two patients have any importance." On the other hand, low prolactin is only an indirect index of brain function, so similar levels do not necessarily imply identical brain processes.

Region	DBH activity.		
	All controls (mean ± S.E.M.)	Controls except one with long D-M time (mean ± S.E.M.)	Schizophrenic (mean ± S.E.M.)
Pons-mesencephalon	77.3 ± 19.5	84.8 ± 20.4	65.0 ± 14.3
Hypothalamus	140.8 ± 26.8	152.4 ± 27.4	118.3 ± 25.6
Hippocampus	39.8 ± 2.72	41.2 ± 2.66	35.5 ± 2.31
Whole rat brain	69.8 ± 2.75		

Fig. 6. Brain dopamine beta-hydroxylase in patients and controls. From Wyatt (8). Wise, Baden and Stein (9) had previously reported very substantial differences in the same direction. While these group means do not differ significantly, the trends suggest that some patients must have been low. Wise and Stein note (8) that the trends appear stronger if paranoid patients are excluded, as they were in their own study.

Subject	Diagnosis	Average MAO activity per sample n/mole/mg protein/20 min	MAO activity order (lowest first)
1	Schizophrenia	0.239	1
2	Schizophrenia	0.455	11
3	Schizophrenia	0.384	6
4	Schizophrenia	0.322	3
5	Schizophrenia	0.533	14
6	Schizophrenia	0.541	15
7	Schizophrenia	0.550	16
8	Schizophrenia	0.603	17 (Tie)
9	Schizophrenia	0.394	7
10	none	0.273	2
11	none	0.490	12
12	none	0.512	13
13	none	0.437	10
14	none	0.603	17 (Tie)
15	none	0.341	5
16	none	0.397	8
17	none	0.329	4
18	none	0.411	9

Fig. 7. Brain monoamine oxidase in schizophrenic patients and controls. From Schwartz et al. (10). The authors note that the subject with the lowest brain MAO, who was schizophrenic, also had low platelet MAO.

Some older hypotheses, which have been more or less discarded, may also still be viable, if account is taken of possible heterogeneity. For example, a study of the hallucinogenic compound dimethyltryptamine in blood of schizophrenics found no significant difference between the means, but several of the patients had high values (Fig. 8). Similarly, another study noted that two out of seventeen psychotic patients had elevated blood dimethyltryptamine levels (12).

The potential importance of deviant cases is not a new idea; it was emphasized as early as Claude Bernard's treatise on experimental medicine. In attempting to produce diabetes in rabbits by a puncture in the floor of the fourth ventricle, he succeeded initially, and then failed nearly ten times because of incorrect placement of the lesion. "Let me assume", he comments, "that, instead of succeeding at once in making a rabbit diabetic, all of the negative facts had first appeared; it is clear that, after failing two or three times, I should have concluded...that puncture of the fourth ventricle did not

produce diabetes. Yet I should have been wrong. How often
men must have been and still must be wrong in this way!" (13).
It is surprising that in biological psychiatry, our methods
are still unable to cope with the potentially informative
deviant case.

Patients and diagnosis	Sex	BPRS			Forrest test	DMT level
		Total	SUSP.	Halluc.		
1 – SAPT	Female	53	5	1	Negative	0.29
2 – SCUT	Male	41	3	4	Negative	0.07
3 – SAPT	Female	46	6	1	Trace	0.29
4 – SAPT	Female	49	4	4	1	0.13
5 – SAUT	Female	58	4	1	2	0.10
6 – SAATD	Female	32	3	3	Negative	0.11
7 – SCUT	Female	57	5	6	Negative	< 0.05
8 – SCATD	Male	45	3	4	Negative	0.13
9 – ALC and DEP	Male	32	3	1	Negative	< 0.05
10 – SAUT	Female	37	1	6	–	< 0.05
11 – SAPT	Female	38	6	1	–	< 0.05
12 – SCT(A)	Female	52	1	1	–	< 0.05
13 – S-LAT	Male	19	1	1	–	< 0.06
14 – Hypomanic	Male	29	1	1	–	0.15
15 – SAPT	Male	40	4	6	Negative	0.07
16 – SAUT*	Male	44	4	5	Negative	< 0.06
17 – Hypomanic**	Male	39	1	1	Negative	0.11
18 – SAATE	Female	67	5	4	–	< 0.05
19 – SCT(A)	Female	unable to rate			–	0.79
20 – SCUT	Male	33	2	1	–	< 0.05
21 – SAUT	Female	40	5	6	–	0.05
22 – SCUT	Female	26	1	3	Negative	< 0.05
23 – SCUT	Male	67	6	4	Negative	0.06

Fig. 8. Blood dimethyltryptamine in psychiatric patients.
From Angrist (11). The mean of the control was .049 ng/ml;
the highest control value was 0.22 ng/ml. SAPT, etc. denote
types of schizophrenia; ALC and DEP--chronic alcoholic, with
endogenous depression.

At the outset, there is no way to know if the deviant
values represent etiological heterogeneity or merely random
variation. Statistical tests for "outliers" will not help us.
A statistical "outlier" might merely reflect a major locus
unrelated to the disease, and conversely an extreme value
could represent a relevant biological deviation even if it
were part of an underlying normal distribution. Our motivation to follow up deviant values, rather than dismiss them
as random variation, rests on the inherent plausibility of
the concept of etiological diversity in schizophrenia.

Suppose, for example, that schizophrenia is indeed
associated with excessive dopaminergic activity in the brain.
This situation could be brought about in a number of ways.
There might be overproduction of dopamine in some patients;
others might have supersensitive dopamine receptors, or
defective inhibitory control of the dopaminergic neurons. In
Parkinson's disease, the treatment of choice until L-Dopa was
blockade of the cholinergic transmitter system, but there was
no actual excess of acetylcholine; rather there was too
little dopamine in the brain, and cholinergic blockade
restored a balance. Consequently, a functional excess of
dopamine could be caused by abnormalities in any of the several
transmitter systems that interact with dopamine, such as
acetylcholine and GABA (14).

Even if the dopamine system were known to be the primary
site of injury, its function could be damaged in a number of
different ways. There might be an insufficiency of any of
several enzymes that act upon dopamine (8-10). There could
be a tumor or vascular lesion in a dopaminergic region; many
cases of psychoses associated with tumors or brain injuries
are known (15). Although anatomical investigations in
schizophrenia have generally been negative, a defect in
neuronal connectivity, dendritic arborization or fine structure would have escaped notice because the histological
methods used were not capable of revealing this level of
detail (16). Purpura has observed dendritic spine abnormalities in Golgi preparations of biopsy tissue from the
brain of a 10-month old retarded infant (Fig. 9); these
techniques have not yet been applied to the psychoses.

Even immune and viral mechanisms could cause defects localized to a particular neurotransmitter system. In the past,
these processes have been discounted as possible causes because they generally damage brain tissue nonspecifically.
The case of myasthenia gravis shows, however, that the autoimmune processes can selectively damage one neurotransmitter
system (viz., the cholinergic system of skeletal muscle).
Antibodies reacting with acetylcholine receptor have been
detected in the sera of myasthenic patients, and the patients'
lymphocytes are stimulated to proliferate in the presence of
the receptor. It is also possible to produce experimental
myasthenia by injection of acetylcholine receptor protein
from other species (18).

Although viruses attacking particular neurotransmitter
systems are not known, it is interesting that bacterial
viruses tend to utilize active transport systems located in

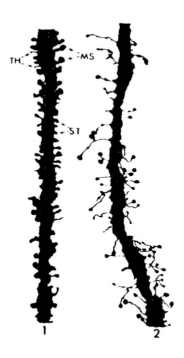

Fig. 9. Dendritic spines in the cerebral cortex of a
retarded infant (right). Note the long thin spines as
contrasted with the normal brain (left). From Purpura (17).

the cell membrane to gain access to the cell. The bacterio-
phage Φ80 attaches to the ferrichrome transport site of
E.coli; similarly, the virus BF23 is carried into the cell by
binding to the vitamin B_{12}carrier; and the phage λ utilizes
the maltose transport system. Each neurotransmitter system
in the brain has its own specific transport mechanisms for
carrying precursors into the nerve ending; in some cases
transmitters are also returned to the nerve ending after
release by an active reuptake process. The neurotoxin
6-hydroxydopamine functions by being transported into the
catecholamine neuron because of its similarity to the naturally occurring neurotransmitter, and once inside exerting a
nonspecific destructive effect. Central nervous system
viruses could, in principle, operate in the same way (18).

The possibility must also be considered that not all
schizophrenia is genetic. Kidd and I have analyzed the incidence data for relatives of schizophrenic patients in terms
of the single major locus model (19), and we conclude that

there is a range of possible gene frequencies. Within this
range, each gene frequency corresponds to a particular
division of the schizophrenic population into homozygotes,
heterozygotes and phenocopies (Fig. 10). Over most of the
permitted range, a substantial proportion of the cases are
predicted to be phenocopies. Homozygous schizophrenics are
estimated to be rare: not more than one in 45, according to
the single major locus model. The rarity of these individuals
may contribute to the difficulty of finding statistically
significant differences in the randomly sampled groups.

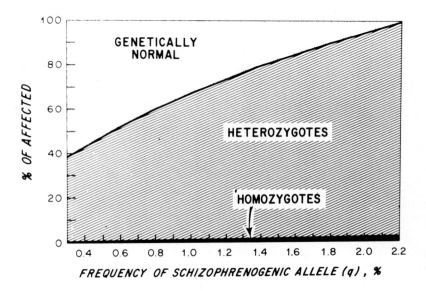

    Fig. 10. Composition of the schizophrenic population,
according to the single major locus model.

The polygenic model gives quite similar results when applied
to the same incidence data (20). Each schizophrenic patient
has a genetic risk, which we define as the probability that
he would develop schizophrenia if he were to start life over
again in a new, randomly selected environment. The probability distribution of genetic risk in the schizophrenic population has a significant peak at 100% risk, with a broad
distribution of lower risks (Fig. 11): 9.1% of the schizophrenic population is estimated to have a genetic risk of
99% or greater. Thus, the polygenic model, like the single
major locus model, predicts wide differences of genetic loading among schizophrenic patients.

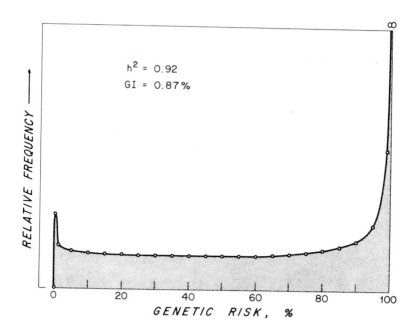

Fig. 11.   Distribution of genetic risk in the
schizophrenic population, according to the polygenic model.
The peak on the left has negligible area.

Additional evidence predisposing us to expect diversity of
etiology in schizophrenia comes from affective disorder, where
the existence of biochemical subtypes is becoming increasingly
likely.   Asberg has noted that cerebrospinal fluid concentration of the serotonin metabolite 5-hydroxyindoleacetic
acid appears to be bimodally distributed in depressed patients
(Fig.12).   There may be clinical differences between the two
subgroups.   40% of the low 5-HIAA group made suicide attempts,
in contrast to 15% of the highs;   the lows used more violent
means, and two of them died from suicide (21).

Patients with low 5-HIAA tend to respond relatively favor-
ably to chlorimipramine (Fig.13).   This drug potentiates biogenic amine transmission in the brain by blocking reuptake of
the released transmitter, and it appears to be particularly
active at serotonin synapses.   There is also some evidence
that the low 5-HIAA group responds to 5-hydroxytryptophan, a
serotonin precursor.   Conversely, the low 5-HIAA patients
are reported to respond relatively poorly to nortriptyline, a
noradrenaline uptake blocker (22).

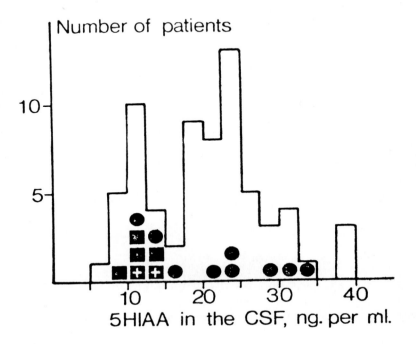

Fig. 12. Cerebrospinal fluid 5-HIAA in depressed
patients. From Asberg (21). Circles represent suicide
attempts with sedative drugs; squares, attempts with other
means; crosses, deaths from suicides.

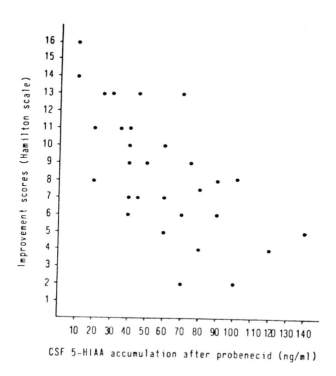

Fig. 13. Relation between cerebrospinal fluid 5-HIAA before treatment and therapeutic response to chlorimipramine. From Van Praag (22).

Another biochemical subgroup of the affective disorders is distinguished by low urinary 3-methoxy-4-hydroxy-phene-thylene glycol (MHPG), a metabolite of noradrenaline which is thought, in substantial part, to reflect brain noradrenaline metabolism. These patients have a relatively favorable response to the noradrenaline reuptake blockers imipramine and desmethylimipramine. Some show a mood brightening response to d-amphetamine (22,23).

The conflicting evidence on X-linkage in manic-depressive illness can also be interpreted as reflecting heterogeneity. Early studies reported absence of father-son transmission, and apparent linkage to colorblindness and to the Xg blood group (although simultaneous close linkage to these markers is inconsistent with the known distance between them). More recently, numerous cases of father-son transmission have been found, as well as pedigrees in which linkage does not appear to be present (24). Conceivably both X-linked and non-X-linked forms exist, and these were for some reason differentially represented in earlier and more recent samples.

The substantial psychological and psychophysiological differences found among schizophrenic patients also lend support to the concept of etiological heterogeneity (25). Gruzelier finds that schizophrenics subdivide into "responders" and "non-responders" in terms of psychophysiological reactivity. The responders habituate more slowly than normal to non-signal stimuli, whereas the non-responders habituate rapidly or may not react at all. There are corresponding differences in behavioral arousal (26). Patients can also be subdivided on the basis of their performance on the "continuous performance test", a measure of sustained attention. Poor performance is associated with a family history of mental illness, as well as with sleep disturbances (27).

So far, we have established that etiological diversity is highly plausible in schizophrenia, and that if it is present, statistically negative results are to be expected in studies of small random samples of patients, even if there are real abnormalities in subgroups. There are two strategies, however, that are capable of coping with heterogeneity.

The first is the systematic study of individuals who are deviant on any given biological variable, without regard to diagnosis. Buchsbaum et.al. have coined the term "biochemical high risk strategy" for this method. They divided a general population sample into deciles based on platelet monoamine oxidase, and compared the upper and lower decile on a number of psychological and familial variables. The families of the lower decile had a higher incidence of suicide. The low -MAO subjects showed increased stimulus seeking and high ego strength scores on psychological tests;

they also reported more active leisure time activities and more time each day socializing (28). Thus they seemed to fall more on the bipolar affective continuum than on the schizophrenia spectrum.

The other strategy is intensive study of pedigrees that include several affected individuals, on the assumption that only one etiological subtype is likely to be present in any one family. It is remarkable that hardly any studies of biological factors in schizophrenia have made use of pedigree methods. The two strategies can effectively be combined, by selecting as subjects schizophrenic patients who deviate on some biological variable of interest and also come from families where there are several affected individuals. Even with large pedigrees, however, statistical comparison of unaffected and affected individuals within the pedigree is not likely to reach a high level of significance. If heterogeneity is present, data from many families will be necessary in order to prove the existence of a biological subgroup. Consequently, if these methods are to be practical, psychiatric journals will have to become accustomed to accepting papers with sound methodology which show interesting trends, even if statistical significance is not reached. Indeed, the publication of complete pedigrees, with each member accurately classified according to research diagnostic criteria, would in itself be a major step forward for genetic analysis.

With those methods, our objective would be gradual delineation of biological subtypes by accumulation of data from many studies rather than confirmation or discomfirmation of a hypothesis applicable to all schizophrenics. Claims will have to be more modest, but methods which take heterogeneity into account may--if I may use a pharmacologist's term--make the process of "release and reuptake" of theories of schizophrenia less frustrating.

Acknowledgements. Supported by Research Scientist Development Award K2-MH-00108 and P.H.S. Grants MH-16674 and MH-25515.

References

1. Matthysse, S. The role of dopamine in schizophrenia. In: Neuroregulators and Psychiatric Disorders (E. Usdin, D.A. Hamburg and J.D. Barchas, Eds.) N.Y.: Oxford University Press, 1977, pp.3-13.

2. Davis, J. Personal communication

3. Seeman, P., Lee, T., Chau-Wong, M., and Wong, K. Antipsychotic drug doses and neuroleptic/dopamine receptors. Nature 261:717-719, 1976.

4. Matthysse, S. Antipsychotic drug actions: a clue to the neuropathology of schizophrenia? Fed. Proc. 32:200-205, 1973.

5. Rotrosen, J. et.al. Thiethylperazine: clinical antipsychotic efficacy and correlation with potency in predictive systems. Arch. Gen. Psychiat. in press.

6. Bowers, M.B., Jr. 5-hydroxyindoleacetic acid (5H1AA) and homovanillic acid (HVA) following probenecid in acute psychotic patients treated with phenothiazines. Psychopharmacologia 28: 309-318, 1973.

7. Meltzer, H.Y., Sachar,E.J., and Frantz, A.G. Serum prolactin levels in unmedicated schizophrenic patients. Arch. Gen. Psychiat. 31:564-569, 1974.

8. Wyatt, R.J., Schwartz, M.A., Erdelyi, E., and Barchas, J.D. Dopamine-β-hydroxylase in brains of chronic schizophrenic patients. Science 187 368-370, 1975.

9. Wise, C.D., Baden, M.M., and Stein, L. Post-mortem measurements of enzymes in human brain: evidence of a central noradrenergic defect in schizophreniz. J. Psychiat.Res. 11: 185-198, 1974.

10. Schwartz, M.A., Aikens, A.M., and Wyatt, R.J. Monoamine oxidase activity in brains from schizo-phrenic and mentally normal individuals. Psychopharmacologia 38: 319-328, 1974.

11. Angrist, B., Gershon, S., Sathananthan, G., Walker, R.W., Lopez-Ramos, B., Mandel, L.R., and Vandenheuvel, W.J.A. Dimethyltryptamine levels in blood of schizophrenic patients and control subjects. Psychopharmacology 47: 29-32, 1976.

12. Lipinski,J.F., Mandel, L.R., Ahn, H.S., Vandenheuvel, W.J.A., and Walker, R.W. Blood dimethyltryptamine concentrations in psychotic disorders. Biol. Psychiat. 9: 89-91, 1974.

13. Bernard, C. An Introduction to the Study of Experimental Medicine. Schuman, 1949, pp. 173-4

14. Matthysse, S., and Sugarman, J. Neurotransmitter theories of schizophrenia. In: Handbook of Psycho-pharmacology, vol. 10 (L.L. Iversen, S.D.Iversen, and S.H. Snyder, Eds.) N.Y. Plenum Press, in press.

15. Davison,K., and Bagley, C.R. Schizophrenia-like psychoses associated with organic disorders of the central nervous system, a review of the literature. Br.J. Psychiat. Special Publication #4, pp.113-184, 1969.

16. Matthysse, S. and Pope, A. The approach to schizophrenia through molecular pathology. In: Molecular Pathology (R.A. Good, S.B. Day, and G. Yunis, Eds.) Springfield, Ill., Charles C. Thomas, 1975, pp.744-768

17. Purpura, D.P. Dendritic spine "dysgenesis" and mental retardation. Science 186:1126-8, 1974.

18. Matthysse,S. and Matthysse,A.G. Virological and immunological hypotheses of schizophrenia. In: Psychopharmacology: A Generation of Progress. N.Y.: Raven Press, in press.

19. Matthysse,S. and Kidd,K.K. Estimating the genetic contribution to schizophrenia. Am. J. Psychiat. 133: 185-191, 1976.

20. Matthysse, S., and Kidd, K.K. Genetic principles in defining homogeneous subgroups of the schizophrenias. In: Psychiatric Diagnosis: Exploration of Biological Predictors (H.S. Akiskal and W.L. Webb, Eds.) Jamaica, N.Y., Spectrum Publications, in press.

21. Asberg, M., Traskman,L., and Thoren,P. 5-HIAA in the cerebrospinal fluid: a biochemical suicide predictor? Arch.Gen.Psychiat. 33: 1193-7, 1976.

22. Van Praag, H.M. Significance of biochemical parameters in the diagnosis, treatment, and prevention of depressive disorders. Biological Psychiat. 12:101-131, 1977.

23. Maas.,J.W. Biogenic amines and depression: biochemical and pharmacological separation of two types of depression. Arch.Gen.Psychiat. 32:1357-1361, 1975.

24. Gershon, E.S., and Bunney, W.E.,Jr. The question of X-Linkage in bipolar manic-depressive illness. J. Psychiat. Res. 13:99-117,1976.

25. Houlihan,J.P. Heterogeneity among schizophrenic patients: selective review of recent findings (1970-75). Schizophrenia Bulletin 3:246-258, 1977.

26. Gruzelier, J.H. Bimodal arousal and lateralised dysfunction in schizophrenia: the effect of chlorpromazine upon psychophysiological, information processing and endocrine measures. In: The Nature of Schizophrenia: New Approaches to Research and Treatment (L.Wynne, R.L.Cromwell and S.Matthysse, Eds.) N.Y., John Wiley and Sons, 1978.

27. Kornetsky,C., and Orzack,M.H. Physiological and behavioral correlates of attention dysfunction in pschiatric patients. J.Psychiat. Res., in press.

28. Buchsbaum,M.S., Coursey,R.D., and Murphy,D.L. The biochemical high-risk paradigm: behavioral and familial correlates of low platelet, monoamine oxidase activity. Science 194:339-341, 1976.

DISCUSSION

CLONINGER: Etiological heterogeneity is a major problem in the study of common diseases and the psychoses are no exception, as Dr. Matthysse's review of the clinical studies clearly illustrates. Available strategies, including those advocated by Dr. Matthysse, are unfortunately limited in their ability to deal with the difficulties presented.

The biochemical high risk paradigm may be really informative in those rare instances where the marker trait is temporally stable and associated with a specific phenotype. However, the comparison of extreme groups from a general population is unlikely to define etiologically or phenotypically homogeneous populations for further study. In general a more robust method is to carry out family studies in which phenotypic and etiological heterogeneity are considered simultaneously as in the multiple threshold method (Reich, Cloninger, Guze, Brit. J. Psych., 127:1-10, 1975). Then variation in important phenotypic factors such as sex, severity, age of onset, or other types of traits (clinical, physiological, or biochemical) can be related to differences in familial aggregation. In this way groups of patients who are more homogeneous etiologically may be identified for further study and no one is in the hopelessly subjective position of trying to distinguish the presence of a few statistical outliers from etiological heterogeneity.

Study of extended pedigrees is a promising method, as Dr. Elston pointed out earlier. However, the assumption that the cause of a common phenotype is homogeneous throughout any given pedigree is unfortunately questionable. Dr. Elving Anderson has recently presented some interesting results about etiological heterogeneity in sibships affected with epilepsy, a disorder occurring at about the same frequency as schizophrenia, i.e., roughly 1% of the population. His simulations indicate that even within single sibships the risk of multiple etiologies for the same phenotype is not negligible. Nevertheless, it seems likely that such heterogeneity is less frequent when large pedigrees are analyzed individually than when many small sibships are pooled to carry out segregation analysis.

ANDERSON: When a condition such as schizophrenia is heterogeneous in etiology there is an inherent difficulty in testing biochemical hypotheses. If a specific metabolite is altered in a small fraction of cases this deviation will be missed whenever data from all cases are pooled.

We are currently working on a study of epilepsy and have been exploring the use of multiplex sibships, those with at least two affected siblings available for further study. This strategy is cost-effective in the sense that it provides a highly screened sample on which to test biochemical and other hypotheses. It also permits an analysis of the results within and between pairs.

Dr. Myra Chern and I have attempted some computer modeling to evaluate in what fraction of such pairs the causes will be the same in both members of the pair. We assume that epilepsy affects 1% of the population and results from a mix of Mendelian, multifactorial, and sporadic (low risk) conditions. Computer modeling using a deterministic approach showed that at least 85% of the pairs would be homogeneous, with the same cause in both members of the pair. We have now completed a stochastic approach generating runs with 100 multiplex pairs in each. There is considerable variation from run to run in the number of pairs with a given etiology, but the number of homogeneous pairs is quite stable, and close to the expected value of at least 85%.

PYLORIC STENOSIS AND THE SIMULATION OF MENDELISM

M. Anne Spence and
Keith Gladstien

Mental Retardation Center
University of California
Los Angeles, California

INTRODUCTION

A shared environmental factor can be solely responsible for the aggregation of a disease within a family. However, when the risk to relatives of probands is elevated up to 50 fold above that for the general population and there is no evidence of a clearly defined environmental cause, the conclusion usually drawn is that genes play at least some role in the etiology of the trait. This partial gene involvement is the current interpretation for the occurrence of pyloric stenosis (1).

The elevated recurrence risks for pyloric stenosis, although varying slightly from study to study, are well documented for a variety of populations (1-5). Numerous papers report series of families with more than one affected individual (6-9), including one set of triplets (10) and occurrences in multiple generations of the same family (11). The most striking pedigree was reported by Snyder in 1943 (12) where 11 individuals were affected in three generations.

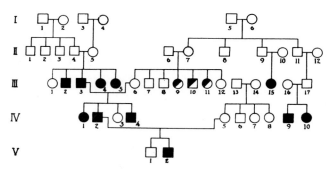

Pedigree of congenital pyloric stenosis:

III—2, Died of pyloric stenosis at 5 months. 3, Recovered from pyloric stenosis. 4, Died of
pyloric stenosis at 5 months. 5, Died of pyloric stenosis at one day. 9, Died at two
months, cause undetermined. 10, Died at three days, cause undetermined. 11, Born
dead. 15, Died in infancy of pyloric stenosis.
IV—1, Died of pyloric stenosis at 8 days. 2, Recovered from pyloric stenosis; father of propositus. 4, Died of pyloric stenosis at 9 months. 9, Died of pyloric stenosis in infancy.
10, Recovered from pyloric stenosis.
V—2, Propositus; operated on for pyloric stenosis; recovered.

Snyder (12)

There were three additional cases of individuals dying in
infancy, cause undetermined. Unfortunately, only one diagnosis was confirmed by surgery. The other diagnoses were
defined by similarity of symptoms including projectile
vomiting and gastric peristalsis. Seven of the ten untreated
cases died prior to five months of age. This family represents an unusually intense concentration of cases, with a sex
ratio of nearly 1:1 (six affected males, five affected females). There is no clear propensity for affected first born,
but the symptoms and mortality rate are clearly compatible
with the diagnosis of pyloric stenosis.

If the occurrence of multiple cases within families is
sufficient to support the idea of gene involvement with
pyloric stenosis, it is not in itself sufficient to indicate
the relative importance of environmental vs. genetic factors
nor the specific type of genetic mechanism.

Earlier genetic studies, notably that of Cockayne and
Penrose (13) suggested that a recessive gene was responsible
for pyloric stenosis. These authors invoked reduced penetrance to explain the failure to observe the expected
Mendelian ratios.

The development of polygenic or multifactorial threshold
models provided an alternate model of gene-environment interaction that might produce a phenotypic trait. In his initial

presentation, Falconer analyzed data on pyloric stenosis and suggested that it represented this type of trait, a multi-factorial disease (14).

Carter in a series of articles (15-17) discussed the various attributes of pyloric stenosis which seem to lend themselves to the multifactorial concept. These aspects included frequency differences between the sexes and among the relatives, environmental contributions to the etiology reflected as possible birth order effects, seasonal variations, and a relation to maternal age. And, maternal-fetal interactions are implicated by changes in gastrin levels during pregnancy in experimental work with dogs (18).

In the late 1960's when the multifactorial threshold model was heralded as the principal explanation for most human malformations, pyloric stenosis was championed as the classic multifactorial trait. However, this explanation of the data has recently been disputed (19). And even in 1969, Carter and Evans (17) suggested that the etiology of pyloric stenosis was best explained by a major gene segregating with a polygenic background.

It is assumed that some genetic factors contribute to the etiology of this disease because of the family aggregation patterns. Several questions remain: (1) Is the genetic contribution many genes each with small, nearly equal, and additive effects? (2) Will this multifactorial threshold model explain all the data? (3) Does a major gene contribute to all cases, with modification by environment? or (4) Does a major gene account for a portion of the cases while environmental factors with or without the action of polygenes account for the remainder?

First we will discuss the epidemiological aspects of this trait which are relevant to all genetic analyses and which must be accounted for in any purported explanation of the data on pyloric stenosis. Then, we will evaluate the evidence from the genetic analyses for each of the possible explanations of the etiology of pyloric stenosis.

EPIDEMIOLOGY

Pyloric stenosis is a disease of infancy resulting from hypertrophy of the pylorus. Symptoms usually begin within the first two months of life and may be present at birth (20). Clinical symptoms include projectile vomiting and weight loss which may lead to malnutrition and alkalosis (21). In the majority of cases, treatment is by surgical procedure although medication may be employed.

Diagnosis is confirmed at surgery by the presence of the pyloric tumor. Radiological evidence is also considered

conclusive (22). There have been some suggestions that
affected individuals could fail to come to medical attention
and therefore not be diagnosed. Very little documentation
exists to support this suggestion.

Incidence

     The incidence of pyloric stenosis varies markedly from
racial group to racial group. The reports for United States
Caucasians are approximately 0.13% (2,23). For the British
Isles, the frequencies are similar, varying from 0.25% in
Oxford (24) to 0.3 to 0.4% in London (17). Figures for
Oriental populations were stated as low (13). The study in
Hawaii failed to detect any cases of pyloric stenosis in
11,274 Chinese births but found a frequency of 0.052% for
Japanese and 0.082% for Koreans. Both of these figures are
higher than the 0.046% reported for American Blacks (23).
     Dodge (3) reported incidence figures for Belfast over the
13 year period 1957-1969 in which it appears the incidence of
pyloric stenosis is declining. No possible explanation for
this observation is suggested. Wallgren (25) also reported a
decline in incidence for Sweden from 4/1000 to 3/1000 live
births. The study in Hawaii (2) covered the period 1942-1966
and gave a statistically significant positive, though small,
regression coefficient for year of birth and incidence. We
attributed this increase partially to better diagnostic
techniques and principally to greatly improved hospital
recordkeeping systems and accessibility of records. These
logistic factors were quite apparent in the Hawaiian retrospective study: a paucity of cases were detected in the first
few years studied. McLean (26) reported an increase in incidence in Northeast Scotland from 1938 to 1953 which was
also attributed to better diagnostic techniques.
     None of the yearly changes in incidence are striking.
Even though they obtain statistical significance, it is not
apparent that they represent basic changes in the occurrence
of pyloric stenosis. Studies over longer periods of time will
be required to determine if these changes reflect long-term
oscillations or new trends in the incidence of pyloric
stenosis.

Sex Differences

     Studies from a number of populations and ethnic groups
report a marked difference in the frequency of pyloric stenosis in the two sexes. For the British Isles, the ratio of
affected males to affected females range from 3.5:1 in

Belfast (3) to 5.5:1 in Oxford (24). The ratio in Japanese in Hawaii was 3.3:1, which was not significantly different from the 4.8:1 in Caucasians in the same population (2). From a larger sample in Japan, Osawa et al. (4) reported an overall ratio of 4.2:1. Their ratio ranged from 3.0:1 in Shikoka District where 16 affected individuals were observed to 7.2:1 in Chubo District where 82 affected individuals were observed.

Reports also exist for several additional population centers within the United States including Louisville (27) 3.3:1, Detroit (20) 3.7:1, and Los Angeles (21) 4.0:1. Reports from other populations include Malta (28) 2.7:1, Hungary (5) 3.1:1, and Iran (29) where the three affected cases were male. No study has failed to find an excess of affected males for pyloric stenosis irrespective of the sample size or the specific diagnostic criteria applied.

Birth Order and Maternal Age Effects

A number of investigators (3,4,13,21,30-40) have reported an association between pyloric stenosis and birth order. The majority of these authors (4,21,32,33,36-38,40) compared the percentage of affected individuals in the early birth ranks and the distribution of birth ranks in the population at large, while others (3,31) used a control population for comparison, and some (13,32,35,36,40) simply state that the percentage of first born for pyloric stenosis infants is higher without making any comparison. A relationship between the etiology of this disease and birth order is widely, but by no means unanimously, accepted.

Several authors (41-49) found no evidence for a birth order effect either by comparing the distribution of birth ranks in the ascertained population with the same distribution in the population at large, or by discounting the importance of one child families. As early as 1933, it was noted by Faxen (44) that any analysis of a birth order effect in pyloric stenosis must not allow the one child families to bias the results. If the distribution of sibship sizes in a study is significantly different from the expected distribution an erroneous conclusion may be drawn with regard to birth order effect. For example, if the number of ascertained small sibships is greater than expected, a disproportionate number of affected individuals in the early birth ranks will be found. Because of this problem, it is difficult to interpret comparisons of the percentage of affected individuals in birth ranks and the distribution of birth ranks in the population.

In order to detect birth order effects, more rigorous methods have been proposed (47,50-54). However, four of these methods (51-54) may be misinterpreted (50) and share the drawback that they lose information by pooling birth rank data. In addition, analyses of birth rank distribution are hindered by the presence of incomplete sibships and by changes in the number of propositi ascertained in certain stages during the compilation of the data.

Barker and Record (55) address these and other problems and demonstrate that the results of birth rank analysis depend upon factors largely, if not entirely, ignored by the investigators studying pyloric stenosis. Using their method of related frequencies, Barker and Record claim the data of MacMahon et al. (56) give evidence for a birth order effect. To simplify the explanation of their procedure we discuss families with sibship size two, exactly one of whom is affected. We assume probands are ascertained from years i to k, and π_j and n_j are the ascertainment probability and the number of these families in the population at large in year j, respectively. Then if there were no birth order effect, the number of affected individuals in the first birth rank of families perceived as having sibship size two is expected to be $\pi_i n_i + \ldots + \pi_{k-1} n_{k-1}$ while the number in the second birth rank is expected to be $\pi_i n_i + \ldots + \pi_k n_k$. To correct for this bias due to incomplete sibships, Barker and Record suggest analyzing the families which result from the elimination of all sibs born outside the period of ascertainment. They would then find no birth rank effect if the number of families, still with sibship size two, ascertained at the beginning and end of the study were equal.

Their first analysis produced no evidence for a birth order effect, but they noted an increase in ascertained incidence over the ten years 1940-1949 of the study. A second analysis using families ascertained during the first six years of their study and eliminating sibs born before 1936 and after 1949 revealed evidence for a firstborn effect, but the authors failed to justify their use of families ascertained from 1940 to 1945 by citing the appropriate ascertained incidence figures.

The statistical problems are now sufficiently understood so that a definitive analysis could be undertaken. However, most of the data sets published do not contain the necessary details on sampling procedures, birth dates and family size. At this point, the issue of a birth order effect has not been adequately resolved.

Other factors complicate the issue of a birth order effect and should be considered in the final analysis. For example, some investigators have advocated an overall birth order effect and some only when consideration is restricted to infants with onset later than three weeks after birth (Wright, personal communication). If the latter is true and if a birth order effect is present, then this would produce a criterion for subdividing the data to search for factors associated with the birth order effect.

In our extensive family interviews in the Hawaii study, it became apparent that affected first born children come to medical attention later. This is due both to the mother's uncertainty about feeding problems and the simple diagnoses which are pursued first, e.g., milk allergies (2). Therefore, the fact that first born affected individuals appear to have later onset and surgery is most likely due to sociological factors.

If first born prove to be at increased risk for contracting this disorder, then one might be tempted to hypothesize that first born males represent a group of individuals with a markedly increased liability for pyloric stenosis. However, both McKeown et al. (30) and Campbell (2) failed to detect any additional deviations in the sex ratio of the first born affected infants.

Although correlated with birth order, maternal age factors are another variable to be examined with respect to the frequency of occurrence for pyloric stenosis. Dodge (3) reported an age distribution for mothers of affected children not greatly different from the distribution in the general population of Belfast. There was, however, a slight tendency towards younger mothers. McKeown et al. (20) in their extensive study failed to detect a maternal age factor associated with pyloric stenosis. In addition to a birth order effect, Osawa et al. (4) report maternal age effect in their series of 773 affected individuals from eight districts of Japan. The male patients exhibited both an increased frequency among first born and from mothers over 30 years of age. Although female patients did not show the birth order effect, they were born to older mothers more frequently than expected. None of the reports detail a striking maternal age effect and it would appear to be of minimal consequence.

Birth Weight

Shim et al. (22) reported a statistically significant increase in mean birth weight for infants who develop pyloric stenosis. This finding was consistent within the Caucasian, Japanese, and hybrid Caucasian/Japanese samples of their Hawaiian study. Cziezel (5) confirmed this finding for males in his Hungarian sample. The tendency was also present in females in his study, but perhaps due to small sample size,

failed to achieve statistical significance. Analysis in both
studies confirmed the difference was due to increased birth
weight independent of influence due to sex or birth order.
Cziezel also demonstrated that gestation time was not responsible for the different weights.

Dodge (3) comments on a slight excess of larger infants
which he attributes to possible bias toward higher social
classes in his series. Gordon et al. (21) in their study of
over 1000 infants in Los Angeles indicate an increased mean
birth weight for the pyloric stenosis infants on a graph but
neglect further comment. Adelstein and Federick (24) report
no differences in birth weight between their 220 affected
infants and a matched control series of 615 infants.

There is evidence from several studies that babies with
pyloric stenosis tend to have heavier birth weights than
normal infants. However, support for this view is not unani-
mous and it is not yet clear whether this phenomenon varies
from population to population or merely reflects differences
in the ability to detect the increase based on study design
and sample size.

Seasonal Variation

Studies on pyloric stenosis also vary markedly in their
ability to detect evidence for a seasonal variation in the
occurrence of the disease. An early report by Kwok and Avery
(57) described a marked seasonal variation for data from
Washington, D.C. Campbell (58) replied to their study by
pointing out that the authors analyzed date of admission
instead of date of birth. In fact, their sample of affected
individuals showed a pattern in distribution of month of birth
similar to the normal population but with about a six week
delay. The average time from birth to surgery is approximately
six weeks. Campbell failed to detect any evidence for seasonal variation in the Hawaii study (58).

Cziezel (5) failed to detect a significant alteration in
the distribution for month of birth for pyloric stenosis infants in his Hungarian study. However, two recent studies by
Dodge in Belfast (3) and Adelstein and Federick in Oxford
(24) report statistically significant peak periods in births
for pyloric stenosis, winter months and July, respectively.
It is not clear what biological interpretation could accompany
these results. A study in the United States undertook extensive virological workups on affected infants, with negative
results (59).

GENETIC ANALYSES

Twin Studies

A large number of twin pairs with one or both members affected with pyloric stenosis have been reported. Kidd and Spence (19) were able to collect 92 monozygotic twin pairs from the literature. Of these, 62 of the 72 male pairs and 14 of the 20 female pairs were concordant. Analysis of these data is difficult and the interpretations complex. Little information is available on how the pairs were ascertained, i.e., whether one or both twins should be designated probands. In fact, this distinction may not ever be easy to assign. Very little information is reported on the criteria used for determining zygosity. Many of these pairs are from older reports in the literature when undoubtedly fewer tests, particularly blood tests, could have been applied to determine zygosity (60-62). Both genetic models analyzed by Kidd and Spence (19) predicted a rate of concordance much lower than observed in this pooled sample. Concerns about sampling bias led to the twin data being excluded from our final analyses.

Without a complete series of twins from a sufficiently large study with good zygosity determination, the interpretation of any concordance figures is tentative at best. We have no idea of the extent of the bias in reporting twin pairs either because of the status in concordance or zygosity. It is a simple matter to derive incorrect ideas from such data, a topic discussed in detail by Smith (63).

Data on twins can provide valuable insight into the importance of genetic contributions to disease, at least to the degree of defining the range of possible involvement. Good information on like and unlike sexed dizygotic twins might provide a measure of the importance of interuterine environmental factors in producing such a different frequency of pyloric stenosis in the two sexes. At this point, however, almost no rigorous interpretation of the available data is warranted with the possible exception that pyloric stenosis can and will occur in twins.

Segregation Analysis

Cockayne and Penrose (13) proposed a recessive Mendelian factor for pyloric stenosis on the basis of the definite familial incidence and the increased proportion of patients with consanguineous parents. They invoked reduced penetrance, supported by environmental influence in birth order effects and sex frequency differences, to explain the failure to observe the expected Mendelian ratios.

Data from our Hawaiian study were subjected to segregation analysis (9) as developed by Morton (64), to test the
major gene hypothesis for pyloric stenosis. The models
employed were those for incomplete selection, i.e., ascertainment through an affected child (64,65), as programmed for
a CDC 3100 computer (66). In these models, three parameters
are estimated:

     (i) p, the segregation frequency, e.g., for
          recessive genes in normal by normal
          matings, p = 1/4.

    (ii) x, the proportion of sporadic cases.

   (iii) π, the probability of ascertainment

The data were grouped by sibship size and the distribution of affected individuals and probands within sibships was
analyzed. Parents and children were classified as affected
(with pyloric stenosis) or normal. The number of affected
sibs, r, plus the number of normal sibs, c, sum to the sibship
size s. The number of probands within a family is designated
a where a is less than or equal to r.

The probability distribution of r affected among s sibs
is used to provide information about the segregation frequency p. The probability for the distribution of a probands
among r affected provides information about π free of assumptions concerning p and x when the probands are independently
ascertained. Specific forms for these distributions are
given by Morton (64) and the summary sr and ra tables are
specified in the original study (2).

The analysis was applied to a pooled data set consisting
of 249 families reported by Carter (15), 476 families detailed by McKeown et al. (67), and 111 Caucasian families
from the Hawaiian study (2). Several tests for heterogeneity
among the three data sets, based on the estimates of the
parameters, were not significant (2). Families with one or
more affected parents were deleted and the maximum likelihood
estimates for the parameters over the remaining 828 families
gave the following estimates and their standard errors:

$$\hat{p} = 0.196 \pm 0.117$$
$$\hat{x} = 0.789 \pm 0.105$$
$$\hat{\pi} = 0.597 \pm 0.084$$

When x was set equal to zero and held constant during the
iterations for estimating p and π, the following estimates
were obtained:

$$\hat{p} = 0.036 \pm 0.006$$
$$\hat{\pi} = 0.594 \pm 0.084$$

A comparison of these two sets of estimates was used to test if the proportion of sporadic cases in the data is significant, i.e., if the families can be divided into a group with a high risk of recurrence and a group with a low risk. Such a division would result if x differed significantly from zero (65). Three chi-square tests are available from the analysis, one from the $UK^{-1}U$ scores, one from the likelihood, and one from the chi-square goodness-of-fit test. All three achieved statistical significance being 11.9, 5.7 and 18.0, respectively, with one degree of freedom.

These studies would indicate that a major gene with an approximately recessive segregation frequency could account for pyloric stenosis if 79% of the cases were attributed to sporadic, low risk causes, e.g., mutation and phenocopies.

Multifactorial Threshold Model Analyses

The failure to detect a major gene which could account for a significant portion of the data on pyloric stenosis stimulated interest in the suggestion of Falconer (14) that pyloric stenosis was a multifactorial threshold trait.

Under Falconer's model (14), the theoretical liability for a trait is assumed to be normally distributed and is attributed to random environment and to the action of genes with small, nearly equal, and additive effects. A threshold, presumably set by physiological constaints, divides the distribution into affected and unaffected individuals. Any individual with a sufficient number of alleles for the trait and/or a sufficient number of environmental factors will exceed the threshold and be classified as affected, resulting in a dichotomous trait. Utilizing the properties of a normal distribution, incidence of the trait in the general population and the incidence among different classes of relatives of probands, it is possible to estimate heritability in the narrow sense, i.e., the proportion of the total variance of liability attributed to additive gene effects.

The preliminary analyses of pyloric stenosis by Falconer (14) and Carter (15-17) consisted of compiling recurrence frequencies for different classes of relatives of probands and estimating the heritability of the liability for pyloric stenosis. These estimates, as summarized by Carter and Evans (17), are 76%, 27%, and 50% for first, second, and third degree relatives, respectively. The lower estimate for second degree relatives was attributed to incomplete diagnoses among aunts and uncles in an earlier generation. The authors emphasized that these weighted estimates of heritability below 100% indicate that there is no major gene effect on the liability for the disease. And they added that this interpretation is strengthened by the fact that the estimates remain low for second and third degree relatives, since a major gene would have inflated the heritability markedly. Their estimates of heritability for probands and relatives of unlike sex versus those of probands and relatives of like sex appear to be consistent.

In 1972, Reich et al. (68) generalized the multifactorial model to include more than one threshold. The resulting model extended the analyses from estimation of heritability to permit a statistical testing of goodness of fit. The only additional requirement was some basis for subdividing the data into at least two categories of affected status. Although there have been suggestions of differences in severity for pyloric stenosis, these are not sufficiently well documented to serve as criteria for subdividing the data. However, Kidd et al. (69) have shown that the same statistical benefits as the Reich et al. generalization are present when the data can be characterized by different frequencies in the two sexes, a fact well documented for pyloric stenosis. The multifactorial multiple threshold model of Kidd et al. (69) was applied to pyloric stenosis by Kidd and Spence (19), using essentially the same pooled data set as that analyzed under segregation analysis. This model yielded estimates of 0.0048 and 0.0011 for the male and female general population incidences, respectively, and 0.442 for the correlation coefficient of liability for sibs and parent-offspring data classes. These estimates are reasonable, and in good agreement with expectation. However, the predicted frequencies for the data classes based on these estimates led to the rejection of the hypothesis that the multifactorial model could account for the data, $\chi^2_6 = 15.01$, p $\sim$ 0.02.

Comparative risks for pyloric stenosis data,
utilizing the multiple threshold model

(Kidd and Spence, J. Med. Genet., 1976)

Multifactorial Model

Probands

| | Male | | Female | |
	Obs.	Exp.	Obs.	Exp.
Brothers	.061	.075	.106	.109
Sisters	.024	.025	.042	.040
Sons	.055	.075	.194	.109
Daughters	.024	.025	.073	.040
Population Incidence	.0048	.0048	.0012	.0010

Having rejected the multifactorial model, we applied a similar threshold model to test for a single major locus (70,71) with the same data set, and reported that this model could not be excluded (19).

Comparative risks for pyloric stenosis data,
utilizing the multiple threshold model

(Kidd and Spence, J. Med. Genet., 1976)

Single Major Locus

Probands

	Male		Female	
	Obs.	Exp.	Obs.	Exp.
Brothers	.061	.060	.106	.124
Sisters	.024	.024	.042	.051
Sons	.055	.060	.194	.124
Daughters	.024	.024	.073	.051
Population Incidence	.0048	.0051	.0012	.0010

$$\chi_5^2 = 8.02, \; p \sim 0.15$$

The major locus could account for only 37% of the cases, requiring environmental factors to account for the remainder. This finding is not strikingly different from that reported from segregation analysis (2).

In an attempt to confirm the rejection of the multifactorial model for pyloric stenosis, Gladstien et al. (72) developed a goodness-of-fit test designed to include ascertainment probabilities, particularly if the frequency of the trait differs in the two sexes. The test requires computing the theoretical distribution of nuclear families with more than one affected sib conditioned on several family dependent variables. These include whether the family was ascertained via only affected males or via at least one affected female, and the affected versus normal status of both parents. Ultimately, a direct measure of the probability of observing the data set is obtained.

This test for the multifactorial model was applied to the families with more than one sib, from the published data of McKeown et al. (67). No other data were appropriate for analysis because determination of proband status within each sibship is critical; this could not be reconstructed from the data of Carter and Evans (17).

The calculations for this data set were done using population incidences for males and females of 5/1000 and 1/1000, respectively. A realistic range of values for both the ascertainment probability π, and the narrow sense heritability, h^2, was used. The estimate of π directly from the data was 0.77 ±0.08. Carter and Evans (17) estimate h^2 to lie between 0.65 and 0.85. With these values of π and h^2, the p values range from 0.45 to 0.001 for the data set of McKeown et al. Without a more explict determination of these two parameters, it is not possible to reject the multifactorial hypothesis based on this set of data:

Computed p-values for pyloric stenosis data given ascertainment is sex dependent. Eighteen families with recurrences out of 319 families.

Values of h^2	Ascertainment Probability, π					
	.5	.6	.7	.8	.9	1.0
.85	.6	.5	.4	.3	.2	.1
.80	.4	.3	.2	.1	.1	.04
.75	.3	.2	.1	.07	.04	.017
.70	.1	.1	.05	.03	.014	.006
.65	.06	.04	.02	.01	.005	.002

Since no alternate hypotheses are specified with this model, the power of the method cannot be determined theoretically. It is difficult to assess what weight to give to the result that the multifactorial model could not be rejected.

A better approach statistically, is to consider both single major locus and multifactorial inheritance as subhypotheses under a general model. In the most recent analysis, Lalouel et al. (73) fit the mixed segregation analysis model of Morton and MacLean (74) to data on pyloric stenosis. This model assumes that a major locus, a polygenic component and the environment contribute independently to the underlying theoretical liability for a trait. Since both a single locus and the multifactorial concept can be treated as subhypotheses of this general mixed model, it provides a more rigorous test of these two alternate modes of inheritance. In their analysis, Lalouel et al. completely reject the major locus hypothesis to explain all the data but find they cannot reject the multifactorial hypothesis. The mixed model hypothesis, that is both a major gene and a polygenic component present, affords only a slightly better fit to the data than the multifactorial hypothesis and, in addition, the gene frequency for the major locus is quite small, 0.001. This study would suggest that the multifactorial hypothesis provides the most complete yet simple explanation of the data on pyloric stenosis.

Both the analysis of Kidd and Spence (19) advocating a role for a single gene and that of Lalouel et al. (73) advocating the polygenetic explanation, clearly defined the situation that offspring of affected women constitute a special class of individuals. Neither model can adequately account for the frequency of occurrence of pyloric stenosis in both sons and daughters of women who themselves were affected. This recurrence pattern was first observed by MacMahon and his colleagues and by Carter (15). The finding suggests a specific maternal effect restricted to women who have been affected. This does not necessarily mean that affected males fail to produce affected offspring. In one of the first summaries of cases of pyloric stenosis in two generations in families, Carter and Powell (11) reported 12 families, six with an affected father and six with an affected mother. Simply, the frequency of affected infants among offspring of mothers who were affected exceeds the predictions of any of the genetic models tested to date.

SUMMARY

The situation with environmental factors is perhaps more clearly outlined for pyloric stenosis than any of the other congenital disorders. Even here, however, there has been confusion and failure to respect the complexity of the issues involved. A maternal effect has been documented. However, critical analyses for birth order effect are almost entirely lacking and we do not yet know whether being first born increases the risk of pyloric stenosis. There does appear to be evidence for birth weight differences and maternal age effects in some but not all of the populations. These environmental factors, where present, have the role of clouding the basic segregation patterns which are the essential criteria for defining gene action. It is, therefore, necessary to resolve as many of these environmental issues as possible before the genetic analyses can hope to be conclusive.

It would appear that several areas for fruitful epidemiological research have been defined through conflicting results from the studies of environmental factors. For example, one important area of research not yet addressed is the isolation of the maternal factors in women who have had pyloric stenosis. An obvious starting point for the experimental investigators is gastrin level determinations in these women. The experimental work with dogs clearly indicates that gastrin crosses the placental barrier and may evoke the

formation of a pyloric tumor (18). Two studies do report
gastrin levels in infants affected with pyloric stenosis, one
study of 10 infants reported an increased level (75) but the
other study of 15 infants reported no differences (76).
Neither study was of sufficient size to test whether males and
females differed. No study has yet been reported testing
women of child bearing age who had pyloric stenosis, nor
testing whether gastrin levels are increased in pregnant
females.

The next step for the genetic analyses is not nearly so
apparent. All studies agree that a single major locus cannot
account for all of the data on pyloric stenosis, even if one
invokes reasonable levels of environmental involvement. However, the other questions concerning the presence of a major
gene and the degree of its involvement remain unanswered.

The analyses of Kidd and Spence (19), which utilized only
the information from summary data on pairs of relatives, rejected the multifactorial model as the explanation for all of
the data on pyloric stenosis. The same multiple threshold
approach failed to reject a single locus contributing to a
portion of the cases. With this approach the two hypotheses
are not tested as subhypotheses of the same general parameter
space. And, some information from the data is lost through
the pooling process which ignores family structure. No
allowances are made for ascertainment bias with the multifactorial threshold models.

Gladstien et al. (72) properly accounted for
ascertainment bias but the power of this test cannot be
specified. It failed to reject the multifactorial hypothesis.

Lalouel et al. (73) had the benefits of a large sample
and a model with the two relevant subhypotheses available for
direct testing. These investigators were unable to exclude a
major gene responsible for a portion of the affected individuals on the multifactorial hypothesis. They chose the multifactorial model as the most parsimonious explanation of the
data, citing the small gene frequency for the major locus.
Their answer provides certain philosophical satisfaction but
leaves us with the dilemma: is there a small group of high
risk families with pyloric stenosis for which genetic counseling should provide recurrence risk figures different from
those predicted under the multifactorial model. Nor should we
be content that we have settled the issue of the etiology of
pyloric stenosis when two such biologically divergent hypotheses remain in contention as potential explanations.

Pyloric stenosis may yet serve as the classic example of
a multifactorial trait, perhaps not in the sense of the mathematical model of Falconer as much as in the sense of a trait

where many factors, environmental and genetic, require careful study.

REFERENCES

1. Carter, C. O., <u>Brit. Med. Bull</u>. 32, 21-26 (1976).

2. Campbell, M. A., Dissertation, University of Hawaii, Honolulu. Dissertation Abstracts 31, order no. 70-19, 506 (1970).

3. Dodge, J. A., <u>Arch. Dis. Child</u>. 50, 171-178 (1975).

4. Osawa, M., Yamamoto, Y., Mitsuya, Y., Tsukamoto, A., Fukuyama, Y., and Tanaka, K., <u>Jap. J. Hum. Genet</u>. 20, 35-53 (1976).

5. Czeizel, A., <u>Arch. Dis. Child</u>. 47, 978-980 (1972).

6. Meyer, B. P., <u>Pediatrics</u> 48, 826-827 (1971).

7. Cameron, A. L., <u>AMA Arch. Surg</u>. 70, 877-894 (1955).

8. Coleman, H. J., <u>Journal AOA</u>. 75, 1049-1051 (1976).

9. Carter, C. O., and Savage, T. R., <u>Arch. Dis. Child</u>. 26, 50-51 (1957).

10. Spitz, L., <u>Arch. Dis. Child</u>. 49, 325 (1974).

11. Carter, C. O., and Powell, B. W., <u>Lancet</u> I, 746-748 (1954).

12. Snyder, L., <u>Ohio Journal of Science</u> 53, 49-50 (1943).

13. Cockayne, E. A., and Penrose, L. S., <u>Ohio Journal of Science</u> 43, 1-16 (1943).

14. Falconer, D. S., <u>Ann. Hum. Genet</u>. 29, 51-76 (1965).

15. Carter, C. O., <u>Brit. Med. Bull</u>. 17, 251-254 (1961).

16. Carter, C. O., in "Progress in Medical Genetics." (A. G. Steinberg and A. C. Bearn Eds.), Vol. IV, pp. 59-84, Grune and Stratton, New York, 1965.

17. Carter, C. O., and Evans, K. A., <u>J. Med. Genet</u>. 6, 233-239 (1969).

18. Dodge, J. A., Nature 255, 284-285 (1970).

19. Kidd, K. K., and Spence, M. A., J. Med. Genet. 13, 290-294 (1976).

20. Benson, D., Mustard, W., Ravitch, M., Snyder, W., and Welch, K., Am. J. Surg. 107, 429-433 (1964).

21. Gordon, H. E., Pollock, W. F., Norris, W. J., and Hart, J. C., West. J. Surg., Obst. & Gynec. 67, 139-146 (1959).

22. Shim, W.K.T., Campbell, M. A., and Wright, S. W., Hawaii Med. Journ. 28, 201-204 (1969).

23. Laron, Z., and Horne, L., AMA J. Dis. Child. 94, 151-154 (1957).

24. Adelstein, P., and Frederick, J., J. Med. Genet. 13, 439-448 (1976).

25. Wallgren, A., Acta Paediat. 49, 530-535 (1960).

26. McLean, M. M., Arch. Dis. Child. 31, 481-482 (1956).

27. Bell, M. J., Surgery. 64, 983-989 (1968).

28. Cachia, E. A. and Fenech, F. F., J. Med. Genet. 3, 49-50 (1966).

29. Gharib, R., J. Ped. 65, 622-624 (1964).

30. McKeown, T., MacMahon, B., and Record, R., Ann. Hum. Genet. 16, 249-259 (1951).

31. Danis, A., Acta Paediat. 11, 248-252 (1957).

32. Dodge, J. A., Clinics in Gastroenterology 2, 523-538 (1973).

33. Ford, N., Ross, M. A., and Brown, A., Am. J. Dis. Child. 61, 747-751 (1941).

34. Ladd, W. E., Pickett, L. K., and Ware, P. F., J. Amer. Med. Assoc. 131, 647-651 (1946).

35. Malmberg, N., Acta Paediat. 38, 472-483 (1949).

36. McQuad, J.N.W., and Porrit, B. E., Lancet 1, 201-204 (1950).

37. Pollack, W. F., Norris, W. J., and Gordon, H. E., Am. J. Surg. 94, 335-348 (1957).

38. Salmi, T., Acta Paediat. 21, 362-379 (1937).

39. Schaefer, A., and Erbes, J., Surg. Gynec. Obst. 86, 45-53 (1948).

40. Shim, W. K., Campbell, A., and Wright, S. W., J. Pediat. 76, 89-93 (1970).

41. Benson, C. D., and Warden, M. J., Surg. Gynec. & Obst. 105, 348-354 (1957).

42. Delprat, G. D., and Pflueger, O., Calif. Med. 68, 76 (1948).

43. Dougall, J., Scot. Med. J. 14, 156-161 (1969).

44. Faxen, N., Acta Pediat. 14, 388-403 (1933).

45. Gerrard, J. W., Waterhouse, A. H., and Maurice, D. G., Arch. Dis. Child. 30, 493-496 (1955).

46. Grimes, O. F., Bell, H. G., and Olney, M. B., J. Pediat. 37, 522-529 (1950).

47. Huguenard, J. R., Sharples, B. S., and Sharples, G. E., J. Ped. 81, 45-49 (1972).

48. Miller, D. R., and Friesen, S. R., Am. Surg. 22, 108-118 (1956).

49. Rinvik, R., Acta Paediat. 27, 296-333 (1940).

50. Barker, D.J.P., and Record, R. G., Appl. Stat. 16, 13-16 (1967).

51. Bennett, B. M., Ann. Hum. Genet. 27, 11-15 (1963).

52. Greenwood, M., and Yule, U., J. Roy. Stat. Soc. 77, 179-197 (1914).

53. Haldane, J.B.S., and Smith, C.A.B., Ann. Eugen. 14, 117-124 (1948).

54. Slater, E., Lancet 1, 69-71 (1962).

55. Barker, D.J.P., and Record, R. G., Am. J. Hum. Genet.
     19, 433-449 (1967).

56. MacMahon, B., Record, R. G., and McKeown, T., Brit. J.
     Soc. Med. 5, 185-192 (1951).

57. Kwok, R. H., and Avery, G., J. Ped. 70, 963-964 (1967).

58. Campbell, M. A., J. Ped. 74, 1006-1007 (1969).

59. Herwig, J. C., Middelkamp, J.N.M., Thornton, H. K., and
     Reed, C. A., J. Ped. 61, 309-310 (1962).

60. Powell, B. W., and Carter, C. O., Arch. Dis. Child. 26,
     45-49 (1957).

61. Welsh, J. B., J. Indiana State Med. Assoc. 44, 762
     (1951).

62. Metrakas, J. D., Arch. Dis. Child. 27, 351-358 (1953).

63. Smith, C., Am. J. Hum. Genet. 26, 454-466 (1974).

64. Morton, N. E., Am. J. Hum. Genet. 11, 1-16 (1959).

65. Morton, N. E., in "Genetics Today," (S. J. Geerts, Ed.).
     Vol. 3, pp. 935-951, Pergamon Press, Oxford, 1965.

66. Yee, S., and Morton, N. E., in "Applications of Computers
     in Human Genetics," (N. E. Morton, Ed.). Vol. II, pp.
     129-139, University of Hawaii Press, Honolulu, 1969.

67. McKeown, T., MacMahon, B., and Record, R. G., Ann. Hum.
     Genet. 16, 260-281 (1951).

68. Reich, T., James, J. W., and Morris, C. A., Ann. Hum.
     Genet. 36, 163-184 (1972).

69. Kidd, K., Reich, T., and Kessler, S., Genetics 74, 137
     (1973).

70. Campbell, M. A., and Elston, R. C., Ann. Hum. Genet. 35,
     225-235 (1971).

71. Kidd, K., and Cavalli-Sforza, L., Soc. Biol. 20, 254-
     265 (1973).

72. Gladstien, K., Lange, K., and Spence, M. A., Am. J. Med.
     Genet. in press.

73. Lalouel, J. M., Morton, N. E., MacLean, C. J., and Jackson, J., <u>J. Med. Genet.</u> in press.

74. Morton, N. E., and MacLean, C. J., <u>Am. J. Hum. Genet.</u> 26, 489-503 (1974).

75. Spitz, L., and Zail, S. S., <u>J. Ped. Surg.</u>, 11, 33-35 (1976).

76. Rogers, I. M., Drainer, I. K., Moore, M. R., and Buchanan, K. D., <u>Arch. Dis. Child.</u> 50, 467-471 (1975).

DISCUSSION

LALOUEL: In our recent analysis on pyloric stenosis, we certainly did not 'completely reject' the possible role of a major locus in the transmission and occurrence of this affection. Rather, likelihood calculations, lending equivalent support to both the mixed model and its multifactorial sub-hypothesis (q = 0), did not provide evidence in favor of the segregation of a major gene; hence we could not infer the existence of such a major gene and, in the absence of support for a major locus from other evidence, we retained the multifactorial model as a description of the observed familial aggregation. This provisional model may reasonably be assumed for calculation of recurrence risks until more is known about this affection, particularly with regard to the suggested maternal effect, possibly by taking into consideration a quantitative trait such as gastrin.

ROTTER: I would like to make two comments. The first deals with the possible existence of heterogeneity within this disorder, a concern which Dr. Spence has addressed. The existence of an adult form of hypertrophic pyloric stenosis is still being defined. There have been several reports of adult and congenital pyloric stenosis occurring in the same family, usually in multiple generations. Also a relation between peptic ulcer and pyloric stenosis has been claimed, either as a complication, or as an association in families. (These points are reviewed in Dodge, J.A., Clinics in Gastro-enterology, 2:523, 1973). Both are an area that needs further study. But this clinical evidence of potential heterogeneity must be added to the difficulty of trying to fit pyloric stenosis to either the multifactorial or single gene model.
    The second comment relates to the hypothesis that maternal hypergastrinemia may be a pathogenetic factor in a certain proportion of pyloric stenosis cases. This is an eminently testable hypothesis. There are two ways that it could be readily tested. One is to utilize an experiment of nature,

the Zollinger-Ellison syndrome. This syndrome consists of
tumors of non-beta pancreatic islet cells that produce gastrin
in the highest quantities known to man. They present clinically with a severe, intractable ulcer diathesis. It would be
of great interest to know what the outcome of any pregnancies
have been in mothers who are afflicted with this syndrome.
Secondly, since it is the sibs and offsprings of affected
females that are at the highest risk empirically for pyloric
stenosis, these at-risk pregnancies could be monitored by
measuring maternal serum gastrin values. Since there is a
wide range of normal fasting serum gastrin, these studies
should probably include the gastrin response to a protein meal.
This has been documented to be abnormal in a certain proportion of duodenal ulcer patients.

SPENCE: I completely agree with the thrust of Dr. Rotter's
first point, a possibility does exist that pyloric stenosis
may result from one or more genetic or environmental causes.
It is important to emphasize the point, however, that none of
the analyses discussed in this paper used any data other than
patients with onset in infancy. The existence of a syndrome
in adults with symptoms similar to early onset pyloric stenosis
suggests that more than one causal factor may result in the
same phenotype, but it is not evidence that the early onset
form is heterogeneous in its etiology.

KIDD: Dr. Spence's results for pyloric stenosis can be
used to illustrate several general points about the inheritance of many congenital malformations and common diseases.
In the late 60's and the first half of the 70's the "poly-
geneticists" used the simple multifactorial model with polygenes as the genetic component to explain the inheritance of
virtually all disorders that showed familial aggregation in
the absence of any clear Mendelian pattern of inheritance.
One medical genetics textbook even listed 10 criteria for
identifying traits with polygenic inheritance; pyloric stenosis
met most, if not all, of the criteria. Among the many other
diseases which also met most of the "expectations" were celiac
disease (gluten-sensitive enteropathy) and ankylosing spondylitis. While the emphasis for pyloric stenosis is still on
testing mathematical hypotheses, segregation at a single locus
has now been shown to be the primary genetic component in
susceptibility to both ankylosing spondylitis (1) and celiac
disease (2). The association of these two diseases with
marker alleles at the HLA locus is responsible for this clearer
understanding. The general point illustrated by these recent

discoveries is that there is no qualitative aspect of
inheritance patterns that is unique to polygenic inheritance.
Only in the precise quantitative expectations do the models
involving a major (or megaphenic) locus differ from polygenic
inheritance. As Dr. Spence has shown, available mathematical
methods may not be powerful enough to discriminate between
these hypotheses. Thus, we must consider alternatives for
the disorders that have been labelled "multifactorial-
polygenic". Each of them could also be heterogeneous, as
emphasized by Dr. Matthysse (reference his paper this conference).

Contrary to the opinions of some, I feel that the
distinction between a polygenic and a major locus explanation
is not trivial. In the design of biochemical and physiological experiments for the study of these disorders the distinction may have major importance. More important, however, is
the question of genetic counseling. A point often overlooked
in using multifactorial expectations for genetic counseling
is that the single locus expectation may differ considerably
in some specific familial situations. For example, Chung
et al. (3) could fit both a general single locus model and a
polygenic model to the available family data on cleft lip
(with or without cleft palate). They tabulated the risk to
the next offspring for various types of families as predicted
by the two models. When both parents are normal and all
existing offspring are affected, the risks can differ to a
degree that would be highly significant in genetic counseling:

Number of Affected Sibs	Risk to Next Sib Monogenic	Polygenic
0	0.1%	0.1%
1	5.5	4.4
2	6.1	12.3
3	7.3	19.4
4	9.0	24.9
5	11.4	29.1

Of course, not all predictions depend so strongly on the model,
but the degree to which risks are model dependent is not
generally known.

In conclusion, I think we must consider the multifactorial-
polygenic and the major locus models equally likely explanations for all of these common disorders until specific tests
of hypotheses or specific biological/biochemical data indicate
otherwise. The equivalence as hypotheses, however, does not
imply an equivalence in prediction for genetic counseling or
of utility in experimental design. Efforts should continue to

be made to discriminate between these classes of hypotheses
both through testing of sophisticated models and through
innovative new biological experimentation.

References

1. Kidd, K.K., Bernoco, C., Carbonara, A.O., Daneo, V.,
    Steiger, U., and Ceppellini, R., in "HLA and Disease,"
    (J. Dausset and A. Svejgaard, Eds.) Munksgaard,
    Copenhagen, 1977.
2. Strober, W., ibid.
3. Chung, C.S., Ching, G.H.S., and Morton, N.E.,
    Am. J. Hum. Genet. 26, 177-188 (1974).

GENETIC EPIDEMIOLOGY AND POPULATION STRUCTURE

Peter L. Workman

Dept. of Anthropology
University of New Mexico
Albuquerque, New Mexico

As discussed by Morton (1), genetic epidemiology is
primarily concerned with distinguishing the biological and
cultural causes of family resemblance. That is, the major
focus of this hybrid discipline is on intra-population variation in disease manifestation. Consequently, the primary
methodological developments have been directed toward improving estimates of the components of phenotypic variation (e.g.,
by path analysis) and refining the specification of the underlying genetic model: single locus, polygenic, or a mixed
model (by segregation analysis of nuclear families or genealogies). Such techniques are, however, not suitable for dealing
with inter-population variation in prevalence rates, an area
of major importance in epidemiologic studies. Recent work on
the genetic structure of populations suggests that, under the
appropriate restrictions, it should also be possible to
distinguish cultural and biological contributions to inter-
population differences.

Basically, estimation of the genetic contribution to
phenotypic variation, whether within or between populations,
involves comparing phenotypic resemblances between pairs of
individuals or groups with a measure of the genetic correlation
between members of each pair. For individuals within a

population, kinship taken from genealogies provides the appropriate genetic correlation. For pairs of populations, various measures could be used: correlations among gene frequencies, measures of genetic distance which are also measures of divergence, or multivariate measures of biological distance. Such inter-population analyses are clearly restricted to those instances of population subdivision for which a single population ancestral to every sub-population can be postulated and for which the genetic distances actually reflect the degree of similarity in the gene pools. Thus, comparisons among groups only distantly related (such as racial comparisons) could not be made by this procedure; there are, on the other hand, numerous instances of population structure which do seem to be suitable for this approach. When the genetic contribution to interpopulation differences is quite small, as evidenced by a gross discordance between genetic structure and the pattern of phenotypic variation, no sophisticated techniques need be utilized. Such a situation is exemplified by the pattern of variation in hyperglycemia among southwestern United States Indian tribes as can be seen by a comparison of genetic and epidemiologic variation among these groups.

In recent years, several studies have documented the high prevalence of diabetes in southwestern Indian tribes (e.g., 2, 3). A diagnostic test for hyperglycemia, based on examination of plasma glucose levels one or two hours after a 75 gram glucose equivalent load, has provided a useful comparative measure for defining prevalence rates for "diabetes" in a number of populations. Unfortunately, genetic data sufficient to characterize the phylogenetic relations among these groups exist only for the Pima (4), Papago (5), and Zuni (6). Published data on hyperglycemia in the Pima (3) and previously unpublished data on the Papago and Zuni provide the epidemiologic characterization of these three tribes.

Table I shows the distribution of two-hour plasma glucose levels in the Zuni. Using 160 mg per 100 ml as a threshold above which individuals are said to be hyperglycemic, the prevalence rates for Zuni males and females 35 years of age or older are, respectively, 16 and 48 percent. For the Papago, limitations of the field situation necessitated utilization of one hour-plasma glucose levels; for such results, a value of 180 mg per 100 ml is used to obtain roughly comparable prevalence rates. For the Papago data shown in Table II, the male and female rates were 21 and 20 percent, respectively. The Zuni and Papago data was collected by the Human Genetics Branch of the National Institute of Dental Research under the direction of J. D. Niswander.

TABLE   I

Distribution of Two Hour Plasma Glucose Levels (mg per 100ml)
in Zuni Indians by Age and Sex

Glucose Level	Males 13-14	15-24	25-34	35-44	45-54	55-64	65+
<80	0	25	0	3	0	1	1
80- 99	10	44	6	3	3	1	5
100-119	3	21	5	10	3	6	6
120-139	0	7	4	3	3	4	6
140-159	0	0	1	2	0	1	8
160-179	0	0	2	0	0	1	1
180-199	0	0	0	1	0	1	2
200-299	0	0	2	0	2	1	1
300+	0	0	1	0	0	2	1
Total	13	97	21	22	11	18	31

Glucose Level	Females 13-14	15-24	25-34	35-44	45-54	55-64	65+
<80	1	18	1	0	0	0	0
80- 99	16	81	10	4	2	2	1
100-119	2	67	28	9	5	7	1
120-139	4	27	16	7	10	6	8
140-159	0	9	6	4	1	2	4
160-179	0	4	3	6	2	5	7
180-199	0	0	3	2	0	1	1
200-299	0	1	2	5	7	4	8
300+	0	0	0	2	4	7	6
Total	23	207	69	39	31	34	36

Table II summarizes the prevalence rates in each of the three
tribes.

The genetic relationships among these tribes, discussed
by Niswander et al. (5) and Workman et al. (6), show complete
agreement with inference on their phylogenetic origins from
archaeological, linguistic and ethnohistorical material.   The
Pima and Papago, members of the Piman linguistic subfamily of

TABLE II

Distribution of One Hour Plasma Glucose Levels (mg per 100 ml) in
Papago Indians by age and sex

Glucose Level	Males					Females				
	9-14	15-34	35-54	55-64	65+	9-14	15-34	35-54	55-64	65+
<80	15	5	1	1	2	21	9	0	1	0
80- 99	48	23	10	2	4	55	26	6	2	1
100-119	40	15	13	2	2	47	33	18	2	1
120-139	15	12	12	1	2	11	22	19	2	1
140-159	0	3	6	1	2	3	8	9	4	1
160-179	0	8	5	1	2	1	4	9	2	3
180-199	0	1	4	1	0	0	3	1	1	1
200-299	0	4	6	2	1	0	2	2	3	0
300+	1	3	2	2	0	0	1	7	3	2
TOTAL	119	74	59	13	15	138	108	71	20	10

the Uto-Aztecan group, are closely related descendants of the Hohokam culture, dominant in southern Arizona for many centuries.   These tribes are geographically close, have a long history of mate exchange, and are exceedingly similar from most anthropological perspectives.   Their gene frequencies are very similar; indeed, genetic drift and isolation by distance among Papago subgroups has given rise to far greater intra-tribal variation than exists between the Pima and Papago.   For 14 alleles at 8 loci, the average inter-tribal difference in allelic frequency is .037.   The Zuni appear to represent an amalgam of indigeneous southwestern Indians (Anasazi and Mogollon) but have remained relatively isolated for several centuries.   Any common phylogenetic origin for the Zuni, Pima and Papago would reflect a much more distant time period than that relating to the divergence of the Pima and Papago. Genetic distances are very similar for the Zuni-Pima and Zuni-Papago comparison, and much smaller for the Pima-Papago.

    The pattern of hyperglycemia in these tribes, shown in Table III is very clearly not a reflection of the genetic relationships and no sophisticated mathematical analysis is called for.   The marked difference in disease rates between Pima and Papago occur in genetically very similar groups. The Zuni show an atypical extreme difference in sex-specific rates and no concordance with phylogenetic relations.   Thus

TABLE III

Prevalence of Hyperglycemia in Papago, Pima, and
Zuni Indians, 35 Years or Older

	Male			Female		
	Number	Affected	Percent	Number	Affected	Percent
Papago	87	18	20.7	101	20	19.8
Pima[1]	342	138	40.3	407	235	57.8
Zuni	82	13	15.9	140	67	47.9

[1]Diagnosis by plasma glucose test and clinical exams.

an explanatory model for the tribal differences in hyper-glycemia need not invoke genetic differentiation as an important causal factor.   Factors which do merit future

investigation include variation in diet, level of physical
activity, and for the Zuni in particular, differences in the
sexual division of labor (and diet).

Two specific features of this approach to genetic
epidemiology should be mentioned. First, for both intra-and
inter-population studies, an important outcome of a genetic
analysis may be the elimination of genetic factors from
consideration in an explanatory model of disease variation.
In such situations, research can confidently proceed with a
focus on environmental factors. Similar studies are now in
progress in Finland where the genetic structure of the entire
country (7) can be compared to patterns of variation of heart
disease·occurrence; a preliminary examination of the data
suggests that genetic variation among sub-populations shows
essentially no concordance with epidemiologic patterns.
Second, it should be stressed that there is no logical relation between the components of intra-population phenotypic
variation and those contributing to inter-population variation.
Present inference indicating no genetic contribution to
differential diabetes rates among Indians in the southwest
provides absolutely no inference for questions about why one
member of a tribe develops the disease and another does not.

References

1. Morton, N.E., in "Gene-Environment Interaction in Common
    Diseases," pp 21-40, Univ. of Tokyo Press, Tokyo, 1977.
2. Henry, R.E., Burch, T.A., Bennett, P.H., and Miller, M.,
    Diabetes 18, 33 (1969)
3. Bennett, P.H., Burch, T.A., and Miller, M., in "Diabetes
    Mellitus in Asia, 1970," p. 33, Excerpta Medica Inter-
    national Congress Series No. 221, 1970.
4. Matson, G.A., Burch, T.A., Polesky, H.F., Swanson, J.,
    Sutton, H.E., and Robinson, A., Am. J. Phys. Anthrop.
    29, 311 (1968).
5. Niswander, J.D., Brown, K.S., Iba, B.Y., Leyshon, W.C.,
    and Workman, P.L., Am. J. Hum. Genet. 22, 7 (1970).
6. Workman, P.L., Niswander, J.D., Brown, K.S., and
    Leyshon, W.C., Am. J. Phys. Anthrop. 41, 119 (1974).
7. Workman, P.L., Mielke, J.H., and Nevanlinna, H.R.,
    Am. J. Phys. Anthrop. 44, 341 (1976).

SPENCE: Dr. Workman has clearly delineated the differences
between intra-and inter-population studies. The inclination
of most geneticists is not to consider the question of the
genetic contribution to the etiology of a trait sufficiently
resolved until the underlying genetic mechanism is specified.
As stressed in the papers of Morton (1), Lange (2) and others,

estimating the components of variation is simply the first step toward applying the more refined techniques of segregation analysis. Therefore, the question that comes to mind is what information is provided by the inter-population studies which contributes to our understanding of the genetic basis for any particular trait?

My difficulty in agreeing completely with Dr. Workman's interpretation of his results stems from two questions: the accuracy of the genetic distance measures, and the acceptance of the simple direct relationship of one phenotype to a general genetic measure of similarity. For the first question, our measures of genetic distances suffer from certain ambiguities, and their strict interpretation is subject to differences of opinion. Discussions of these points are available in most population genetics texts. The more basic question is that the differences in frequency in glucose phenotype between Papago and Pima Indians, while their genetic distance is less than that of the Zuni, leads directly to the result that the differences indicate "no genetic contribution". Either population could have different alleles or loci for the trait in question through new mutation, drift, bottle-neck effects or differential selection, any or all of which could reasonably be expected to have effects in these small populations with stressful environmental situations. In other words, the extrapolation seems strong given the assumptions underlying this basic approach. And, as Workman suggests, these results "provide absolutely no inference" regarding questions on why one individual develops the disease and another does not. Although the variance component estimations and path analyses do not specify the genetic mechanisms, they do lead directly to estimates of gene versus environmental contribution and therefore directly to the next step of the analysis. If our goal is to understand the relative roles of the genetic and environmental components and to specify the genetic mechanisms then it would seem that the inter-population studies contribute no progress toward that goal. An appropriate epidemiological study would be to examine these populations for associations of diabetes with HLA haplotypes. Associations are reported for some forms of diabetes in other populations (3).

A study of glucose tolerance in the Pimas using the combined approach of path analysis and segregation analysis has been initiated by several of us (Spence, Rao and Morton, in preparation).

References

1. Morton, N.E., <u>Am. J. Hum. Genet.</u> 26, 318 (1974).
2. Lange, K.L., Westlake, J., and Spence, M.A. <u>Ann. Hum. Genet.</u> 18, 11 (1976).
3. Christy, M., Nesup, J., Bottazzo, G.F., Doriach, D., Platz, P., Svejgaurd, A., Ryder, L.P., and Thomsen, M., <u>Lancet</u> 142 (1976).

GENETIC EPIDEMIOLOGY

AN APPROACH TO THE INVESTIGATION OF MATERNAL FACTORS

IN CONGENITAL MALFORMATIONS

Ntinos C. Myrianthopoulos

National Institute of Neurological and Communicative
Disorders and Stroke, National Institutes of Health,
Bethesda, Maryland 20014

Families from the Collaborative Perinatal
Project (NCPP) which contained children born to the
same mother by more than one father have been used to
study the role of maternal factors in the occurrence
of congenital malformations. The rationale is that
if a malformation appeared in half siblings of the
same family with a frequency higher than that in the
general population, it is most likely to be due to
maternal influences, genetic or environmental. Among
informative malformations, clubfoot, umbilical and
inguinal hernias, polydactyly, congenital heart defects
and café au lait spots occurred with significantly
higher frequency in half siblings than in the NCPP
population. The recurrence risks of these malformations were the same in full and half siblings. While
this approach cannot differentiate between genetic
and environmental maternal factors, it provides clues
for formulating and testing biological hypotheses.

I.   INTRODUCTION

One important determinant of familial resemblance is
maternal influence, genetic and environmental. The latter is
presumed to operate especially in traits which show familial
aggregation but do not mendelize. Maternal effects have been
demonstrated in the occurrence of several such abnormalities
-- Rh hemolytic disease, low birth weight, chromosomal aberrations, -- and is strongly suspected in others. The investigation of maternal factors in such disorders falls within
the realm of genetic epidemiology which Morton (1) defined as
the science that deals with the etiology, distribution and
control of disease in groups of relatives or with genetic
causes (biological or cultural) of disease in populations.
This paper describes briefly our attempt to investigate

the role of maternal factors in the occurrence of congenital malformations.

The material for this investigation comes from the Collaborative Perinatal Project (NCPP), a cooperative endeavor of 12 institutions throughout the United States, and the National Institute of Neurological and Communicative Disorders and Stroke. The broad objective of the NCPP is to observe and study events which affect the parents, particularly the mother, before and during pregnancy, and to relate these events to the outcome of pregnancy. To this end, about 55,000 pregnant women have been followed from the first months of their pregnancy through labor and delivery, and their study children have been followed to age 8 years. The collection of information, medical examinations and laboratory tests have been done in uniform fashion and according to preestablished protocols.

The population of the NCPP has several advantageous features for epidemiologic-genetic investigations. One is that it is a prospectively collected, though, it should be pointed out, not an entirely representative, sample of the general population. Another is its fairly large size. Still another, which prompted us to undertake this investigation, is that a large proportion of participating women have had children by more than one mate, both before they enrolled in the NCPP, and after their study child was born.

It should be possible to utilize information about these families to study the role of maternal factors in the occurrence of abnormalities in the children. The rationale is that if an abnormality appeared in half sibships of the same family with a frequency higher than that in the general population, it is most likely due to maternal influences, genetic or environmental.

Congenital malformations are particularly attractive candidates for such an investigation because a large proportion of them show familial aggregation but do not mendelize. This investigation is part of a continuing study of congenital malformations which occurred in study children born to NCPP mothers.

II. MATERIALS AND METHODS

Two kinds of information are needed for this investigation: information about the reproductive performance of the mother; and information about malformations in the children.

Information about past reproductive history and occurrence of malformations in children born prior to the study pregnancy, was obtained during lengthy and detailed inter-

views with the mother by specially trained interviewers. This
information was verified by repeat interviews and, in many
cases, by examination of medical and other records. The study
children were closely followed and repeatedly examined during
the 8-year follow-up period. The reproductive history of the
mothers and health histories of non-study children were up-
dated in a final interview which was part of the 7-year
battery of examinations of the study children.

The use of anamnestic information always raises some concern about its quality, but efforts at verification and the
results of frequent quality control trials gave us fair assurance of its accuracy and reliability. Unfortunately, information about the reproductive history of the mother and
malformations in non-study children is coded only to general
categories and is not retrievable in useable form except by
painstaking and time-consuming review of the voluminous individual records. And while such review has added an extra
measure of accuracy, the constraint of time has not allowed
more than a preliminary analysis of the data to date.

From the NCPP population we ascertained families which
contained children born to the same mother by more than one
father, and in which a malformation had occurred in at least
one of the children. Four hundred and fifty eight families,
the great majority of them black, were identified as fulfilling these criteria. Their characteristics are described in
Table I. These were big families; they comprised 1,195 sibships with 2,685 children, 2,352 of whom were liveborn and
333 fetal deaths. The mean number of pregnancies per woman
was 5.9, the mean number of mates per woman 2.6, and the mean
number of children per sibship 2.2.

TABLE I   Families with Children Born to the Same Mother
by Different Father

Number of families	458
Number of sibships	1,195
Total number of pregnancies	2,685
Number of fetal deaths	333
Number of live births	2,352
Mean number of pregnancies per woman	5.9
Mean number of mates per woman	2.6
Mean number of children per sibship	2.2

A large number of malformation types was found in these children but most of them occurred only once or twice. For a preliminary look we selected 14 malformations which occurred with sufficient frequencies to merit consideration. These were found in 631 liveborn children, and their distribution is shown in Table II.

TABLE II Distribution of Selected Malformations
in 631 Liveborn Malformed Children Born to the
Same Mother by More Than One Father

Malformations	No. of families	No. affected
Clubfoot	88	106
Umbilical hernia	83	98
Polydactyly	61	72
Congenital heart defects	60	69
Inguinal hernia	51	60
External ear malformations	47	51
Café au lait spots	36	41
Undescended testes	37	38
Supernumerary nipples	23	23
Neural tube defects	17	18
Hydrocephaly	15	15
Cavernous hemangioma	14	14
Cong. dislocation of hip	14	14
Cleft lip and/or palate	12	12
Total	558	631

The various diagnostic categories of clubfoot have been pooled since only a little over half the cases carried a specific diagnosis; and anyway, not without justification, for the clinical picture is not always clear, and there is no agreement on the definition of the various categories even among orthopedists. Polydactyly includes only the postaxial type. Congenital heart defects comprise mostly septal defects and abnormalities of the valves and great vessels. External ear malformations include malformations of the ear pinna and the primordial branchial clefts. Café au lait spots were included only if they were multiple or more than 3x3 cm in diameter. The cleft lip/palate category does not include isolated cleft palate.

All syndromic malformations have been excluded. For example, congenital heart defects found in children with Downs syndrome are not included in Table II. Multiple malformations, therefore, have been counted as many times as they were observed in an individual.

III. RESULTS AND DISCUSSION

Two kinds of comparisons are relevant to our problem. First, a comparison of the recurrence risk of a particular malformation in half siblings with the risk in the general population; and second a comparison of the risk for a particular malformation in proband and half sibships, or in full and half siblings.

A proband is the first affected child with a particular malformation through whom the family was ascertained, whether or not the child was a study child. A proband sibship is the sibship containing the proband, irrespective of its order in the family. Siblings in the proband sibship are considered full siblings; all other siblings are considered half siblings.

It is evident from inspection of Table II that supernumerary nipples, hydrocephaly, cavernous hemangioma, congenital dislocation of the hip and cleft lip/palate will not be informative since these malformations did not recur either in the full or in the half siblings. Undescended testes and neural tube defects recurred only once and they, too, are not likely to be informative. These malformations therefore, will not be considered further. The recurrence frequencies of the remaining malformations do not look very encouraging. Thus, in spite of the relatively large numbers of NCPP mothers and half sibships, we are confronted again with a perennial problem in human population genetics, to use a favorite expression, the tyranny of small numbers.

Table III shows the distribution of malformations in the half sibships by order of sibship without any reference to proband siblings or sibships. It merely gives an idea of the size of these sibships and the frequency of the affected children within them. The first and second sibships are by far the largest. Sibships subsequent to the second are fairly small and they have been pooled. The distribution of the various malformations in these sibships, with one exception, does not reveal any serious underreporting or any parity or birth order trends. The exception, café au lait spots, is much more frequent in the second and subsequent sibships than in the first, indicating that it was underreported in chil-

TABLE III Distribution of Malformations in Half Siblings by Order of Sibship

Malformations	First Sibship			Second sibship			All subsequent sibships		
	No. of sibs	No. affected	% affected	No. of sibs	No. affected	% affected	No. of sibs	No. affected	% affected
Clubfoot	188	44	23.40	160	40	25.00	101	22	21.78
Umbilical hernia	178	40	22.47	159	40	25.16	97	18	18.56
Polydactyly	144	39	28.08	123	24	19.51	62	9	14.52
Congenital heart defects	134	35	26.12	123	26	21.14	57	8	14.03
Inguinal hernia	107	28	26.17	94	19	20.21	38	13	34.21
External ear malformations	81	15	18.52	83	25	30.12	40	11	27.50
Café au lait spots	64	5	7.81	76	27	35.53	40	9	22.50

dren of the first sibships, who most likely were born prior to the study children.

The comparison of malformation recurrence risks in half siblings with the risks in the NCPP population (2) is shown in Table IV. Recurrence risks have, of course, been calculated after the probands have been removed from the number of sibs and the number affected. Except for external ear malformations, the differences for all other malformations are highly significant. Clearly, these malformations have been repeated with a frequency far exceeding that expected in the general population, indicating the possibility of some maternal effect.

The finding that polydactyly has a higher recurrence risk in half siblings than in the general population is surprising. Postaxial polydactyly is inherited as a dominant trait though it shows lack of penetrance and may be genetically heterogeneous (3, 4). The explanation for this unexpected finding may lie in the racial distribution of the malformation and the sample: postaxial polydactyly is over 12 times as frequent among blacks as among whites (5), and there is a disproportionate number of black families in the sample. A comparison, however, of recurrence risks by race failed to remove the difference in blacks (p < 0.001).

Café au lait spots also have a significantly higher incidence among blacks than among whites (2) but, again, comparison by race failed to remove the difference in blacks (p < 0.01). There were no recurrent cases of either postaxial polydactyly or café au lait spots in white families.

We now turn to the comparison of malformation risks in full and half siblings. If the recurrence risk of a malformation is about the same in full and half siblings, it is reasonable to attribute its occurrence to maternal factors, mostly other than classic single gene effects. If, however, the recurrence risk is significantly different in full and half siblings, then the maternal effect is presumably diluted by paternal influences, most probably of genetic origin.

Table V shows these comparisons. In no case is the malformation recurrence risk different in full and half siblings.

Some of these results are quite confusing and difficult to interpret. Although genetic factors have been postulated for some types of clubfoot (6, 7, 8), simple inheritance has not been established. It is possible that maternal uterine factors such as overcrowding may be deciding in the production of this malformation, though the evidence is conflicting (9).

Umbilical and inguinal hernias are fairly common developmental defects and autosomal dominant inheritance has been reported in some cases of inguinal hernia (10, 11). It is difficult to envision what kind of maternal influences might

TABLE IV   Malformation Risks in Half Siblings and the NCPP Population

Malformations	No. of families	No. of sibs	No. affected	Risk of recurrence	Birth incidence in NCPP population
Clubfoot	88	449	106	0.0499	0.0276**
Umbilical hernia	83	434	98	0.0427	0.0012****
Polydactyly	61	329	72	0.0410	0.0074****
Congenital heart defects	60	314	69	0.0354	0.0076****
Inguinal hernia	51	239	60	0.0479	0.0134****
External ear malformations	47	204	51	0.0255	0.0160 N.S.
Café au lait spots	36	180	41	0.0347	0.0075***

**   p < 0.01

***   p < 0.001

TABLE V Risk of Malformations in Proband and Half Sibships

| Malformations | Proband sibships | | | | Half sibships | | | | x^2 |
	No.	No. of sibs	No. of affected	Risk	No.	No. of sibs	No. of affected	Risk	
Clubfoot	88	224	97	0.0661	137	225	9	0.0400	0.64
Umbilical hernia	83	204	90	0.0578	130	230	8	0.0348	0.48
Polydactyly	61	171	65	0.0364	100	158	7	0.0443	≈0
Congenital heart defects	60	153	62	0.0215	86	161	7	0.0435	0.25
Inguinal hernia	51	118	57	0.0984	69	121	3	0.0248	1.99
Café au lait spots	36	90	39	0.0556	47	90	2	0.0223	0.34

play a role in the occurrence of these malformations.

Polydactyly still remains a puzzle. It is interesting that in an earlier preliminary study using a small number of the then available half sibships we came up with exactly the same finding (12). It is possible that most of the mothers of affected children were themselves affected. Information in existing records shows that less than half of the mothers reported having polydactyly. Unfortunately, this does not resolve the question one way or the other because the malformation is usually corrected in infancy and the mother may have not been aware that she was born with the malformation.

The evidence for genetic factors in congenital heart defects, mainly from twin studies, is conflicting. Some studies report no or very little concordance in MZ twins (13, 14) while others report concordance from 25-45% (15). If maternal factors operate in these malformations, they are likely associated with exposure of the mother to teratogens, though no such teratogens have been convincingly demonstrated to date.

Café au lait spots are embryologically early malformations and are associated with disturbances of neural crest cell migration and/or differentiation. Again, here, it is impossible to envision what maternal factors may influence the forces that control cell migration in the early stages of neuroectodermal development.

Now, when we speak of maternal factors, most of us understand either genetic factors due to single gene loci, or factors of the intrauterine environment, hormonal and metabolic disturbances, and other factors intrinsic to the mother. Sometimes we include sociocultural factors such as nutritional deficiencies, smoking and drinking which may directly or indirectly have biological significance. But rarely do we consider the extremely important though largely undefined factors which regulate gene-environment interaction, rendering some individuals and some populations genetically susceptible to the adverse action of the environment, but not others. Examples that come to mind are the genetic inability of mothers to metabolize cortisone, which is related to the HLA complex in man and the H-2 locus in mice, and which in A/J mice results in high incidence of clefting in the offspring (16, 17); the recently discovered Ah locus in the mouse (18) and its human analogue, the AHH locus (19), which control the metabolism of the highly carcinogenic and mutagenic aromatic hydrocarbons whose degradation products are also teratogenic; and the remarkable differences in birth incidence of neural tube defects between populations of different ethnic ancestry in highly polluted environments, and of the same ethnic ancestry in highly polluted and relatively unpolluted environments

(20, 21, 22, 23), which suggests differential genetic susceptibility to the action of these environmental pollutants.

These are factors that the half sib approach, or any
other descriptive epidemiologic approach cannot sort out. All
we can expect from these approaches and models is clues as to
how to proceed next. And as is the case with epidemiology in
general, genetic epidemiology should have a dual function,
descriptive and investigative. Once a problem is defined,
measurements are taken, estimates are made and trends are detected, then biological hypotheses should be made and tested
in experimental situations. Only then we shall fulfill the
definition and the objective, that is, come to grips with
etiology.

IV. REFERENCES

1. Morton, N.E., in "Gene-Environment Interaction in Common
    Diseases" (E. Inouye and H. Nishimura, Eds.), p. 21.
    Univ. of Tokyo Press, Tokyo, 1977.
2. Myrianthopoulos, N.C., and Chung, C.S., "Congenital Mal-
    formations in Singletons: Epidemiology Survey". Birth
    Defects: Orig. Art. Series, Vol. X, No. 11, 1974.
3. Walker, J.T., Ann. Hum. Genet. 25, 65 (1961).
4. Woolf, C.M., and Woolf, R.M., Am. J. Hum. Genet. 22, 75
    (1970).
5. Woolf, C.M., and Myrianthopoulos, N.C., Am. J. Hum.
    Genet. 25, 397 (1973).
6. Wynne-Davis, R., J. Bone Joint Surg. 46B, 445 (1964).
7. Alberman, E.D., Arch. Dis. Child. 40, 548 (1965).
8. Juberg, R.C., and Touchstone, W.J., Clin. Genet. 5, 127
    (1974).
9. Chung, C.S., Nemechek, R.W., Larsen, I.J., and Ching,
    G.H.S., Hum. Hered. 19, 321 (1969).
10. Edwards, R.H., in "Clinical Delineation of Birth Defects"
    (D. Bergsma, Ed.), Vol. XVI, p. 329. Williams and
    Wilkins, Baltimore, 1974.
11. Simpson, J.L., Morillo-Cucci, G., and German, J., in
    "Clinical Delineation of Birth Defects" (D. Bergsma,
    Ed.), Vol. XVI, p. 332. Williams and Wilkins, Balti-
    more, 1974.
12. Myrianthopoulos, N.C., abstract, 3rd International Con-
    ference on Congenital Malformations, p. 66. Excerpta
    Medica, Amsterdam, 1969.
13. Hay, S., and Wehrung, D.A., Am. J. Hum. Genet. 22, 662
    (1970).
14. Myrianthopoulos, N.C., "Congenital Malformations in
    Twins: Epidemiologic Survey". Birth Defects: Orig.
    Art. Series, Vol. XI, No. 8, 1975.

15. Nora, J.J., Gilliland, J.C., Sommerville, R.J., and
     McNamara, D.G., <u>N. Engl. J. Med</u>. 277, 568 (1967).
16. Becker, B., Shin, H.D., Palmberg, P.F., and Waltman,
     S.R., <u>Science</u> 194, 1427 (1976).
17. Bonner, J.J., and Slavkin, H.C., <u>Immunogenetics</u> 2, 213
     (1975).
18. Nebert, D.W., and Gielen, J.E., <u>Fed. Proc</u>. 31, 1315
     (1972).
19. Kellermann, G., Luyten-Kellermann, M., and Shaw, C.R.,
     <u>Am. J. Hum. Genet</u>. 25, 327 (1973).
20. Laurence, K.M., <u>Develop. Med. Child Neurol</u>. Suppl. 11,
     10 (1966).
21. Stevenson, A.C., Johnston, A.H., Stewart, M.I.P., and
     Golding, D.R., "Congenital Malformations. A Report of
     a Study of Series of Consecutive Births in 24 Centres",
     Bull. WHO 34 (Suppl.) 1969.
22. Neel, J.V., <u>Am. J. Hum. Genet</u>. 10, 399 (1958).
23. Colmann, R.D., and Stroller, A., <u>J. Ment. Def. Res</u>. 12,
     22 (1968).

DISCUSSION

KIDD: Several of the presentations at this meeting have
dealt with "maternal effects." Because that term has been
used in different ways by different authors, it seems important
to point out that there are at least two types of maternal
effects that must be distinguished. The type of "maternal
effect" discussed by Drs. Nance and Myrianthopoulos in their
papers would result either from cytoplasmic inheritance
through the egg, from the intrauterine environment, or from
the neonatal (or possibly even childhood) environment provided
by the mother. The effect is produced by the maternal genotype or is environmental, it is not a function of the
children's genotypes (at least not their nuclear genotype).
Thus, siblings and maternal half-siblings will both show
similar effects because they have the same biological mother
and the same maternal care during infancy and childhood;
paternal half-siblings would not show any effect. The type
of "maternal effect" referred to by Drs. MacMahon and Spence
in their respective discussions of pyloric stenosis has a
different component. The incidence of the disorder is found
to be higher among the offspring of affected females than
among the offspring of affected males. However, the incidences
among siblings of female probands are also higher than among
siblings of male probands while the general incidence of this

disorder is much higher in males than females. This maternal effect may therefore be largely a genetic consequence of this general sex effect, i.e., it may be a form of sex-modified inheritance in which affected females represent a population with, on average, a higher "genetic loading" than affected males such that more of their relatives have the necessary genes and are therefore affected. The genotypes of the children determine their phenotypes.

Drawing this distinction between types of maternal effects is not trivial because sex effects are very prevalent among the common disorders and among birth defects. For many of these disorders the sex-specific incidences are only slightly different, but for several they are quite discrepant. For example, pyloric stenosis, stuttering, and dyslexia all have at least a threefold difference between the incidences. A general sex effect, i.e., a sex-specific incidence ratio that is significantly different from 1:1, has several possible explanations. All are relevant to epidemiology but only some involve a genetic component other than sex determination itself. The effect may be caused by factors that are extrinsic to the individual, intrinsic, or by a combination of both.

Possible extrinsic causes included social and cultural differences between the sexes. For example, social role differences may account for the ratios observed in lung cancer (1) and alcoholism (2); social roles may also be involved in the sex difference in depression (3). Artifacts, such as errors in reporting the correct incidences or biases in sampling or ascertainment are other possible extrinsic "causes". For example, ankylosing spondylitis has always been thought to have a much greater incidence among males; it now appears that the basic malady is equally frequent among females. The traditional opinion seems to have been caused by more frequent ascertainment of affected males as a result of three factors: 1.) a greater average severity among males, 2.) social role differences making males more likely to seek help for this disorder, and 3.) the diagnosis rarely being made in females because of both the medical tradition of the disease being rare in females and a proper reluctance to give the necessary diagnostic pelvic x-rays to females who have not passed through menopause (4,5).

Possible intrinsic causes of a sex effect include physiological and developmental differences between the sexes as well as certain types of genetic inheritance--X-linked, sex-modified, and sex-limited inheritance. Sex-modified inheritance is the type of greatest relevance here because the other two modes of inheritance are readily rejected for most common diseases and birth defects. Sex-modified inheritance has been clearly indicated for pyloric stenosis: compared to male probands, female probands are less frequent but have a higher frequency of affected individuals, of both sexes, among their relatives. This pattern indicates that affected females have, on average, a higher frequency of whatever genes or genotypes determine susceptibility to pyloric stenosis. This interpretation is not dependent on a polygenic mode of inheritance; it is equally compatible with a major locus being involved.

We have recently collected data that provide another very similar example: stuttering (6). Table I presents some data from our family study. The probands were all adult, Caucasian stutterers who have no indication of neurological disorder (epilepsy, cerebral palsy, brain damage). The probands were contacted through two intensive therapy clinics which draw their clients from throughout the nation. Of those attending the clinics during the period of our study we obtained family data from over 95%. In only one case did two members of the same family attend a clinic during the period of this study;

TABLE I   Incidences of "Ever-stuttered" among Relatives of Adult Stutterers

Relationship	Male Probands (N = 215)	Female Probands (N = 49)
Father	30/215 = .140 ± .024	9/49 = .18 ± .06
Mother	8/215 = .037 ± .013	4/49 = .08 ± .04
Brother	42/250 = .168 ± .024	10/49 = .20 ± .06
Sister	6/207 = .029 ± .012	7/56 = .13 ± .04
Son	12/67 = .18 ± .05	7/16 = .44 ± .12
Daughter	5/74 = .07 ± .03	3/17 = .18 ± .09

The incidences of "ever-stuttered" among the relatives of adult stutterers. The numbers are given as ever-stuttered/total relatives = mean ± standard error. For simplicity the binomial sampling errors are given though they are underestimates of the true standard errors.

the other 262 probands were unrelated. Since stuttering is usually outgrown before adulthood and can vary greatly in severity as a result of purely psychological factors (stress, nervousness, etc.), relatives are classified according to whether or not they ever stuttered. As can be readily seen in the table, male relatives are much more frequently affected than female relatives; the difference is significant ($p < .0001$ for relatives of males, $p < .04$ for relatives of females). Though not as large, there is also a significant ($p < .05$) increase in the risk to all relatives, including offspring, when the proband is a female. An almost equally large sample obtained with less clearly defined ascertainment shows no significant differences from these data. The values can be compared to rough estimates of the lifetime incidences: 5% for males and 2% for females (6). Though stuttering is not a life threatening disorder nor one for which individuals would normally seek genetic counseling, these data illustrate the magnitude of the sex-specific risk figures, a point of great importance in both genetic counseling and in genetic epidemiologic studies.

In the case of pyloric stenosis sex-modified inheritance may not be the only factor; there is also evidence for an intrauterine influence as well. The empiric risk to offspring of affected females is even higher than the available genetic models can explain. Studies in dogs (7) suggest a plausible hypothesis involving maternal gastrin concentrations, although the effect seen in dogs has not yet been studied in humans. That hypothesis and the genetic analyses suggest that the maternal effect in pyloric stenosis is actually composed of both types of effects--a genetic effect that accounts for a higher risk for all relatives of female probands and an environmental effect that increases the risk for offspring of certain females.

The data on both pyloric stenosis and stuttering show how an intrinsic sex effect resulting from sex-modified inheritance might appear as a maternal effect if the data collection and analysis procedures proposed by Dr. Nance were used. Studies of a continuous quantitative trait based on the twin-families strategy should not be affected when no selection is involved in picking families for the study. For a discrete disorder, however, the effect could be large. Consider a study in which the ascertainment criterion is that the disorder occur in at least one member of the twin pair. If the disorder were like stuttering or pyloric stenosis there would be more affected individuals among the descendants of the female twin pairs. Dr. Nance's analytic methods would explain this as a "maternal effect" instead of as a generalized sex effect. Some disorders are much more common among females than among males--idiopathic scoliosis is an example (8). If such disorders also show sex-modified inheritance and a higher incidence among the offspring of male probands, Dr. Nance's methods would apparently estimate a negative "maternal effect."

Even in the absence of sex-modified inheritance, a real, even if extrinsic, sex effect for a disease or a birth defect has important statistical consequences for studies such as Dr. Myrianthopoulos'. It is mandatory to consider the sex composition of the sample since the risk of a random individual in the sample changes as the sex composition of the sample changes. Since one is actually sampling from two different subsamples to estimate two sex-specific risks, the variance of the estimated risk to an individual, ignoring sex, is also a function of the sex composition of the sample. Moreover, because the variance actually has two components, one for the risk to males and one for the risk to females, the actual variance is always larger than the variance estimated when sex is ignored in the risk and variance calculations. Even though the risks in the two sexes may not be as dramatically different as with stuttering and pyloric stenosis, there is still an appreciable increase in the variance of the sexless risk estimate.

In summary, I feel it is important to be more alert to the possibilities of a generalized sex effect in epidemiologic genetic studies. Such sex effects appear to be more nearly the rule, rather than the exception, among common diseases and birth defects. Whether there will be a confounding of a general sex effect with a specific maternal effect will depend on the data collection procedure and on the nature of the trait. Attention to sex-specific risks should be sufficient to preclude confusion of these different phenomena.

REFERENCES

1. Harley, H.R.S., Thorax 31, 254-264 (1976).
2. Reich, T., Winokur, G., and Mullaney, J., in "Genetic Research in Psychiatry" (R.R. Fieve, D. Rosenthal, and H. Brill, Eds.), pp. 259-271. Johns Hopkins University Press, Baltimore, 1975.
3. Weissman, M., and Klerman, G., Archives of General Psychiatry 34, 98-111 (1977).
4. Calin, A., and Fries, J.F., New England Journal of Medicine 293, 835-839 (1975).
5. Kidd, K.K., Bernoco, D., Carbonara, A.O., Daneo, V., Steiger, U., and Ceppellini, R., in "HLA and Disease"

  (J. Dausset, and A. Svejgaard, Eds.), Munksgaard,
  Copenhagen, 1977.
6. Kidd, K.K., Kidd, J.R. and Records, M.A., Journal of
    Fluency Disorders, in press, (1978).
7. Dodge, J.A., Nature (Lond.) 225, 284-285 (1970).
8. Cowell, H.R., Hall, J.N., and MacEwen, G.D. Clinical
    Orthopaedics and Related Research 86, 121-131 (1972).

GENETIC EPIDEMIOLOGY

GENETIC HETEROGENEITY IN DIABETES MELLITUS AND PEPTIC ULCER

Jerome I. Rotter
David L. Rimoin

Division of Medical Genetics
Harbor General Hospital
UCLA School of Medicine
Torrance, California 90509

I. Michael Samloff

Division of Gastroenterology
Harbor General Hospital

It has become increasingly apparent that most clinical disorders are etiologically heterogeneous. While this heterogeneity is often readily apparent in rare disorders, such as the skeletal dysplasias (1), it is frequently difficult to have this concept accepted in the approach to the genetics of common diseases in spite of the fact that over the past 100 years the history of medicine has been characterized by the delineation of heterogeneity in such "diseases" as anemia and jaundice (2). As a result, it is only within the last few years that genetic heterogeneity within diabetes mellitus has been generally accepted (3,4) and is being explored within peptic ulcer (5). This heterogeneity has important implications. If what is termed a "disease" is in reality a number of disorders that are grouped together because of some common clinical feature, these distinct disorders may differ markedly in genetics, pathogenesis, natural history, and response to therapy or prophylactic measures. This heterogeneity must, therefore, be considered in our genetic and epidemiologic studies, and furthermore these studies must be designed to uncover as yet unrecognized heterogeneity.

I. THE PROBLEM - GENETICS OF COMMON DISEASES

The recognition of this potential genetic heterogeneity and the utilization of clinical tools to uncover it has made clinical genetics an increasingly productive area of investigation. However, genetic studies utilizing clinical techniques alone have their limits, since clinically normal individuals with the mutant genotype will not be recognized. These studies may be greatly aided, however, by the use of

381

subclinical markers which are closer to the basic defect and
thus likely to detect more individuals with the abnormal genotype.

In this paper the evidence for heterogeneity in both diabetes mellitus and peptic ulcer will be discussed, focusing
on the use of subclinical markers to delineate this heterogeneity. For the purpose of this discussion, subclinical
markers will be defined broadly to include all studies that
are not part of physical and routine radiologic exams, including 1) genetic markers such as ABO or HLA antigens; 2) biochemical measurements, such as serum insulin and pepsinogen
levels; 3) physiologic measurements, such as gastric acid secretory capacity or rate of gastric emptying; and 4) immunologic studies, such as insulin and pancreatic islet antibodies. Diabetes will be discussed first since genetic heterogeneity has now been well established in this syndrome (3,6)
and led us to propose the hypothesis of heterogeneity within
peptic ulcer (5).

From an epidemiologic-genetic point of view, diabetes
mellitus and peptic ulcer share many features in common. Both
are among the commonest of chronic diseases, occurring in 2 to
10% of the population in their lifetime (depending on such
factors as geography, population, level of health care, nutritional status) (7,8,9,10). This leads to a number of problems
for genetic epidemiologic studies. Is a relative affected because he has the same genotype, shares the same environment,
or has a chance occurrence of a common disorder? These disorders are sufficiently common that different forms of them
may occasionally occur in the same family by chance alone.
Both are chronic diseases increasing in frequency with increasing age, although both can occur throughout life. Both
are characterized by marked clinical variability and marked
variability of age of onset. Therefore, it is impossible to
say at any given point in time whether a clinically unaffected
individual carries the mutant genotype. Both have suffered
from the confusion engendered by the use of varying definitions of "affected" by different investigators - e.g. "affected" varying from an individual with mildly abnormal glucose
tolerance to a clinically affected individual in diabetes, and
from abdominal pain to an endoscopically demonstrated crater
in peptic ulcer. The greatest obstacle to genetic epidemiologic studies has been our ignorance concerning the basic de-
fect(s) in each disorder, and hence our inability to detect
individuals with the genotype prior to its clinical manifestation. The study of diabetes has been sufficiently frustrating that Neel called it the "geneticist's nightmare" (11).
In an analogous fashion, Rimoin has referred to the study of
peptic ulcer genetics as the "geneticist's heartburn".

II. DIABETES MELLITUS

Clinical heterogeneity and the importance of genetic factors have long been recognized in diabetes. For example, the Hindu physicians Charaka and Sushruta, over 2,000 years ago, commented on "honey urine" of two causes - genetic, i.e. passed from one generation to another in "the seed", and environmental, i.e. injudicious diet; and also the existence of two types of disease, one associated with emaciation, dehydration, polyuria and lassitude, and the other associated with stout build, gluttony, obesity, and sleepiness (quoted in 12,8).

A. The Heterogeneity Hypothesis

As the familial aggregation of diabetes became appreciated during the past half century, numerous studies were done which led to a variety of genetic hypotheses - autosomal recessive, autosomal dominant, X-linked, multifactorial, homozygosity for juvenile diabetes and heterozygosity for maturity onset, etc. (reviewed in 12,13,14). In 1967, Rimoin proposed the hypothesis of genetic heterogeneity based on several lines of evidence (15). Indirect evidence included: 1) the existence of over 30 distinct, mostly rare disorders that have glucose intolerance as one of their features (15,16,17); 2) ethnic variability in prevalence and clinical features (13,18); 3) genetic heterogeneity in diabetic animal models (19,20); 4) clinical variability between the thin ketosis prone, insulin dependent juvenile onset diabetic versus the obese, non-ketotic insulin resistant adult onset diabetic; and 5) physiologic variability - the demonstration of decreased plasma insulin in juvenile versus the hyperinsulinism of maturity onset diabetics (21,22). In addition, some direct evidence for heterogeneity came from clinical genetic studies by Harris (23,24), Simpson (25,26), and the working party of the British College of General Practitioners (27), all of which suggested that juvenile and adult onset diabetes differed genetically.

1. Genetic syndromes associated with glucose intolerance

The recognition of the association of glucose intolerance with over 30 distinct genetic syndromes due to mutations at different loci is important, not just for the obvious implications for genetic heterogeneity, but because they illustrate the wide variety of pathogenetic mechanisms that can result in glucose intolerance. As such, these rare disorders suggest that similar heterogeneity, both genetically and pathogenetically, may exist in "idiopathic" diabetes mellitus. It should be pointed out that the majority of these syndromes result in glucose intolerance alone, without frequent vascular complications asso-

ciated with diabetes. But many individuals diagnosed as diabetic are similarly mildly affected. The different syndromes
are classified in table 1 by pathogenetic mechanism or associated features (reviewed in 13,17). The mechanisms range from
absolute insulin deficiency due to pancreatic degeneration in
such disorders as hereditary relapsing pancreatitis, cystic
fibrosis, polyendocrine deficiency disease, and hemochromatosis, to insulin antagonism in the various hereditary syndromes associated with pheochromocytomas and the multiple endocrine adenoma syndromes; to nonketotic insulin resistance
in such disorders as ataxia telangectasia, myotonic dystrophy,
and the lipoatrophic diabetes syndromes. Even within these individual categories, further division can be made, either by
mechanism or by genetic criteria. For example, the lipoatrophic syndromes - characterized by the total or partial absence
of adipose tissue, hyperlipidemia, insulin resistance, nonketotic diabetes mellitus, increased basal metabolic rate, and
hepatomegaly - can be further subdivided into a recessive,
several dominant, and nongenetic forms (28). Even within what
is currently felt to be one genetic entity, multiple endocrine
adenoma type 1, an autosomal dominant disorder characterized
by pituitary, parathyroid, and pancreatic adenomas, a variety
of different hormonal mechanisms can result in insulin antagonism. That is, eosinophilic adenomas of the pituitary may
secrete growth hormone, adenomas of the adrenal gland can
secrete cortisol, and non beta islet cells of the pancreas can
produce glucagon (29,30,31). Each of these hormones individually is an insulin antagonist and their excess can lead to
marked glucose intolerance.

Table 1   Genetic Syndromes
Associated with Glucose Intolerance

Syndromes associated with pancreatic degeneration
Hereditary relapsing pancreatitis
Cystic fibrosis
Polyendocrine deficiency disease
Hemochromatosis

Hereditary endocrine disorders with glucose intolerance
Isolated growth hormone deficiency
Hereditary panhypopituitary dwarfism
Pheochromocytoma
Multiple endocrine adenomatosis

Inborn errors of metabolism with glucose intolerance
Glycogen storage disease type I
Acute intermittent porphyria

Hyperlipidemias

Syndromes with nonketotic insulin resistant early-onset diabetes
    Ataxia telangiectasia
    Myotonic dystrophy
    Lipatrophic diabetes syndromes

Hereditary neuromuscular disorders with glucose intolerance
    Muscular dystrophies
    Late-onset proximal myopathy
    Huntington's chorea
    Machado's disease
    Herrmann's syndrome
    Optic atrophy-diabetes mellitus syndrome
    Friedreich's ataxia
    Alstrom's syndrome
    Laurence-Moon-Biedl syndrome
    Pseudo-Refsum's syndrome

Progeroid syndromes with glucose intolerance
    Cockayne's syndrome
    Werner's syndrome

Syndromes with glucose intolerance secondary to obesity
    Prader-Willi syndrome
    Achondroplasia

Miscellaneous syndromes with glucose intolerance
    Steroid-induced ocular hypertension
    Mendenhall's syndrome
    Epiphyseal dysplasia and infantile-onset diabetes

Cytogenetic disorders with glucose intolerance
    Trisomy 21
    Klinefelter's syndrome
    Turner's syndrome

From Rimoin (reference 6)

2. Ethnic variability

The marked ethnic variability in the prevalence and especially in the clinical features of diabetes also suggests heterogeneity (reviewed in 13). A large part of the differences in prevalence rates can be attributed to environmental factors such as overnutrition e.g., the rise in diabetes among the Kurdish and Yemenite Jews following their migration to Israel. But not all of this variability in prevalence appears to be environmental, as exemplified by the high frequency of diabetes in individuals whose origin is the Indian subcontinent, regardless of current nationality. The marked ethnic variability in clinical features cannot be explained by diet alone (table 2). With similar high fat, high carbohydrate diets, Europeans and Ashkenazi Jews have a form of diabetes in which ketosis and vascular complications are common, the Pima Indians and Rhodesian Sephardic Jews have rare ketosis and common vascular complications, and in the Navajo Indians both complications are rare. Similarly, with a low fat, high carbohydrate diet, ketosis and vascular complications are rare in the Japanese, ketosis is rare but vascular complications common in the South African Indian, and ketosis is common but vascular complications are rare in the South African Zulus.

Table 2   Ethnic Differences in Diabetes Mellitus

Ethnic group	Diet		Ketosis	Vascular complications
	Fat	Carbohdyrate		
European	High	High	Common	Common
Ashkenazi Jew[100]	High	High	Common	Common
Rhodesian Sephardic Jew[57]	High	High	Uncommon	Common
Pima Indian[107,108]	High	High	Rare	Common
Alabama-Coushatta Indian[109]	High	High	Rare	Common
Seneca Indian[110]	High	High	Rare	Common
Lebanese[111,112]	High(vegetable)	–	Uncommon	Common
Navajo Indian[113,114]	High	High	Rare	Uncommon
Eskimo[115-117]	High	Low	Rare	Rare
Japanese[118-120]	Low	High	Rare	Uncommon
Ceylonese[121]	Low	High	Rare	Uncommon
Indian[101]	Low	High	Rare	Common
South African Indian[102,103,122]	Low	High	Rare	Very common
South African Zulu[102,103,122]	Low	High	Common	Rare
Rhodesian African[123]	Low	High	Common	Rare

From Rimoin & Schimke, numbers in the table refer to this reference (13).

B. Direct Evidence

Between 1967 and 1975 the concept of heterogeneity in diabetes mellitus gained increasing acceptance (3,4), due to accumulation of numerous new lines of evidence directly supporting the heterogeneity hypothesis.

1. Family studies

The first line of evidence consisted of various family studies that indicated that juvenile and adult onset diabetes appeared to be separate disorders genetically: 1) Cammidge's studies in the 20's and 30's in which he claimed that early age of onset diabetics most often had recessive appearing family histories and late onset more often had dominant appearing family histories (32,33); 2) Harris (23,24) found increased parental consanguinity among the parents of juvenile but not adult onset cases and a six fold increase of juvenile diabetes among the sibs of juvenile as opposed to adult propositi (23,24); 3) Simpson, in her extensive Canadian studies, reported a greater frequency of juvenile diabetes among the sibs (10 fold) and offspring (20 fold) of juvenile diabetic probands compared to adult onset and control probands, and no increased incidence of adult onset diabetes among the parents of juvenile probands (25,26,34); 4) A survey by the British College of General Practitioners found an increased relative risk for diabetes to siblings of young (<30) vs. old diabetics (>50) (27); 5) Harvald and Degnbol demonstrated that the morbid risk before age 40 for relatives (siblings and offspring) of late onset diabetics was not different from the general population, while the before age 40 risk to the relatives of juvenile onset diabetes was increased 5 to 10 times (35); 6) Kobberling found a 25 fold increased frequency of juvenile onset diabetes among the siblings of juvenile onset diabetics as opposed to the siblings of maturity onset diabetics, and a incidence of adult onset diabetics among the parents of juvenile probands similar to that expected in controls (36,37); 7) LeStradet studied the families of juvenile diabetic probands and found the incidence of non-insulin dependent diabetics in the parents and grandparents of such cases to be equal to that of controls, with a contrasting significant increase in insulin dependent diabetics in these families (38); 8) MacDonald reported similar results, i.e., the incidence of maturity onset diabetes (onset >45) in the grandparents of diabetic children was same as that in the grandparents of control children (39).

2. Twin studies

The second line of new evidence was the extensive monozygotic twin studies of the British group (40,41,42,43), in-

cluding over 100 MZ twin pairs. 71 of these pairs were concordant, 35 discordant. But when the pairs were classified
according to age of onset, only 50% of the pairs whose age of
onset in the index twin was below age 40 (32/64, mostly juvenile insulin dependent) were concordant, as opposed to 100% of
those whose onset in the index twin was over age 50 (26/26,
maturity onset insulin independent). Similar results could
be derived from a reevaluation of previous smaller studies
(44,45). Of the discordant pairs, most had remained so greater than 10 years and in these there was no trend toward increasing concordance with time (42,46,47). These findings
provide further evidence for separating juvenile and maturity
onset diabetes. A further difference between the juvenile and
adult twin pairs could be found by comparing the frequency of
affected first degree relatives in the two groups; 70% of the
first degree relatives of the adult onset diabetics (>40 y.o.)
were affected as opposed to only 15% of the relatives of the
juvenile onset diabetics (< 40y.o.).

3. Maturity onset diabetes of the young (MODY)
        The third piece of evidence was the delineation of a dis-
tinct autosomal dominant form of juvenile onset diabetes with
a maturity onset phenotype by Tattersall and Fajans (48,49,50).
This group of patients have an early age of onset but have few
symptoms, no ketonuria, and can be controlled without insulin,
with little progression in severity of carbohydrate intolerance over 20 years. These "maturity onset diabetics of young
people" (MODY patients) are clearly phenotypically different
from the classical juvenile onset diabetic (JOD). Genetic
studies provided further evidence that these are separate entities. Of the MODY propositi, 85% had a diabetic parent,
usually with a similar phenotype, 53% of sibs tested had diabetes, and 46% of the families showed three generations of direct vertical transmission of the trait, suggesting autosomal
dominant inheritance. In contrast, only 11% of JOD parents
were diabetic, 8 of 74 sibs were diabetic, 6 with similar JOD
phenotypes and only 6% of the families showed three-generation
transmission. This study most clearly demonstrates the need
to carefully dissect out the phenotypic differences among diabetics before genetic analysis is possible. If these MODY patients had been classified by either age of onset or by diabetic phenotype alone, they would have been lumped together
with "classic" JOD's or MOD's respectively, and their distinctive pattern of inheritance would have been obscured. Physiologic studies of these patients support this phenotypic differentiation, as these patients have insulin responses to glucose
loads much more characteristic of maturity onset diabetes
(51,52).

4. Insulin requirements and response

The evidence alluded to thus far has been largely clinical. What about various subclinical markers? As already mentioned, the study of insulin response to a glucose load provided evidence for physiologic heterogeneity in diabetes. The insulinopenic response of juvenile onset diabetics (21) and the hyperinsulinemic response of maturity onset diabetics parallels therapeutic observations of the absolute insulin requirement of the juveniles (insulin dependent) versus the ability to manage most adult onset cases with oral hypoglycemics and/or diet (insulin independent). In fact, this has led Irvine to propose that insulin dependence and independence, rather than age of onset, should be used as a basis of classification (53). His group has also presented evidence supporting this classification in family studies (54).

5. HLA association

The clear and consistent association of juvenile insulin dependent, but not maturity onset insulin independent diabetes, with HLA antigens B8 and BW15, has been a major argument for etiologic differences between these disorders (55,56, 57,58,59,60,61,62,63,64,65,66). The relative risk for a B8 or BW15 individual for insulin dependent diabetes ranges from 2 to 3 depending on the specific study. The most likely explanation for the relatively low order of magnitude of this type of HLA association is linkage disequilibrium (67,68,69, 70). The B8 and BW15 antigens are felt not to be directly responsible for juvenile insulin dependent diabetes themselves, but are linked in disequilibrium to other genes of the HLA loci, such as immune response genes, which may be directly responsible for the individual's susceptibility to diabetes. Linkage disequilibrium is known to occur between alleles of the various HLA loci (69,70,71).

6. Pancreatic islet cell antibodies

The ability to type for pancreatic islet cell antibodies has provided another line of evidence supporting an autoimmune pathogenesis for at least some forms of diabetes, as well as a potential marker for genetic studies. While these antibodies were first detected only in insulin dependent diabetics with coexistent autoimmune endocrine disease (72,73), it soon became clear that they were common (60 to 80%) in newly diagnosed juvenile diabetics (74,75,76,77). Furthermore they might serve as a preclinical marker for certain types of diabetes (78,79). Islet cell antibody studies supported the differentiation of insulin dependent from insulin independent diabetes as antibodies were present in 30-40% of former group as opposed to 5 to 8% of the latter (75,77,80). Of interest, the majority of the insulin independent yet anti-

body positive patients appeared to become insulin dependent
with time (77,79). They also have flat insulin responses to
a glucose load (80). This has suggested that physiologically
they belong in the insulin dependent category (that is, they
are just an intermediate state in the development of insulin
dependence).

C. Further Heterogeneity

By 1977 there was clear evidence that juvenile insulin
dependent diabetes mellitus and maturity onset insulin independent diabetes mellitus were separate genetic disorders.
This was based on clinical genetic studies, such as the family
and twin studies which separated juvenile from maturity onset
diabetes, the delineation of a third entity, maturity onset
diabetes of the young (MODY); and on the use of physiologic
(insulin response to a glucose load), immunologic (antipancreatic islet cell antibodies) and genetic (HLA antigens) markers.

1. Heterogeneity within juvenile insulin dependent diabetics,
   based on HLA association

On the basis of an analysis of recent immunologic and
metabolic studies, we have been able to uncover further heterogeneity among the JOD form of diabetes, that has led us to
postulate that the HLA B8 and BW15 associated forms of diabetes are distinct diseases (81).

a. Additivity of HLA risks. This further heterogeneity
was first suggested by the reports that the relative risks for
HLA antigens B8 and BW15 were additive; i.e., the risk for individuals who had both B8 and BW15 was greater than for individuals with only one of these antigens (table 3) (58,59,61,
68,82).

Table 3   Additive Risk of B8 and BW15

Reference	Relative Risk		
	B8	BW15	B8 & BW15
1) Cudworth & Woodrow [58,59]	2.54	2.00	5.82
2) Svejgaard et al.[68] & Nerup et al.[61]	2.69	2.45	6.16
3) Barta & Simon[82]	2.03	1.17	18.25
Pooled relative risks +standard error	2.43+.11	1.83+.13	7.24+.28

(Relative risk calculated by method of Woolf (83,84))

When we pooled the data from these three studies, it was
clear that this increase in the relative risk for the individual with both B8 and BW15 was statistically significant.
Furthermore, the relative risk for diabetes was not increased

by homozygosity for either B8 or BW15; that is, it made no
difference whether an individual had one or two B8 genes or
one or two BW15 genes (68). Only the compound B8-BW15 heterozygote was at increased risk. As a clinical correlate of this
additivity, Ludviggson et al., reported that B8-BW15 diabetics
had a younger age of onset and had a decreased incidence of
detectable C-peptide (presumably indicating greater pancreatic islet cell destruction) than individuals with only one of
these antigens (62). Differences between B8 and BW15 were
also seen in the examination of HLA types in the British monozygotic twin study (60). The concordant pairs had an increased frequency of both B8 and BW15, while only BW15 was increased in the discordant pairs.

b. Linkage disequilibrium. Another line of evidence for
heterogeneity in JOD relates to the concept of linkage disequilibrium as an explanation for the HLA-disease association:
the B locus alleles, B8 and BW15, may not themselves be responsible for the predisposition to diabetes, but are in linkage disequilibrium with other closely linked genes in the major histocompatibility complex which are more directly related
to diabetes susceptibility. For example, it is well known
that antigens A1 at the A locus and B8 at the B locus are in
linkage disequilibrium in Caucasian populations (69,70,71).
A1 has been found to be associated with insulin dependent diabetes, with a relative risk of 1.65(59). Since this is lower
than the relative risk of 2.5 for B8, the A1 association with
diabetes can be said to be secondary to its linkage disequilibrium with B8 (70). Thomsen, et al., have found a marked
increase in the D series antigen DW3 (formerly Ld-8a), among
insulin dependent diabetics, resulting in a relative risk of
4.5 for DW3 as compared to 2.4 for the B8 antigen (85). Furthermore,
whereas all B8 individuals were DW3 positive, there were DW3 diabetics who were B8 negative . These data suggest that the
association of B8 with diabetes is merely secondary to its
linkage disequilibrium with DW3. The DW4 antigen (formerly
LDw15a) was also increased in the diabetics, but not significantly. However, there were more patients who were BW15 positive and DW4 negative than BW15 negative and DW4 positive,
suggesting that the increase in DW4 was only secondary to the
BW15 association. Schernthaner, et al., have found an increased frequency of the CW3 antigen (formerly T3) of the C
locus in insulin dependent diabetics (63). Among the diabetic patients, there was an increased frequency of CW3 in the
absence of BW15 and the frequency of BW15 was almost identical
in CW3 negative patients and controls. They concluded that
the increased frequency of BW15 in diabetics was secondary to
its linkage disequilibrium with the CW3 allele. Thus, the B8
antigen appears to serve as a marker for a diabetogenic gene

closer to the D locus, while the BW15 allele serves as a marker for a diabetogenic gene closer to the C locus. Since the C and D loci are on opposite sides of the B locus, these results indicate that different genes are responsible for the susceptibility to diabetes in B8 and BW15 individuals.

c. Insulin antibodies. The anti-insulin antibody response to exogenous insulin therapy also appears to differ between the B8 and BW15 associated juvenile onset diabetes. Bertrams, et al., studied 112 insulin dependent diabetics treated with bovine and/or porcine insulin (64). On the basis of their titers of anti-insulin antibodies, the patients were classified into three groups: 39 non-responders with no detectable insulin antibodies; 41 medium responders with titers of 1 in 5 to 1 in 30; and 32 high responders with titers greater than 1 in 30. As a total group, they had an increased frequency of B8 and BW15 and a decreased frequency of B7. However, when the group was broken down into antibody responders and nonresponders, major differences in HLA associations were found. The antibody nonresponders had an increased frequency of B8, but a normal frequency of BW15; whereas, in contrast, the responders (medium and high) had a normal frequency of B8 and an increased frequency of BW15. Ludvigsson, et al., have confirmed this observation by finding increased insulin antibodies, by insulin binding capacity of IgG, among the BW15 positive diabetics (62). On the other hand, their B8 diabetics had more individuals with low insulin antibody titers than any other antigen group. Thus, the immune response gene associated with the production of anti-insulin antibodies appears to be associated only with the BW15 allele.

d. Diabetic complications. The frequency and severity of diabetic complications may also differ between the B8 and BW15 forms of juvenile onset diabetes. In the British monozygotic twin study, the concordant pairs were said to develop complications of diabetes, such as retinopathy, more frequently and severely than the discordant pairs (41,43), and it was only the concordant pairs that had an increased frequency of B8 (60). Barbosa, et al., studied HLA antigens in 110 juvenile onset diabetics with terminal glomerulonephritis and retinopathy, who required kidney transplantation (86). They found a significant increase in the frequency of B8 among those patients with severe microangiopathy, but the frequency of BW15 was similar to that of the controls. This suggests that the B8 antigen and not the BW15 antigen appears to be associated with an increased predilection to diabetic microangiopathy.

e. Pancreatic islet cell antibodies. The presence or absence of pancreatic islet cell antibodies also appears to distinguish between the B8 and BW15 forms of juvenile onset diabetes. Nerup et al. found that the frequency of islet cell antibodies was more common among juvenile onset diabetics who were positive for HLA B8 than among those who had other HLA types (61). Morris, et al. assembled a large group of juvenile onset diabetics who had islet cell antibodies and found a significantly increased frequency of HLA B8 (61%) among them in comparison to the control group, but not of HLA BW15 (87). Interestingly, maturity onset diabetics who were islet cell antibody positive also had a similarly increased frequency of B8. This is in accord with the observation that many of these islet cell antibody positive patients became insulin dependent with time (77,79) and Irvine's hypothesis that islet cell antibody positive patients have the same disorder regardless of age of onset and that classification by age of onset is at least partly artifical (53). The increased frequency of B8 in the islet cell antibody positive diabetics was accentuated when the duration of the disease was considered, as 71% of those diabetics who were positive for islet cell antibodies five or more years after the diagnosis of their disease also had the B8 antigen. In addition, Nerup found that 89% of B8 positive juvenile onset diabetics had evidence of pancreatic autoimmunity, as defined by the presence of islet cell antibodies and/or antipancreatic cell mediated immunity, as compared to 58% of other HLA types (61). Thus, the B8 form of juvenile onset diabetes appears to be associated with islet cell autoimmune disease.

f. B8 associations. Several other lines of evidence support the concept that the B8 form of insulin dependent diabetes is of autoimmune origin. It has long been known that insulin dependent diabetes is associated with other autoimmune endocrine disorders, such as Hashimoto's thyroiditis, pernicious anemia and Addison's disease (88,89,90,91). In addition, serological studies have revealed that insulin dependent diabetics have a higher incidence of organ specific antibodies to thyroid, gastric parietal cells, intrinsic factor, and adrenal cortex (88,89,90,91). Finally, Schmidt's syndrome, a constellation of autoimmune disease of the adrenal cortex and thyroid, is often associated with insulin dependent diabetes (92,93). Hence, there is good evidence on clinical and serological grounds for an autoimmune form of juvenile onset diabetes. Like juvenile onset diabetes, a variety of autoimmune endocrine disorders, such as Addison's disease (94,85), Grave's disease (95,96,97,98), and hypergonadotrophic hypogonadism (99), have been found to have an increased frequency of HLA B8 and DW3. However, none of these other autoimmune endocrine diseases has been associated with BW15. Thus, autoimmune islet cell disease, as well as other forms of autoimmune endocrine disease, appear to be associated with HLA B8 and not with BW15 or other HLA types.

g. B7 Protection. HLA antigen B7 has been found to be decreased in frequency in juvenile onset insulin dependent diabetics; it has been said to have a "protective effect" (100). A review of the literature indicates that this decreased prevalence of B7 only occurs in the presence of the B8 form of the disease. For example, B7 frequency was decreased in Bertrams' insulin antibody nonresponder group, the group with the increased prevalence of B8, but not in the antibody responder group, the group which had an increased prevalence of BW15 and not B8 (64). This same distinction was found in the microangiopathy study of Barbosa, et al. (86). Those individual who had severe angiopathy and an increased prevalence of B8 also had a decreased prevalence of B7. It is also of interest that persons with other B8 associated autoimmune disorders, such as coeliac disease (101, 102) and Grave's disease (96) have been found to have a decreased frequency of B7.

h. Isolated pedigrees. Studies of two large families have also suggested marked differences between the B8 and BW15 forms of diabetes. The first family studied by Nerup, et al., and Thomsen, et al., consisted of 21 individuals in 4 generations, 7 of whom had diabetes (61,85). All affected members of the pedigree who were typed shared a common HLA-A2, BW15, CW3 haplotype. All of the family members who were not BW15 positive were found to be nondiabetic. Among those BW15 positive relatives who did not have clinical diabetes, all that were examined showed a decreased early insulin response to intravenous glucose. The authors suggest that this might imply the presence of an inherited insensitivity to glucose, an inherited reduced beta cell mass, or an impaired regeneration capacity to subclinical islet damage among BW15 positive individuals. In another family, reported by Van Thiel, et al. an apparent autoimmune genetic disorder associated with B8 juvenile onset diabetes has been described (103). This family had a syndrome consisting of diabetes mellitus, immunoglobulin A deficiency, malabsorption, and a common HLA haplotype. All affected individuals shared a haplotype consisting of HLA A2, B8 and DW3. Other members of the family who had this same haplotype, but did not have diabetes, had evidence of other autoimmune disorders, such as vitiligo, Grave's disease and other antiendocrine antibodies.

i. Distinct forms of juvenile diabetes. This accumulated evidence strongly suggests that genetic heterogeneity exists even within the typical insulin dependent juvenile onset form of diabetes. We conclude that there are at least two clearly distinct forms of juvenile onset diabetes, one of which is associated with HLA B8 and the other with BW15 (table 4). The HLA-B8 form of the disease may be called the autoimmune form. It is characterized by an increased prevalence of the DW3 allele of the HLA D locus, a decreased frequency of HLA B7, an increased prevalence of pancreatic islet cell antibodies and antipancreatic cell mediated immunity, a lack of antibody response to exogenous insulin, and increased susceptibility to microangiopathy. The second form of juvenile onset insulin dependent diabetes is associated with HLA BW15 and is less well characterized. It appears to be associated with the CW3 allele of the HLA C locus, it is not associated with autoimmune disease or islet cell antibodies, and it is accompanied by an increased antibody response to exogenous insulin.

It is quite likely that even further heterogeneity will be encountered among "classic" juvenile onset diabetes. For example, it has been recently suggested that HLA B18 is increased in insulin dependent diabetics (59, 97). Measurable plasma C peptide was found to be increased in the B18 patients, but not in B8 and BW15 diabetics (62). This may indicate yet another distinct form of juvenile onset diabetes and Ludvigsson et al., have suggested that the B18 antigen may result in a milder form of the disease. Obviously this group of patients needs to be studied in greater detail.

2. Heterogeneity within juvenile diabetes based on pathogenesis

It should also be mentioned that other classifications of insulin dependent diabetes have been proposed. Both Battazo and Doniach (104) and Irvine (53) have proposed that insulin dependent diabetes can be subdivided into autoimmune and viral induced types (with an intermediate category included in the Irvine classification). The autoimmune type is fairly well delineated and is characterized by pancreatic islet cell antibodies, which may occur years before the onset of clinical diabetes and persist for years after its onset, by the presence of other associated autoimmune endocrinopathies and antibodies, by an onset at any age, by a higher incidence in females, and by its association with HLA B8. In contrast, the hypothesized viral induced type has transient islet cell antibodies at the

Table 4   Heterogeneity within Juvenile Insulin
            Dependent Diabetes Mellitus

Evidence	B8	BW15
1) Relative risk diabetes	-ADDITIVE-	
2) Linkage disequilibrium with other HLA loci	Increased association with DW3	Increased association with CW3
3) Twin studies	↑ in concordant twins only	↑ in concordant and discordant twins
4) Insulin antibodies	Nonresponder (no antibodies)	High responder (produce antibodies)
5) Diabetic complications	↑ microangiopathy	Not increased
6) Islet cell antibodies	Increased	Not increased
7) Antipancreatic cell mediated immunity	Increased	Not increased
8) HLA B7	Decreased	Normal frequency
9) Isolated pedigrees	Autoimmune disorder	Defect in insulin release

onset of disease which disappeared within the next year, is
not associated with autoimmunity, tends to have an age of onset less than 30 (but may occur later), has equal sex incidence and its association with any specific HLA antigens is
unclear. There are clear areas of overlap with our HLA classification, specifically, the B8 associated type of juvenile
insulin dependent diabetes.   It is unclear at this time in
what manner the proposed viral induced category overlaps with
our HLA classification.

3. Racial differences
     There are also racial differences in the HLA diabetes
association which may partially account for some of the ethnic
variability referred to earlier. In the Japanese, initial
reports have indicated that antigens B22J and B12 are increased in insulin dependent but not insulin independent diabetics, and that antigen B5 is decreased in this group (105,
106,107). These results parallel the B8, BW15 increase and B7
decrease in the Caucasian group (Northern European and North
American), but with different antigens. This finding provides
strong evidence for linkage disequilibrium as a basis for the
HLA diabetes association. An important consequence of the
linkage disequilibrium theory is that since the association
between the HLA antigens themselves has been found to be different among racial groups (70,71), one then expects that the
association between the antigens and the disease should also be
different in different races (68,70). That is, if the antigens are on the average linked (in disequilibrium) to different immune response genes in different races and it is these
immune response genes that are responsible for the predisposition to a given disease, then the association of different
antigens in different races with the same disease is the expected finding. On the other hand, if the disease is associated with the antigen itself, and not merely as a marker for
another part of the major histocompatibility complex genome,
then the expected finding would be that the same association
between antigen and disease would occur in different races, as
seems to be the case for B27 and ankylosing spondylitis (68,
70). These different associations might herald phenotypic
differences that have not been clearly defined, and so detailed studies are going to be required for each racial group.

4. Heterogeneity within maturity onset diabetes
     Thus heterogeneity within the juvenile insulin dependent
group seems well documented. What about heterogeneity within
the adult onset or insulin independent group?

     a. Pancreatic islet cell antibodies. One example of well
documented heterogeneity is the maturity onset (regardless of

insulin status) pancreatic islet cell antibody positive, B8
associated group (87,53,77,79); that is, diabetics who though
they have a late age of onset (>40), are insulin dependent,
also have an increased frequency of B8 (59) and have the same
prevalence of islet cell antibodies as younger diabetics with
the same duration of diabetes (77). In addition, a certain
fraction, up to 8% of those diabetics intially classified as
insulin independent i.e., managed on oral hypoglycemics, are
islet cell antibody positive (80,75,77). These have a flat
insulin response to a glucose load reminiscent of insulin dependent diabetes (80). The majority of these patients progress to insulin dependence within a few years (79).
Several investigators consider this group as equivalent to the
insulin dependent juveniles with simply a later age of onset
(53,104). In that sense, these data would provide the basis
for the reclassification rather than heterogeneity. Whether
these patients comprise a further genetic subgroup (of either
maturity onset diabetes or insulin dependent diabetes depending on one's classification) or are just one end of the spectrum of insulin dependent diabetes, still needs additional
evaluation.

b. Clinical studies. Clinical genetic studies have also
suggested heterogeneity within the adult onset type. For example, Kobberling (108,37) divided his adult onset probands
into low, moderate, and markedly overweight categories, using
an index consisting of degree of overweight (in percent) times
number of years overweight before the onset of diabetes. He
then compared the frequency of diabetes among the siblings of
insulin independent (treated by diet and oral hypoglycemics)
probands in the various categories. He found a significantly
higher frequency of affected siblings in the light proband
category (38%) and a significantly lower frequency in the
heavy proband category (10%). Similar results were
obtained when he used as his index criteria the number of
pregnancies in the affected diabetic; that is those diabetics
with a lower number of pregnancies (0 to 2) had a higher frequency of diabetic siblings (29%), and those with many pregnancies (>5) had a significantly lower frequency of affected
siblings (10%). However, these divisions did not seem
to matter if he used insulin dependent cases as his probands.
The percentage of affected siblings was constant regardless of
the weight or parity of the insulin dependent diabetic proband. Kobberling comments that one explanation for these
findings could be an additive gene model. Obesity or multi-
parity would be an additional pathogenetic risk factor. Therefore, individuals with higher degrees of obesity would require
fewer disease predisposing genes to progress to clinical diabetes. However, this could also be explained by different

monogenic forms with different susceptibilities, i.e., different dependence on exogenous predisposing factors. The data of Irvine, et al., (54) also suggest a difference between the non-obese and obese insulin independent propositi. They observed a different clinical range of diabetes in the relatives of the non-obese and obese propositi, but the numbers in this study were too small to attain statistical significance.

c. Insulin responses. Finally Fajans and co-workers have described heterogeneity of the insulin response to a glucose load in non-obese (latent) insulin independent patients (109, 110,111,52). They described both insulin under-responders and insulin over-responders. A few of the insulin under-responders progressed to a requirement for insulin in order to control fasting hyperglycemia (not to prevent ketosis). Excluding those few, as time progressed, both groups on the average "improved". That is, the under-responders increased their insulin output and the over-responders decreased their insulin output. However, neither group approached the norm, as both were still clearly distinguishable as high and low output groups. Fajans suggests that in the under-responder category, the lack of insulin is one of the principal determinants of abnormal glucose tolerance. On the other hand, he suggests that in the over-responder category, the hyperinsulinemia is secondary to other factors which cause glucose intolerance.

Thus heterogeneity within diabetes mellitus appears to be extensive and well documented. A summary of the various well delineated disorders and a proposed classification is included in table 5 below.

Table 5   Classification of Documented Heterogeneity
Within Diabetes Mellitus

I. Juvenile Onset (JOD), insulin dependent

   A.   Classification by HLA association
       1. B8 - autoimmune
       2. BW15 - immune response to insulin
       3. ? B18 - ? milder

   B.   Classification by proposed pathogenesis, overlaps with IA
       1. Autoimmune
       2. Virus induced
       3. Both 1 and 2
       4. ? others

II. Juvenile onset, insulin independent - maturity onset diabetes of the young (MODY)

III. Maturity onset (MOD)

    A.   Insulin dependent, B8, islet cell antibody associated

    B.   Insulin independent, pancreatic islet cell antibody positive, ? progress to insulin dependence

    C.   Insulin independent
        1. Non-obese
           a. Decreased insulin response
           b. Supernormal insulin response
        2. Obese

Note: Some investigators lump IA1, III A & B

III PEPTIC ULCER

Now let us turn to peptic ulcer disease. Here the heterogeneity is not so well defined nor acknowledged. Though the familial aggregation of peptic ulcer disease had been well established in the 1950's, as had the association of duodenal ulcer with the genetic markers blood group 0 and nonsecretor status (112), no substantial progress had been made in our understanding of the genetics of this disorder for 20 years. Polygenic inheritance has been the prevailing hypothesis to explain the genetics of peptic ulcer. We have proposed that genetic heterogeneity within peptic ulcer disease would explain both the familial aggregation and the lack of a simple Mendelian pattern of inheritance (5).

A. Gastric versus Duodenal Ulcer

Some degree of heterogeneity already had been demonstrated in peptic ulcer disease. In 1950, Doll and Buch showed that peptic ulcers occurred 2 to 2-1/2 times as frequently among the sibs of peptic ulcer patients as among sibs of controls (113). In 1951, Doll and Kellock demonstrated the independent segregation of gastric and duodenal ulcers (114). Their data indicated that the relatives of gastric ulcer propositi had a 3 fold increased prevalence of gastric ulcer compared to the general population, whereas duodenal ulcer occurred no more frequently among these relatives than in the general population. Likewise, the relatives of duodenal ulcer patients had 3 times as much duodenal ulcer compared to the control population, but no increased risk of gastric ulcer. These data provide strong evidence, from a genetic point of view, that gastric and duodenal ulcer are independent disorders. Other genetic studies have supported this independence. In the vast majority of like sex twins reported as concordant for peptic ulcer (115), the ulcer site was found to be identical. Also, blood group O and nonsecretor status were found to be associated with duodenal ulcer (with or without associated gastric ulcer) but not with primary gastric ulcer (112). Since then, a great mass of clinical and physiologic data has supported the concept that duodenal and primary gastric ulcer are separate entities. It is well established that, on the average, patients with gastric ulcer tend to secrete subnormal amounts of acid while those with duodenal ulcer tend to secrete more acid than normal individuals (116). Even further heterogeneity was suggested by Doll and Kellock, in that there was an increased prevalence of combined gastric and duodenal ulcer in the relatives of patients with combined ulcer disease (4/18), as compared to the relatives of probands with either isolated gastric or duodenal ulcer (2/111). Although the numbers are small, they suggest even further genetic heterogeneity within clinical ulcer disease; that is, does combined (gastric and duodenal) ulcer disease segregate independently from isolated gastric and duodenal ulcer, as they do from each other?

B. Genetic syndromes with peptic ulceration

Additional evidence of genetic heterogeneity within peptic ulcer disease is provided by the existence of two distinct autosomal dominant disorders that feature peptic ulceration as a prominent part of their phenotype. The first is multiple endocrine adenoma syndrome, type I (MEA I, Werner syndrome), characterized by pituitary, parathyroid, and pancreatic adenomas (117,29). The pancreatic adenomas, when composed of non beta islet cells, have been shown to secrete gastrin, resulting in a severe ulcer diathesis (Zollinger-Ellison syndrome) (118). Until the association of ulcer disease with these tumors was recognized, its pattern of inheritance elucidated, and the biochemical marker of increased plasma gastrin levels characterized, this specific entity was lost among the mass of peptic ulcer patients. The second condition was described recently by Neuhauser et al. in a family of Swedish-Finnish ancestry in which an autosomal dominant gene appears to result in a tetrad of abnormalities - essential tremor, congenital nystagmus, a narcolepsy like sleep disturbance, and severe duodenal ulceration (119). Twelve of 17 affected members had essential tremor, 12 of 17 had nystagmus, and 8 of 17 had duodenal ulcers, the latter occurring almost exclusively in individuals with the neurologic syndrome and sometimes preceding the onset of neurologic symptoms.

C. Heterogeneity within duodenal ulcer

1. Clinical studies

Lam and Sircus (120) and Lam and Ong (121) have classified duodenal ulcer patients on clinical grounds, using different criteria in each study. Lam and Sircus (120) using the criteria of maximum acid secretory capacity (corrected for body weight), proposed that people with duodenal ulcer could be divided into two types: 1) patients with a stimulated acid output within the normal range, who had an increased likelihood of being blood group O, who were prone to the complications of bleeding and perforation, whose peak age of onset fell within the 4th decade, who had mild symptoms of gastroesophogeal reflux, and who usually did not have a family history of ulcer disease; and 2) patients with a stimulated maximal acid output greater than two standard deviations above the mean, who were predominantly of blood groups A, B and AB, who less commonly had complications such as bleeding and perforation, whose peak onset was in the third decade, who had more frequent symptoms of gastroesophogeal reflux, and who had a strong family history of peptic ulcer disease. Lam and Ong (121), in a geographically different study population, classified duodenal ulcer into two subgroups on the basis of age of onset of the disease. Their early-onset group (onset below age 20 years) had a significantly stronger family history, a frequency of blood group O similar to that of controls, more frequently presented with gastrointestinal bleeding as the first manifestation of the disease, and rarely had complications such as perforation, obstruction, intractable pain or secondary gastric ulcer. In contrast, their late onset group (onset after age 31 years) infrequently had a family history of ulcer disease, were more likely than controls to be blood group O, presented less frequently with gastrointestinal bleeding, and had an increased frequency of complications such as perforation, pyloroduodenal stenosis, severe pain, virulent ulcer, and secondary gastric ulcer. In an earlier study, Kubickova and Vesely found that family history could be used to separate a "genuine" duodenal ulcer group (positive family history), having an increased frequency of blood group O, from a "solitary" duodenal ulcer group (negative family history), who did not have an increased frequency of blood group O (122). Furthermore, Eberhard reported that concordant monozygotic twins with ulcer disease, when compared to discordant monozygotic twin pairs, appeared to have an increased family history of ulcer and an increased frequency of blood group O (123). Like the reports of Lam and Sircus and Lam and Ong, these latter two studies suggest heterogeneity within duodenal ulcer disease, but come to different conclusions about

the association of a positive family history and increased
frequency of blood group O. These differences may be due in
part to the different populations included in each study.

2. Physiologic studies

Biochemical evidence for heterogeneity is provided by the
data of Samloff et al. on quantitative immunoreactive serum
group I pepsinogen concentrations (124). They described a
bimodal distribution of serum pepsinogen concentrations in
duodenal ulcer patients, suggesting that those individuals
with markedly elevated pepsinogen levels had one or more distinct disorders.

Byrnes et al. have also presented evidence that duodenal
ulcer patients may be subdivided on physiologic grounds (125).
They found one group to be characterized by normal acid secretion and increased gastrin response to meals (both integrated gastrin and peak gastrin response elevated). The second group of patients was characterized by acid hypersecretion
and normal gastrin response to meals. Fritsch et al. have reported similar results (126). When we compared the peak acid
output to integrated gastrin response in Byrnes' two groups
and controls, an additional distinction became apparent. In
comparison to controls, the acid normosecretor group seems to
have lost the normal feedback relation between acid output and
gastrin release. Acid hypersecretors, on the other hand, retained the inhibition of gastrin release by acid, but the level of inhibition occurred at a higher level; that is, it took
more acid to inhibit their gastrin release. This latter phenomenon occurs in patients with increased maximum acid output,
and by inference, increased parietal cell mass (127).

Additional evidence for physiologic heterogeneity comes
from the work of Howlett et al. who studied gastric emptying
of a solid meal in duodenal ulcer patients (128). Applying
the mathematical technique of principal component analysis to
their results, they were able to separate their duodenal ulcer
patients into two groups without overlap - one group whose
rate of emptying was similar to that of controls and the other
with an increased rate of gastric emptying. Further support
for this finding is provided by the study of Creutzfeldt et
al., who examined the oral glucose tolerance of duodenal ulcer
subjects (129). A majority of their duodenal ulcer patients
had a normal oral glucose tolerance test (OGTT) and only a
slightly elevated gastric inhibitory polypeptide (GIP) response to a meal. However, a large subgroup was characterized
by an elevated OGTT and a markedly increased GIP response.
They speculate that these findings may be another reflection
of the gastric emptying difference described by Howlett's
group.

3. Further heterogeneity demonstrated by the use of sub-clinical markers.

Under the auspices of the Center for Ulcer Research and Education at UCLA, we have initiated a number of collaborative projects to test for further heterogeneity. A major difficulty in the study of the genetics of peptic ulcer has been the lack of subclinical markers of the ulcer diathesis. A sensitive radioimmunoassay to determine the concentration of pepsinogen I (PG I) in serum has recently been developed (130). PG I is synthesized only by the peptic cells in the fundic mucosa (131,132). PG I levels have been found to correlate with gastric secretory capacity (133), to serve as a marker for the ulcer diathesis (being elevated in approximately two-thirds of unrelated duodenal ulcer patients), and as mentioned previously, to demonstrate heterogeneity within duodenal ulcer patients, i.e. PG I levels follow a bimodal distribution (124). We have utilized this new assay for genetic studies of peptic ulcer disease and have identified autosomal dominant transmission of an elevated serum PG I level in two large familes with a prominent history of duodenal ulcer (134,135,136).

Studying 120 members of the two families over 3 generations, we found apparent autosomal dominant inheritance of hyperpepsinogenemia I, as 50% of the offspring of affected individuals (affected defined as elevated PG I) were also affected, and none of the offspring of unaffected individuals was affected. Furthermore, only those individuals with an elevated PG I level appeared to be susceptible to clinical duodenal ulcer disease. Although both families had marked familial aggregation of clinical duodenal ulcer disease, there were instances of skipped generations, and the percent of individuals affected did not conform to any simple pattern of inheritance. When segregation analysis was done with hyperpepsinogenemia I as the trait in question, all individuals transmitting the trait were found to be affected, and the segregation ratios fit the simple autosomal dominant model.

Preliminary data from sibling and twin studies indicate that in most families with duodenal ulcer, PG I levels are concordant among affected members of ulcer sibships or twin pairs (137). Thus duodenal ulcer appears to be divisible into hyperpepsinogenemic I and normopepsinogenemic I forms on a familial basis, providing further evidence for genetic heterogeneity within this group of disorders. The autosomal dominant form of hyperpepsinogenemic I duodenal ulcer disease may be fairly common, as 50% of an unselected series of sibships with one or more individuals affected with duodenal ulcer disease had segregating hyperpepsinogenemia (137).

Thus, as in diabetes, evidence for genetic heterogeneity within peptic ulcer has now been provided by both direct and indirect methods.

Table 6   Genetic Heterogeneity
in Peptic Ulcer Disease

I. Duodenal ulcer vs. primary gastric ulcer

 A. Clinical Studies
  1. Family studies
     Demonstrated familial aggregation and independent
     segregation of duodenal and gastric ulcer.
  2. Twin studies
     Ulcer site concordant in vast majority of like
     sexed twins
 B. Subclinical Markers
  1. Blood group O and nonsecretor status associated
     with duodenal ulcer.
  2. Acid secretion
     a. Increased in duodenal ulcer patients (on the
        average)
     b. Normal or decreased in primary gastric ulcer
  3. Serum pepsinogen I
     a. Increased in duodenal ulcer (on the average)
     b. Normal or decreased in gastric ulcer

II. Genetic syndromes with peptic ulceration as a prominent
    feature

 A. Multiple endocrine adenoma type I and Zollinger
    Ellison

 B. Dominant syndrome of tremor, congenital nystagmus and
    duodenal ulceration

III. Heterogeneity within duodenal ulcer

 A. Evidence for subdivision of duodenal ulcer on clinical
    grounds
  1. Acid hypersecretors vs. normosecretors
  2. Early age of onset vs. late age of onset
  3. Positive family history vs. negative family history
  4. Concordant vs. discordant monozygotic twins

 B. Physiologic evidence for heterogeneity
  1. Bimodal distribution of serum pepsinogen I con-
     centrations
  2. Acid normosecretors with elevated gastrin response
     vs. acid hypersecretors with normal gastrin re-
     sponse
  3. Increased rate of gastric emptying vs. normal rate
     of gastric emptying

    4. Normal glucose tolerance vs. abnormal glucose
      tolerance

C. Genetic studies utilizing subclinical markers - serum
  pepsinogen I (PG I)
    1. Three generation families with autosomal dominant
      inheritance of an elevated PG I
    2. Sibship studies
      a. Segregation of PG I in hyper-PG I sibships
      b. Normopepsinogenemic I and hyperpepsinogemic I
        sibships
    3. Twin studies
      a. Concordance for PG I greater than for clinical
        ulcer
      b. Hyperpepsinogenemic I and normopepsinogemic I
        twin pairs

When the nature of the inheritance of diabetes mellitus was still a matter of controversy, it was speculated that hyperglycemia was no more specific than anemia, and insulin therapy no more specific than a blood transfusion (13). The same speculation can be made today about the specificity of peptic ulcer disease and antacid therapy (5). In order to substantially advance our knowledge of these groups of disorders, future genetic epidemiologic studies must take this documented heterogeneity into consideration, and must devise means to uncover the as yet unrecognized heterogeneity.

Acknowledgements
    This work was supported by a USPHS Peptic Ulcer Center Grant (AM 17328) and a USPHS Fellowship Award to Dr. Rotter (AM 050602)
    The authors would like to thank Ellen Bruce, Alycia Bittick, and Rachel Rubin for their assistance in preparing this manuscript.

IV.   REFERENCES

1.   Rimoin, D.L., "The Chondodystrophies, Advances in Human
     Genetics,"Vol.5, (H. Harris and K Hirschhorn, Eds.), Plen-
     um Pub. Corp., New York, 1975, pp. 1-118.
2.   McKusick, V.A., in "Medical Genetics" (V.A. McKusick and
     R. Clairborne, Eds.), pp.211-220. H.P. Pub. Co., Inc.,
     New York, 1973.
3.   "The Genetics of Diabetes Mellitus" (W. Creutzfeldt, J.
     Kobberling, J.V. Neel, Eds.). Springer-Verlag, New York,
     1976.
4.   Report of the workgroup on genetics of the Committee on
     Scope and Impact to the National Commission on Diabetes,
     Report of the National Commission on Diabetes to the Cong-
     ress of the U.S., Vol.3, Part 2 (DHEW Pub. No. (NIH) 76-
     1022), Government Printing Office, Washington D.C., 1976,
     pp. 163-170.
5.   Rotter, J.I. and Rimoin, D.L., Gastro. 73, 604-607 (1977).
6.   Zonana, J., and Rimoin, D.L., N.E.J.M. 295, 603-605 (1976).
7.   Grossman, M.I., in "Textbook of Medicine" (P.B. Beeson and
     W. McDermott, Eds.), Vol. II, pp. 1198-1202. W.B. Saunders
     Co., Philadelphia, 1975.
8.   ibid., pp. 1599-1619.
9.   Langman, M.J.S., Clin. in Gastro. 2, 219-226 (1973).
10. Williams, R.H. and Porte, D., in "Textbook of Endocrinolo-
     gy" (R.H. Williams, Ed.), 5th Ed., pp. 502-627. W.B.
     Saunders Co., Philadelphia, 1974.
11. Neel, J.V., Fajans, S.S., Conn, J.W. and Davidson, R.T. in
     "The Genetics and Epidemiology of Chronic Diseases" (J.V.
     Neel, M.W. Shaw, W.J. Schull, Eds.), A Symposium, pp. 105-
     132. PHSP No. 1163, Feb., 1965.
12. Simpson, N.E., in "The Genetics of Diabetes Mellitus" (W.
     Creutzfeldt, J. Kobberling and J.V. Neel, Eds.), pp. 12-
     20. Springer-Verlag, New York, 1976.
13. Rimoin, D.L. and Schimke, R.N., in "Genetic Disorders of
     of Endocrine Glands", pp. 150-194. C.V. Mosby Co., St.
     Louis, 1971.
14. Neel, J.V., in "The Genetics of Diabetes Mellitus" (W.
     Creutzfeldt, J. Kobberling and J.V. Neel, Eds.), pp. 1-11.
     Springer-Verlag, New York, 1976.
15. Rimoin, D.L., Diabetes 16, 346-351 (1967).
16. Rimoin, D.L., Med. Clin. North Am. 55, 807-819 (1971).
17. Rimoin, D.L., in "The Genetics of Diabetes Mellitus" (W.
     Creutzfeldt, J. Kobberling and J.V. Neel, Eds.), pp. 43-
     63. Springer-Verlag, New York, 1976.
18. Rimoin, D.L., Arch. Int. Med. 124, 695-700 (1969).
19. Dickie, M.M., Adv. Metab. Dis. 1, 23 (1970).
20. Stauffacher, W., Kikkawa, R., Amherdt, M. and Orci, L., in

"The Genetics of Diabetes Mellitus", pp. 155-164.

21. Parker, M.L., Pildes, R.S., Chao, K.L., Cornblath, M, Kipnis, D.M., Diabetes 17, 27-32 (1968).

22. Berson, S.A. and Yalow, R.S., Diabetes 14, 549-572 (1965).

23. Harris, H., Ann. of Eugenics 14, 293-300 (1949).

24. Harris, H., Ann. of Eugenics 15, 95-119 (1950).

25. Simpson, N.E., Ann. of Human Genetics 26, 1-12 (1962).

26. Simpson, N.E., Diabetes 13, 463-471, (1964).

27. College of General Practitioners, Brit. Med. J. i , 960-962 (1965).

28. Kobberling, J., in "The Genetics of Diabetes Mellitus", pp. 147-154.

29. Rimoin, D.L. and Schimke, R.N., in "Genetic Disorders of the Endocrine Glands", pp. 200-205.

30. Schimke, R.N., Adv. Int. Med. 21, 249-265 (1976).

31. Boden, G. and Owen, O.E., N.E.J.M. 296, 534-538 (1977).

32. Cammidge, P.J., Brit. Med. J. 2, 738-741 (1928).

33. Cammidge, P.J., Lancet i, 393-395 (1934).

34. Simpson, N.E., The Canadian Med. Assn. J. 98, 427-432 (1968).

35. Harvald, B., Acta Med. Scand. Supplement 476, 17-27 (1967).

36. Kobberling, J., Diabetologia 5, 392-396 (1969).

37. Kobberling, J., in "The Genetics of Diabetes Mellitus", pp. 79-87.

38. Lestradet, H. Battistelli, J. and Ledoux, M., Le Diabete 2, 17-21 (1972).

39. MacDonald, M.J., Diabetologia 10, 767-773 (1974).

40. Tattersall, R.B., Pyke, D.A., Lancet ii, 1120-1124 (1972).

41. Pyke, D.A., Tattersall, R.B., Diabetes 22, 613-618 (1973).

42. Pyke, D.A. and Nelson, P.G., in "The Genetics of Diabetes Mellitus", pp. 194-202.

43. Nelson, P.G. and Pyke, D.A., in "The Genetics of Diabetes Mellitus", pp. 215-223.

44. Then Berg, H., reported in JAMA 112, 1091 (1939).

45. Gottlieb, M.S. and Root, H.F., Diabetes 17, 693-704 (1968).

46. Pyke, D.A., Theophanides, C.G. and Tattersall, R.B., Lancet ii, 464 (1976).

47. Rimoin, D.L. and Rotter, J.I., N.E.J.M. 295, 1321 (1976).

48. Tattersall, R.B., Quarterly J. of Med. XLIII, No. 170, 339-357 (1974).

49. Tattersall, R.B. and Fajans, S.S., Diabetes 24, 44-53 (1975).

50. Tattersall, R., in "The Genetics of Diabetes Mellitus", pp. 88-94.

51. Johansen, K., Acta Med. Scand. 193, 22-33, 1973.

52. Fajans, S.S., Floyd, J.C., Pek, S. and Taylor, C.I., in "The Genetics of Diabetes Mellitus", pp. 224-233.

53. Irvine, W.J., Lancet ii, 638-642 (1977).

54. Irvine, W.J., Holton, D.E., Clarke, B.F., Toft, A.D.,

Prescott, R.J. and Duncan, L.J.P., <u>Lancet</u> ii, 235-238 (1977).

55. Singal, D.P. and Blajchman, M.A., <u>Diabetes</u> 22, 429-432 (1973).

56. Nerup, J., Platz, P., Ortved Andersen, O., Christy, M., Lyngsoe, J., Poulsen, J.E., Ryder, L.P., Staub Nielsen, L., Thomsen, M., Svejgaard, A., <u>Lancet</u> ii, 864-866 (1974).

57. Cudworth, A.G. and Woodrow, J.C., <u>Diabetes</u> 24, 345-349, (1975).

58. Cudworth, A.G., Woodrow, J.C., <u>Brit. Med. J.</u> ii, 133-135 (1975).

59. Cudworth, A.G., Woodrow, J.C., <u>Brit. Med. J.</u> ii, 846-848 (1976).

60. Nelson, P.G., Pyke, D.A., Cudworth, A.G., Woodrow, J.C. and Batchelor, J.R., <u>Lancet</u> ii, 193-194 (1975).

61. Nerup, J., Platz, P., Ortved Anderson, O., Christy, M., Egeberg, J., Lyngsoe, J., Poulsen, J.E., Ryder, O.P., Thomsen, M and Svejgaard, A., in "The Genetics of Diabetes Mellitus", pp. 106-114. 1976.

62. Ludvigsson, J., Safwenberg, J. and Heding, L.G., <u>Diabetologia</u> 13, 13-17 (1977).

63. Schernthaner, G., Mayr, W.R., Pacher, M., Ludwig, H., Erd, W., Eibl, M., <u>Hormone Metab. Res.</u> 7, 521-522 (1975).

64. Bertrams, J., Jansen, F.K., Gruneklee, D., Reis, H.F., Drost, H., Beyer, J., Gries, F.A., Kuwert, E., <u>Tissue Antigens</u> 8, 13-19 (1976).

65. Landgraf, R., Landgraf Lewis, M.M.C., Lander, T., Scholz, T.S., Kuntz, B., Albert, E.D., <u>Lancet</u> ii, 1084-1085 (1976).

66. Patel R., Ansari, A., Covarrubias, C., <u>Metab.</u> 26, 487-492 (1977).

67. McDevitt, H.W., Bodmer, W.F., <u>Lancet</u> i, 1269-1275 (1974).

68. Svejgaard, A., Platz, P., Ryder, L.P., Staub Nielsen, L., and Thomsen, M., <u>Transplantation Rev.</u> 22, 3-34 (1975).

69. Svejgaard, A., Hauge, M., Jersild, C., Platz, P., Ryder, L.P., Staub Nielsen, L., Thomsen, M., "Monographs in Human Genetics", Vol. 7. Basel S. Karger (1975).

70. McMichael, A and McDevitt, H., in "Progress in Medical Genetics", Vol. II (A.G. Steinberg, A.G. Bearn, A.G. Motulsky and B. Childs, Eds.), pp. 39-100. W.B. Saunders Co. 1977.

71. Ward, F., Biegel, A.A., <u>Amer. J. of Human Genetics</u> 28, 1-8 (1976).

72. Bottazzo, G.F., Florin-Christensen, A., Doniach, D., <u>Lancet</u> ii, 1279-1282 (1974).

73. MacCuish, A.C., Irvine, W.J., Barnes, E.W., Duncan, L.P.J. <u>Lancet</u> ii, 1529-1531 (1974).

74. Lendrum, R., Walker, G. and Gamble, D.R., <u>Lancet</u> i, 880-883 (1975).

75. Lendrum, R., Walker, G., Cudworth, A.G., Theophanides, C.,

Pyke, D.A., Bloom, A., Gamble, D.R., Lancet ii, 1273-1276 (1976).

76. Cudworth, A.G., Gamble, D.R., White, G.B.B., Lendrum, R., Woodrow, J.C., Bloom, A., Lancet i , 385-388 (1977).

77. Irvine, W.J., McCallum, C.J., Campbell, C.J., Duncan, L. J.P., Farquhar, W., Vaughan, H., and Morris, P.J., Diabetes 26, 138-147 (1977).

78. Irvine, W.J., Gray, R.S., McCallum, C.J., Lancet ii, 1097-1102 (1976).

79. Irvine, W.J., Gray, R.S., McCallum, C.J., Duncan, L.J.P., Lancet i , 1025-1027 (1977).

80. Del Prete, G.F., Betterle, C., Bersani, G., Romano, M., Tiengo, A., Lancet ii, 1090 (1976).

81. Rotter, J.I. and Rimoin, D.L., Evidence for further genetic heterogeneity within juvenile onset insulin dependent diabetes mellitus, Diabetes, 1978 (in press).

82. Barta, L., Simon, S., N.E.J.M. 296, 397 (1977).

83. Woolf, B., Ann. Human Genetics 19, 251-253 (1955).

84. Emery, A.E.H., in "Methodology in Medical Genetics: An Introduction to Statistical Methods", pp. 98-106. Churchill Livingstone, Edinburgh, 1976.

85. Thomsen, M., Platz, P., Ortved Andersen, O., Christy, M., Lyngsoe, J., Nerup, N., Rasmussen, N., Ryder, L.P., Staub Nielsen, L., Svejgaard, A., Transplantation Rev. 22, 125-147 (1975).

86. Barbosa, J., Noreen, H., Emme, L., Goetz, G., Simmons, R., deLeiva, A., Najarian, J., Yunis, E.J., Tissue Antigens 7, 233-237 (1976).

87. Morris, P.J., Vaughn, H., Irvine, W.J., McCallum, F.J., Gray, R.S., Campbell, C.J., Duncan, L.J.P., Farquhar, J. W., Lancet ii, 652-653 (1976).

88. Ungar, B., Stocks, A.E., Martin, F.I.R., Whittingham, S., MacKay, I.R., Lancet ii, 415-418 (1968).

89. Irvine, W.J., Clark, B.F., Scarth, L., Cullen, D.R., Duncan, L.J.P., Lancet ii, 163-168 (1970).

90. Whittingham, S., Mathews, J.D., MacKay, I.R., Stocks, A. E., Ungar, B., Martin, F.I.R., Lancet ii, 763-767 (1971).

91. MacCuish, A.C., Irvine, W.J., Clin. in Endo. and Metab. 4, 435-469 (1975).

92. Carpenter, C.C.J., Solomon, N., Silverberg, S.G., Bledsoe, T., Northcutt, R.C., Klinenberg, J.R., Bennett, I.L., Harvey, A.M., Medicine 43, 153-180 (1964).

93. Rimoin, D.L., Schimke, R.N., in "Genetic Disorders of the Endocrine Glands", pp. 128-129 and 191-192.

94. Platz, P., Ryder, L., Staub Nielsen, L., Svejgaard, A., Thomsen, M., Lancet ii, 289 (1974).

95. Grumet, C., Konishi, J., Payne, R.O., Kriss, J.P., Clin. Research 21, 493 (1973).

96. Grumet, C., Payne, R.O., Konishi, J. and Kriss, J.P., J.

Clin. Endocrinol. and Metab. 39, 1115-1119 (1974).

97. Seignalet, J., Mirouze, J., Jaffiol, C., Selam, J.L., Lapinski, H., Tissue Antigens 6, 272-274 (1975).
98. Farid, N.R., Barnard, N.M., Marshall, W.H., Tissue Antigens 8, 181-189 (1976).
99. Christy, M., Thomsen, M., Platz, P., Ryder, L., Staub Nielsen, L., Starup, J., Svejgaard, A., Nerup, J., HL-A Antigens and Hypergonadotropic Hypogonadism (in preparation). Referred to in reference 61.
100. Ludwig, H., Schernthaner, G., Mayr, W.R., N.E.J.M. 294, 1066 (1976).
101. Falchuk, Z.M., Rogentine, G.N., Strober, W., J. of Clin. Inv. 51, 1602-1605 (1972).
102. Stokes, P.L., Asquith, P., Holmes, G.K.T., MacKintosh, P., Cooke, W.T., Lancet ii, 162-164 (1972).
103. Van Thiel, D.H., Smith, W.I., Rabin, B.S., Fisher, S.E. and Lester, R., Ann. Int. Med. 86, 10-19 (1977).
104. Bottazo, G.F., Doniach, D., Lancet ii, 800 (1976).
105. Wakisaka, A., Aizawa, M., Matsuura, N., Nakagawa, S., Nakayama, E., Itakura, K., Okuna, A., Wagatsuma, Y., Lancet ii, 970 (1976).
106. Nakao, Y., Funkunishi, T., Koide, M., Akazawa, K., Ikeda, M., Igarashi, T., Yahata, M. and Imura, H., Diabetes 26, 736 (1977).
107. Kawa, A., Nakazawa, M., Sakaguchi, S., Nakamura, S., Kono, Y., Hazeki, H., Kanehisa, T., Diabetes 26, 591(1977)
108. Kobberling, J., Diabetologia 7, 46-49 (1971).
109. Fajans, Stefan, S., Floyd, J.C., Taylor, C.I. and Pek, S. Trans. Amer. Assoc. of Physicians 87, 83-94 (1974).
110. Fajans, S.S., Floyd, J.C., Tattersall, R.B., Williamson, J.R., Pek, S., Taylor, C.I., Arch. Int. Med. 136, 194-202 (1976).
111. Fajans, S.S., in "The Genetics of Diabetes Mellitus", pp. 64-78.
112. McConnell, R.B., in "The Genetics of the Gastrointestinal Disorders", pp. 76-101. Oxford Univ. Press, London,1966.
113. Doll, R. and Buch, J., Ann. of Eugenics 15, 135-146 (1950)
114. Doll, R., Kellock, T.D., Ann. of Eugenics 16, 231-240 (1951).
115. Gotlieb-Jensen, K., in "Peptic Ulcer: Genetic and Epidemiological aspects based on Twin Studies", Munksgaard, Copenhagen, 1972.
116. Wormsley, K.G., Grossman, M.I., Gut 6, 427-435 (1965).
117. Ballard, H.S., Frame, B., Hartsock, R.J., Medicine 43, 481-516 (1964).
118. Isenberg, J.I., Walsh, J.H., Grossman, M.I., Gastro. 65, 140-165 (1973).
119. Neuhauser, G., Daly, R.R., Magnelli, N.C., Barreras, R.F.,

Donaldson, R.M., Opitz, J.M., <u>Clin. Genetics</u> 9, 81-91 (1976).

120. Lam, S.K., Sircus, W., <u>Quarterly J. of Med.</u> 44, 369-387 (1975).
121. Lam, S.K. and Ong, G.B., <u>Gut</u> 17, 169-197 (1976).
122. Kubickova, Z. and Vesely, K.T., <u>J. of Med. Genetics</u> 9, 38-42 (1972).
123. Eberhard, G., <u>Acta Psych. Scand.</u>, Supplement 205 (1968).
124. Samloff, I.M., Liebman, W.M. and Panitch, N.M., <u>Gastro.</u> 69, 83-90 (1975).
125. Byrnes, J.D., Lam, S.K., Sircus, W., <u>Clin. Sci. and Molecular Med.</u> 50, 375-383 (1976).
126. Fritsh, W.P., Hausaman, T.U., Rich, W., <u>Gastro.</u> 71, 552-557 (1976).
127. Card, W.I. and Mark, I.N., <u>Clin. Sci.</u>, 19, 147-173 (1960).
128. Howlett, P.J., Sheiner, H.J., Barber, D.C., Ward, A.S., Perez-Avila, C.A., Duthie, H.L., <u>Gut</u> 17, 542-550 (1976).
129. Creutzfeldt, W., Ebert, R., Arnold, R., Becher, H.D., Borger, H.W., Schafmeyer, A., <u>Gastro.</u> 72, 814 (1977).
130. Samloff, I.M. and Liebman, W.M., <u>Gastro.</u> 66, 494-502 (1974).
131. Samloff, I.M., <u>Gastro.</u> 61, 185-188 (1971).
132. Samloff, I.M., Liebman, W.M., <u>Gastro.</u> 65, 36-42 (1973).
133. Samloff, I.M., Secrist, D.M., Passaro, E., <u>Gastro.</u> 69, 1196-1200 (1975).
134. Rotter, J.I., Gursky, J.M., Samloff, I.M., Rimoin, D.L., in Excerpta Medica, International Congress Series, No. 397, p.96 (1976).
135. Rotter, J.I., Sones, J.Q., Richardson, C.T., Rimoin, D.L. Samloff, I.M., McConnell, R.B., <u>Clin. Res.</u> 25, 325A (1977).
136. Rotter, J.I., Rimoin, D.L., Samloff, M.I., Gursky, J.M. Sones, J.Q., Richardson, C.T. and Walsh, J.H., Hyper-pepsinogenemic I Duodenal Ulcer Disease, An Autosomal Dominant Disorder in Man, submitted for publication.
137. Rotter, J.I., Rimoin, D.L., Samloff, I.M., McConnell, R.B., Gotlieb Jensen, K., Gadeberg, O., Hauge, M., <u>Gastro.</u> 72, 1165 (1977).

DISCUSSION

SING: I am impressed by the extent of the genetic
heterogeneity which you believe exists for diabetes mellitus.
I would like to suggest that although great phenotypic heterogeneity undoubtedly exists for this disease you may have over-
estimated the amount of genetic heterogeneity. For instance,
citing evidence that insulin tolerance is abnormal in 30
distinct inherited disorders may not be evidence for 30
separate causations of diabetes but simply that most of the
major perturbations of the human system will affect metabolism
in some way. Analysis of heterogeneity is fraught with the
problem of mixing measures of the genotype-phenotype link
which are a cause of the disorder with those that are an
effect. It is extremely difficult to conclude from your
presentation which measures are observations on intervening
variables which link the genotype and the disease phenotype
and which measures are simply phenotypic correlates of the
disease phenotype. I would expect that if we were able to
measure enough variables we would find (as expected!!) that
all diabetics are genetically unique. In this case the role
of inheritance in predicting disease would be trivial. I
suggest that we should be looking for commonalities as
vigorously as we pursue the heterogeneity. Then, understanding
the role genes and the environment play in the variability of
these common variables may help us understand the observed
familial aggregation of diabetes and peptic ulcers.

ANDERSON: Dr. Sing has underestimated the relevance of
single locus traits that show glucose intolerance. For most
of these Mendelian traits we do not yet understand the precise
pathway from genotype to phenotype with reference to glucose
metabolism. Thus these Mendelian traits can provide excellent
probes whereby we can seek to understand the variety of ways
in which the symptoms of diabetes can be produced.

ROTTER: Dr. Sing's comment that the existence of glucose
intolerance in 30 distinct inherited disorders may reflect a
general perturbation of human metabolism rather than pathogenetic heterogeneity, is simply not consistent with what is
known about these disorders. As we've indicated in our classification in Table I, these disorders operate through a variety
of separate, distinct pathogenetic mechanisms, ranging from
pancreatic destruction through insulin antagonism. We agree
with Dr. Anderson that these rare disorders provide a powerful

opportunity to delineate the variety of pathophysiologic
derangements that can lead to glucose intolerance and clinical
diabetes.

GENETIC EPIDEMIOLOGY

EPIDEMIOLOGIC AND GENETIC ISSUES IN MENTAL RETARDATION

Zena Stein* [1,2]
Mervyn Susser[1]

Columbia University[1]
New York, N.Y.

New York State Psychiatric Institute[2]
New York, N.Y.

The epidemiology of mental retardation is briefly summarized. Severe mental retardation is rare (prevalence ~ 4 per 1,000 children), but fairly constant in frequency and type across populations. Chromosomal anomalies are involved in about one-fifth of cases, some form of genetic transmission possibly in another third, and known exogenous factors including infections in a smaller fraction. Mild mental retardation is about ten times more common than severe mental retardation. The three-quarters of cases not associated with detectable organic or metabolic defects are invariably concentrated among the poorest classes. In British cities, the relative risk for such cases among them is about fifteen times as high as among the highest social classes.

Next, we discuss anomalous conceptions in the context of studies of spontaneous abortions and give examples of variation with time and with environmental exposures. A model for surveillance of anomalous conceptions is presented, and some problems are illustrated from data on the effects of maternal exposure to smoking and to oral contraceptives.

415

The possibility of a relationship of chromosomal anomalies to unconventional viruses is raised by consideration of a reported link between familial Alzheimer's disease and Down's syndrome. We have collected genealogies of an unconventional virus encephalopathy, Creutzfeldt-Jakob disease, among Libyan Jews. That community has a 40-fold excess of this rare disorder. We show clustering within lineages, and we discuss the implications for a theory of genetic susceptibility to this unconventional virus.

Problems of gene environment interaction and covariance are further considered in a quite different set of circumstances. An epidemiological study of measured intelligence in a complete Warsaw cohort at age eleven was extended to include testing of 600 children who were members of a family set comprising an index child, a sib and a cousin. We outline an attempt to use family set models.

I.   EPIDEMIOLOGY OF MENTAL RETARDATION

A brief general statement of the epidemiology of mental retardation will serve to frame this discussion and explain some directions our research has taken. Mental retardation is not a unitary condition either in its manifestations or its causes. Apart from the existence of social handicap and psychological dysfunction, it is difficult to make a single useful statement about mental retardation that remains true across grades of severity.

Severe mental retardation is here defined by an intelligence test score of less than 50. Severely retarded infants are born with much the same frequency to families in all walks of life, handicap is usually diagnosed in infancy, and with a few exceptions the therapeutic possibilities are extremely limited. The dysfunction and handicap are rooted in persisting organic or physiological impairments of the developing brain. These impairments have some known causes and undoubtedly many unknown causes. Most arise before conception or in the prenatal period. Among the known causes are genetic factors, exposures of the parents to detrimental elements in the physical environment, prenatal and perinatal infections, and birth trauma. It follows that for the prevention of much severe retardation we must look to factors antecedent to conception or birth.

Prevalence rates of severe mental retardation amongst school age children can be reliably determined because, where schooling is universal, the condition is easily ascertained. From many different studies (exemplified by Turner's series (1) of outpatients in New South Wales on which we have based Table 1) it would seem that chromosome

anomalies and genetic factors of one or another kind are
implicated in about half the cases of severe mental retardation. In such a contemporary population, the sequelae of
congenital syphilis and tuberculous meningitis are no longer
found, individuals with Down's syndrome tend to survive, and
those with phenylketonuria are treated. The estimated distribution of **causes** uses some current assumptions, for
example about the frequency of inapparent cytomegalovirus
as a cause of microcephaly, and about the greater frequency
of metabolic errors found with sophisticated chromatography.

TABLE 1   PRESUMED CAUSES OF SEVERE MENTAL RETARDATION

Gross estimated percentage distributions freely adapted from
Turner, 1975 [1]

INHERITED		22.0
Dominant	4.5	
Recessive	9.0	
X-linked recessive	8.0	
Chromosome anomalies	0.5	
GENETIC PREDISPOSITION		13.0
Syndromes with raised		
recurrence risks		
e.g. neural tube		
defects		
CHROMOSOME ANOMALIES		19.0
INFECTIONS		13.0
Perinatal	7.5	
Postnatal	5.5	
PERINATAL FACTORS		10.0
Prematurity, Rh		
Cretinism, Birth		
Injury		
TRAUMA, CHILD BATTERY, ETC.		2.0
UNKNOWN (INCLUDING		21.0
HYDROCEPHALUS, ...)		

---

[1]
   Turner provided the proven and the likely diagnosis of
a consecutive series of 1,000 out-patients, mainly children.
Turner omitted Down's syndrome cases, and we have added them,
allotting a proportion of ∼ 18 percent.

We can compare this modern series of cases with those
Penrose collected in the 1930's from Colchester, England (2).
This series was twice reanalyzed by Morton and his colleagues (3,4) to provide estimates of the proportion attributable to autosomal recessive or sex linked genes. In order
to examine the validity of the reanalyses of the Colchester
data, we must recognize inherent difficulties for an
epidemiological analysis. Incidence and prevalence are
distinguished but not in terms of current epidemiological
conventions. Comparability of frequencies between populations, allowing for unconventional usages, remains extremely doubtful where age-specific prevalence is not given.
The most useful measures are specific to school-age children.
The problem of comparability is compounded where the frequencies are estimated from institutionalized cases alone,
however careful the actual survey may be. With mental retardation selection biases tend to be extreme (5,6). In
general, such rates cited even by the most respectable
sources in the literature must be viewed with a suspicious
eye; most are no better than guesses. Within the population
of cases, the comparability of distributions is rendered
doubtful in the absence of age and sex specific data, and
also by apparently changing definitions for categories of
cases.

To allow us to proceed, we have assumed (in the light of
the original Penrose material) that the Colchester cases were
virtually all of school age, and we have used Lewis' contemporary population prevalence rates (7). Further, we have
equated the "biological" cases of the second reanalysis (4)
with severe mental retardation. We perforce ignore selection biases. In these circumstances extrapolation to population frequencies cannot but be seen as hazardous. We shall
risk them in the interests of furthering a possibly fertile
line of inquiry.

The first reanalysis (3) is limited to severe mental defect with specified exclusions.[2] The series fits current
reports of case distributions reasonably well. Thus the
11 to 12% of the Colchester cases attributed to autosomal recessive genes is close to the 9% identified or suspected
among the same categories in Turner's New South Wales series.

2
   Cases of obvious exogenous origin, and Down's syndrome,
hydrocephalus, and cerebral neoplasm were excluded, as well
as children of mentally retarded parents.

In the second reanalysis of the Colchester series, Morton et al. (4) arrive at what they believe to be a much higher estimate of autosomal recessives. This later analysis relates to a category of cases described as 'biological'. The discrepancy between these two estimates is explained on the grounds that the earlier analysis was limited to the severely retarded. In fact, we find no great discrepancy between the two estimates if as seems likely 'biological' cases are mainly severe. Thus they estimate a population frequency of autosomal recessives associated with mental retardation in children after infancy of 2.3 per 1000 overall. Among the 'biological' cases, population frequency is 0.5 per 1000. This rate is 12.5 to 14% of a total prevalence of 3.5 to 4 per 1000 of severe retardation in childhood, a proportion not incongruent with the 1965 estimate of Dewey et al. of 11 to 12%, also with Turner's of 9%. Mildly retarded children would contribute the remaining 1.8 per 1000 of the estimated overall rate of 2.3 per 1000. We shall return to this figure below.

Even in the absence of directly comparable data over time, from what is known one can reasonably infer that changing patterns of childbearing, standards of living and health practices have increased the expectation of life at birth for severely retarded infants and particularly for those with Down's syndrome. It is a puzzle that in spite of these known changes, the prevalence of severe mental retardation in childhood has changed little and remains at a rate of 3.5 to 4.5 per thousand (8,9,10). This apparent stability must in some part be owed to a balance between declining incidence and increased survival. Although differences across the range of rates for time and place lie between 20 and 30 percent, the small absolute range supports the notion that less variable factors, like genetic conditions, are responsible for a larger proportion of cases than more variable environmental factors. If infections are important, their nature is likely to be endemic (like cytomegalovirus or toxoplasmosis) or rare and sporadic (like subacute sclerosing panencephalitis) rather than epidemic.

Mild mental retardation is up to ten times as prevalent as severe mental retardation. The social handicap and psychological dysfunction of mild mental retardation is rooted in detectable handicap to learning in only a minority of perhaps 25 to 30 percent (11, 12,13). Prevalence rates for mild mental retardation vary markedly with age, circumstances and definition although a rate of about 30 per 1000 is often cited as if it were universal. Mildly retarded children

with no detectable handicap to learning come almost entirely
from families at the bottom of the social scale (7, 11).
They form a homogeneous category drawn from large families
with parents in unskilled manual occupations and of little
education (11, 14, 15). Incompetence at school is their
major social handicap. This handicap is temporary and age-
linked, in large part because it is tied to the school system,
but also because to a degree social and psychological matura-
tion is deferred into young adulthood (11, 15). In families
with a mildly retarded member sibs tend to resemble the proband in intellectual performance (14). (This is not the
case in families with a severely retarded member, in which
unaffected sibs have I.Q.s that are normally distributed.)

In our view, the evidence allows a strong inference that
the origin and prevention of much mild mental retardation
must be sought in postnatal factors that interfere with the
acquisition of functional abilities and social roles.
Because children with mild mental retardation are found predominantly among the poor, causes for the condition may best
be sought in their impoverished social environment. Malnutrition, exposure to pollutants such as lead, infections and
inadequate health care, schooling and rearing patterns are
among many postulated mechanisms.

The genetic determinants of the common forms of the condition have been most plausibly conceptualized as polygenic.
The invariably strong social class distribution of the condition has been seen either in terms of gene-environment interaction or covariance, and with sharply differing emphases.
In terms of gene-environment interaction, the distribution
has been interpreted as a product of the impact of a harsh
environment upon the poorly endowed individuals at the lower
end of a continuous scale of intelligence (7, 11, 14). In
terms of gene-environment covariance, the distribution has
been interpreted as a product of selective social mobility
over generations, a process in which those highly endowed
intellectually move upward, and those poorly endowed move
downward (16).

Simpler patterns of genetic transmission - autosomal and
sex-linked recessives and dominant mutations - could account
for some cases of mild mental retardation. A base-line for
their frequency is perhaps given by the rate of mild mental
retardation in the children of families of high social status:
they have neither been exposed to the harsh environment of
the poorer classes nor to selective downward mobility. The

rarity of mild mental retardation without detectable underlying disorder among families of high social status precludes
a high frequency for these mechanisms. The available data
are congruent, however, with a frequency approximately of
the order estimated by Morton et al. (4). In a search of
schools of the highest social standing in Manchester and
Salford in England, and including those children who were not
in school, we found a prevalence of 0.65 per thousand of
'cryptogenic' cases of mild mental retardation and/or educational subnormality (11). In schools of the poorest social
standing the relative risk for conditions without detectable
handicaps to learning was fifteen times as great. The rate
of 0.65 per 1,000 for 'cryptogenic' cases is not far from
Morton's estimate for autosomal recessives of 1.8, if we
allow for two particular differences. First, in our population the cut-off point for the definition of mild mental retardation yielded a total prevalence among pre-pubertal
children of about 10 per 1,000, in contrast with Morton's
estimate for Colchester of 24.5 per 1,000. Second, our rate
of 0.65 per 1,000 for 'cryptogenic' cases refers to a largely
outbreeding population of higher status families. In the
families of the lowest social status that yield the bulk of
cases, which in the population we studied has features of
a subculture, consanguinity is probably more common than in
higher status families.

With the subject of this conference in mind, we have
chosen three studies, each of which takes us to a meeting-
place of epidemiology with genetics. Their themes, like the
epidemiological array of mental retardation, are heterogeneous. Each involves distinct epidemiologic problems and different aspects of genetics. The first study is based on our
work with spontaneous abortions, and deals with variations,
over time and with environmental exposures, in the type and
frequency of anomalies. The second study deals with Creutzfeldt-Jakob disease, and we consider the interaction of an
unconventional virus with familial susceptibility, and speculate about possible associations with chromosome anomalies.
The third study was designed in the first instance to distinguish between intra-familial and extra-familial influences
in cognitive development and mild mental retardation, and we
report our subsequent efforts to allow for a genetic contribution in estimating the environmental contribution to
the intrafamilial component.

II.   ENVIRONMENTAL CAUSES OF VARIATION IN ANOMALOUS
      CONCEPTIONS.[3]

1.   Evidence of Environmental Causes of Variation.

     We believe that the frequency of anomalous conceptions
varies within fairly narrow limits.   Thus in severe mental
retardation, the causes of which are predominantly prenatal,
we noted above its stable prevalence.   One of the main and
best measured components of severe mental retardation prevalence rates is Down's syndrome, and the rate of Down's
syndrome births among women in given age groups has been
thought to vary little over time, from place to place, and
across populations.   Among spontaneous abortions, too, the
frequency of karyotypic anomalies, both overall and for particular anomalies, has been remarkably similar in series reported from Paris, London, Aarhus and Vancouver.   Nor does
our New York series diverge from these (17).

     On the other hand, there is also evidence of variation.
Latterly, rates of Down's syndrome have shown signs of change.
Among ethnic and cultural groups the rates at birth have been
found to differ (18,19) and recent data suggest a rising
secular trend (20).   A rising trend among older women would
be consonant with the high frequency of trisomy found on
amniocentesis, as compared with the postnatal prevalence of
affected individuals.   Case selection for amniocentesis, unmeasured perinatal loss, and underreporting in prevalence
surveys of Down's syndrome may not be sufficient to reconcile
the discrepancies, although some have attempted to do so.
These data, taken together with the demonstration of an
effect of preconceptional maternal irradiation on the frequency of trisomy and of Down's syndrome among older women,
encourage one to look for environmental sources of variation
in the frequency of Down's syndrome.

     Several years ago, Collman and Stoller (21), demonstrated
a rise and fall in the prevalence of Down's syndrome among

3
     Jennie Kline, Dorothy Warburton and ourselves have been
jointly engaged on the studies of spontaneous abortions
that provide the background for this discussion.

birth cohorts in Victoria, Australia, This they attributed
to an epidemic of hepatitis concurrent with the time of conception. Subsequent efforts to replicate this association
failed. More recently Harlap (22) reported cyclical
fluctuations in Down's syndrome births in Jerusalem. With
due caution the significance of these fluctuations also has
been questioned, because of the possibility of both selective
survival and selective notification between conception and
enumeration, e.g. Leck (23).

We have ourselves now to report another periodic variation
in the frequency of trisomy that is less vulnerable to these
particular selective losses. Figure I shows rates of trisomy
over time in cell cultures from a consecutive series of spontaneous abortions up to 28 weeks gestation. The series comprises aborted fetuses routinely collected from three hospitals in New York City. A cluster of trisomic conceptions
was noted in the winter of 1976. Starting in September,
rates were above the expected for the three fall months,
reached a peak in December, 1976 and January, 1977, and then
returned to their usual level in February, 1977 (Table 2a).

There is no easy way of distinguishing an etiologically
meaningful cluster of events from a random cluster, One test
that argues against randomness is replication of the cluster
in independent data sources. We therefore sought information
from amniocentesis clinics about women who reported conceptions over the period July, 1976 to January, 1977. The
curve for trisomies derived from amniocentesis is also shown
in Figure I. Like the curve for spontaneous abortion cultures, that for amniocentesis cultures also shows a marked
rise for the December and January cohort of conception (Table
2b) (although there is no notable rise for September, October
and November). The amniocentesis curve has the strength of
an independent test of an hypothesis, since the hypothesis
was derived from the prior finding of the spontaneous abortion curve, and both the data sources and the populations
studied are entirely separate. The result strengthens the
case for a true periodic variation.   A further replication of the test of the hypothesis is now being carried
out on the same conception cohorts as they reach term,

More generally, these results show that in a cohort of
conceptions, the finding of an excess of trisomies among
spontaneous abortions with a mean gestational age of 12
weeks can convey information that is predictive for survivors
of the cohort some six weeks later, at gestational age

TABLE 2a

FREQUENCY OF TRISOMY AMONG SPONTANEOUS ABORTIONS BY MONTH OF
LAST MENSTRUAL PERIOD (January 1974-March 1977)

MONTH OF LMP	NUMBER TRISOMIC	NUMBER KARYOTYPED	% TRISOMIC
Jan-Jun 1974	3	15	20.0
Jul-Dec 1974	4	32	12.5
Jan-Jun 1975	6	70	8.6
Jul-Dec 1975	10	86	11.6
Jan-Jun 1976	16	88	18.2
Jul 1976	1	13	7.7
Aug 1976	1	13	7.7
Sep 1976	0	9	0
Oct 1976	2	12	16.7
Nov 1976	3	10	30.0
Dec 1976	7	16	43.8
Jan 1977	5	14	35.7
Feb 1977	1	7	14.3
Mar 1977	1	8	12.5
Total Excluding LMP's in Nov 1976-Jan 1977	45	353	12.7 ± 3.5[1]
LMP's in Nov 1976-Jan 1977	15	40	37.5 ± 15.0[1]
Total	60	393	15.3 ± 3.6[1]

[1]95% confidence limits

TABLE 2b

PERCENTAGE OF TRISOMIES AMONG
SUCCESSFULLY CULTURED AMNIOTIC TAPS IN FIVE
NEW YORK HOSPITALS
(NOVEMBER 1976- May 1977)

MONTH OF LMP	NUMBER OF CASES	NUMBER OF TRISOMIES	% TRISOMIC
Jul 1976	46	0	0
Aug 1976	57	2	3.5
Sep 1976	83	3	3.6
Oct 1976	120	3	2.5
Nov 1976	84	2	2.4
Dec 1976	79	4	5.1
Jan 1977	40	4	10.0
TOTAL	509	18	3.5

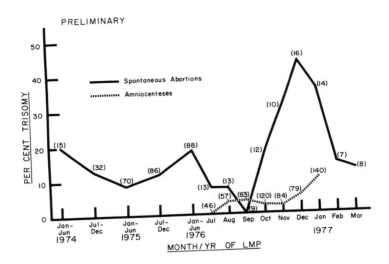

Fig.   1

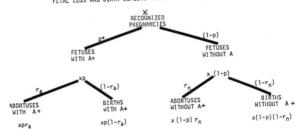

DIAGRAM SHOWING RELATIONSHIPS BETWEEN INCIDENCE OF ANOMALIES,
FETAL LOSS AND BIRTH DEFECTS AMONG RECOGNIZED PREGNANCIES

*p could be taken as a function of gestational time.
+for the moment only one "A" per fetus is assumed.

SOURCE: Stein et al. Spontaneous Abortion as a Screening Device. American Journal of Epidemiology, 1975, 102(4):285-290.

x = number of recognized pregnancies
A   denotes any specific anomaly or group of anomalies
p = probability of A originating either at conception or during pregnancy
xp = number of expected conceptions with anomaly A
r_a = probability that a conceptus with A aborts spontaneously
r_n = probability that a conceptus without A aborts spontaneously

Fig.   2

around 18 weeks when amniocentesis is performed. This prediction could not be taken for granted. Attrition of anomalous fetuses is high and, further, most of the trisomies contributing to the peak observed in spontaneous abortions were
of a type that are not seen among the liveborn, among the
stillborn, or even among later abortions.

To establish the relationships between anomalous conceptions that reach viability and those that fail to come to
notice because they abort is crucial to the elucidation of
causes of developmental disorders including severe mental retardation (24). Figure 2 shows a schema of the probabilities
of anomalous and "normal" conceptuses aborting or being born
that takes account of such selective losses. This is the
working model for our study of spontaneous abortions. With
regard to trisomies, it is already clear that the attributes
of women who abort trisomies are similar to those of women
who carry them to term. In both the women are older, and in
both they more often give a history of past exposure to
irradiation. Also, women who abort a trisomic fetus when
compared to women who abort   karyotypically normal fetuses
have more often had a previous Down's syndrome birth or a
previous trisomic abortus. With regard to all other
anomalies, the evidence about their attributes among abortions
and among births is as yet slender.

2.   Uses of Variation for Surveillance

The recognition of temporal variation in the frequency
of trisomies, together with other evidence of environmental
teratogens, leads naturally to thoughts about the traditional epidemiological function of surveillance (17). A surveillance system in our view would best, if not solely,
monitor both the incidence of spontaneous abortions and the
prevalence of defects in the conceptus in spontaneous abortions. The use of spontaneous abortions for keeping a watch
on teratogens in the environment has advantages over the
current surveillance of birth defects alone in at least four
respects:

  i) lead time is gained for the discovery of the effects
     of teratogenic exposure. A change in the incidence of
     spontaneous abortions or of anomalies in spontaneous
     abortions can be detected, as we have seen, six months
     or more before a change in the incidence of birth
     defects.

ii) abortion specimens, unlike liveborn infants, can be
studied at will and can be preserved for future
studies as well

iii) many anomalies that appear among spontaneous abortions appear rarely or never among live births.
Hence teratogens that cause only such anomalies
could not be detected by studies of birth defects.
The lack of viability of the anomaly caused by a
teratogen in no way detracts from the significance
of the teratogen either for health or for biological
theory.

iv) The great majority of anomalous conceptions is found
among spontaneous abortions. Among the few that
survive to birth, changes in the type and the frequency of defects may be missed unless the exposed
population is very large. Far less widespread exposure to teratogens is needed to produce detectable
incidence changes in spontaneous abortions. Thus
studies of spontaneous abortions are efficient and
precise in providing information about the conceptus,
and parsimonious of the numbers needed to screen for
a suspected teratogen.

(i)   Comparison of Required Sample Sizes

The search for teratogens has been approached through
studies of the frequency of defects, most usually in live
births, and occasionally in perinatal deaths. A more sensitive means of detecting teratogens is to study the incidence
of spontaneous abortions.[4] A considerably more sensitive
means is to combine data on the incidence of abortions and on
the prevalence of anomalies in the aborted conceptions.

---

[4]
The prevalence of anomalies seen in livebirths is a
function both of the incidence of the anomaly at conception,
and of its survival through gestation. The chances of survival can be stated as the probability that a conceptus with
the defect will not be rejected through spontaneous abortion.
The probability of spontaneous abortion is almost always
greater for an anomalous conceptus than for a conceptus of
normal karyotype and morphology. Possible exceptions to this
rule may exist, but must certainly be infrequent. It follows
that a teratogenic agent that causes anomalies will as a rule
produce an increased incidence of spontaneous abortions as
well as an increased incidence of anomalous fetuses among
abortions.

TABLE 3 OUTCOME VARIABLES AND STATISTICAL POWER: ESTIMATES OF RELATIVE RISK AND SAMPLE SIZE NEEDED TO DETECT A CHANGE IN THE INCIDENCE OF A GIVEN OUTCOME IN COHORTS OF PREGNANT WOMEN, WITH A POWER OF .80 AND ASSUMING THAT THE PROBABILITY OF AN ANOMALY AT RECOGNIZED CONCEPTION IS DOUBLED IN THE EXPOSED GROUP.*

	Incidence in exposed	Incidence in unexposed	Relative risk	Sample size needed for each exposed and unexposed group.
Chromosomal defects in newborn: diagnosed on appearance.	.002	.001	2.0	22,843
Chromosomal defects in newborn: diagnosed on systematic karyotyping.	.010	.005	2.0	4,542
Incidence of spontaneous abortions.	.20	.15	1.3	901
Incidence of chromosomal anomalies in abortions (4-28 weeks).	.45	.30	1.5	161
Incidence of chromosomal anomalies in abortions (4-15 weeks).	.63	.46	1.4	133

*
For this table, we have assumed that among 1,000 recognized conceptions in an unexposed population, 50 conceptions are chromosomally abnormal. We assume that 92% of all chromosomally anomalous conceptions abort spontaneously (adapted from Kline et al., (17).

In Table 3 we compare the sample sizes of exposed and unexposed groups that would be needed to detect an agent that
doubles the rate of chromosomal anomalies at conception. The
records of 22,843 exposed newborns must be examined to detect an effect of this size. If all the newborn were to be
karyotyped, a heavy undertaking, the number can be reduced
to 4,542. In order to detect the rise in the incidence of
spontaneous abortions to be expected with the same agent, 901
exposed pregnant women need to be identified. If pathological
and karyotypic examinations of abortuses were to be undertaken, only 161 exposed conceptions would be required to detect the expected rise in incidence. Were all these examinations to be carried out on the early abortions that occur
before 16 weeks of gestation, 133 would suffice.

(ii)   Power and the Specificity of Hypotheses

The more specific the hypotheses to be tested, the greater
the power that the design is likely to attain. Refinement of
the independent study variable and, in this case particularly,
refinement of the dependent variable will help to specify
hypotheses (25).

To illustrate, vinyl chloride provides a possible example
of the teratogenic effect of paternal exposure to a hazardous
agent. A relative risk of 1.8 for spontaneous abortion in
the wives of vinyl chloride workers as compared with the
wives of unexposed controls was recently reported (26). Let
us take this to be a firm result. With this volatile gas,
the likely vehicle is through male germinal cells, damaged
by exposure, that transmit their defect to the conceptus at
fertilization and thereby increase spontaneous abortion rates.
Any one of three mechanisms seems plausible on the basis of
current knowledge:

a.   Vinyl chloride may act as a clastogen in germ cells
     to produce in the chromosomes of the conceptus such
     structural rearrangements as translocations, partial
     deletions, or inversions.

b.   Vinyl chloride may act as a mutagen and cause domi-
     nant or recessive lethal mutations. The outcome of a
     dominant mutation might be a karyotypically normal
     but biochemically incompetent conceptus and produce
     either an intact empty sac, a severely disorganized
     embryo, or a malformed fetus.

c. Vinyl chloride may induce chromosomal abnormalities during gametogenesis or fertilization to produce a trisomic, monosomic or triploid conceptus.

The consequences of each of these postulated mechanisms for the abortus are developed in Table 4. These distributions of morphologic and karyotypic anomalies in spontaneous abortions, when adjusted for maternal and gestational age, have proved highly consistent from series to series (17). Table 4 shows estimates of the sample sizes needed to detect the effect of an agent. The estimates take as given any of the three hypothetical mechanisms described above and our further assumptions about what the sperm-transmitted effects would be. In each instance, the predicted size of the effect is derived from the 1.8 relative risk of spontaneous abortion observed in the wives of vinyl chloride workers.

With clastogenesis, an increased incidence of structural rearrangements could be detected in the distribution of karyotypic anomalies among a mere 12 abortuses. With induction of point mutations, effects could be detected over a range of 16 to 75 abortuses, depending on the specific outcome. With abnormalities of gametogenesis or of fertilization, a rise in the proportion of conceptions with chromosomal anomalies could be detected in a series of 56 abortuses (fewer, if the particular anomaly could be specified).

The power of surveillance methods based on the combinations of measures permitted by our simple model may take us to a new level of environmental monitoring. There are traps for the unwary, however, as we show in the following section.

(iii) The Proportion of Anomalies

In Table 5 we set out preliminary data on maternal smoking and oral contraception from our series of cases of spontaneous abortion. The table shows the relative frequency of aneuploidy for each of the four possible combinations of smoking and oral contraception, taking the overall frequency of 1.0. At first sight, it appears that women who smoke have a lesser frequency of anomalies (.75). By contrast, it also appears that women who have ever used oral contraception and are non-smokers, have a raised frequency (1.20).

These frequencies do not mean that smoking reduces aneuploidy at conception nor that oral contraception increases it. Inferences relating to anomalies at conception need to consider the risks of spontaneous abortion in these categories

TABLE 4   SAMPLE SIZE AND PATHOGENESIS: SAMPLES NEEDED TO DETECT AN ASSOCIATION BETWEEN PATERNAL VINYL CHLORIDE EXPOSURE AND ANOMALIES IN THE ABORTED CONCEPTUS FOR DIFFERENT PATHOGENETIC HYPOTHESES. SIZE OF THE EFFECT CORRESPONDS TO A RELATIVE RISK OF 1.8 FOR SPONTANEOUS ABORTION INCIDENCE IN MATES OF MEN EXPOSED TO VINYL CHLORIDE. (α = .05, TWO-TAILED TEST, POWER = .90).

Pathogenesis	Consequences anticipated	Percent distribution in affected cells Predicted in Exposed	Expected in Unexposed	Sample size required
clastogen	Structural re-arrengement of chromosomes.	45*	.64*	12
point mutation	normal karyotype, growth disorganized embryo.	47	4	17
meiosis, sperm viability, or fertilization	abnormal karyotype	62	32	56
excess normal karyotypes	normal karyotype	82	68	198

*The expected and observed incidence of translocations has been contrasted in these columns and the sample size is calculated for this increase only.

TABLE 5   RELATIVE AND ABSOLUTE (<u>ABNORMAL</u>/TOTAL) FREQUENCY OF ANEUPLOIDY AMONG SPONTANEOUS ABORTIONS, BY SMOKING AND ORAL CONTRACEPTIVE USE. (ALL = 1).

Ever Used Oral Contraception

		Yes		No		Total	
SMOKING DURING PREGNANCY	Yes	.80	$\frac{(16)}{(71)}$	.56	$\frac{(\ 3)}{(19)}$	.75	$\frac{(19)}{(90)}$
	No	1.20	$\frac{(38)}{(113)}$	1.01	$\frac{(19)}{(67)}$	1.13	$\frac{(57)}{(180)}$
	Total	1.04	$\frac{(54)}{(184)}$	.90	$\frac{(22)}{(87)}$	1.00	$\frac{(76)}{(270)}$

5

TABLE 6   RELATIVE FREQUENCY OF SMOKING DURING PREGNANCY AND ORAL CONTRACEPTIVE USE AMONG WOMEN WITH SPONTANEOUS ABORTION AND CONTROLS WITH VIABLE PREGNANCIES (ALL = 1).

Ever Used Oral Contraception

		Yes	No	Total
SMOKING DURING PREGNANCY	Yes	1.48	1.43	1.46
	No	.67	1.19	.82
	Total	.89	1.27	1

(570 spontaneous abortions
316 controls)

5

The table shows the odds of being a case compared to those of being a control.

of women, as well as of anomalies among their infants carried
to a viable stage of gestation. In Table 6, taken from our
case-control study, we show the association of smoking during
pregnancy and of any previous oral contraception use with
spontaneous abortion. The expected ratio in each cell refers
to the total series of cases and controls. Smokers are over-
represented among women with spontaneous abortions (1.46).
By contrast again, women who have ever used oral contraceptives, and are non-smokers, are underrepresented among women
with spontaneous abortions (.67).

In the literature, smoking and prior oral contraceptive
use have generally not been associated with anomalies at
birth (27). There is a parsimonious explanation for the data
presented here. These karyotype and case-control data, taken
together, suggest that both smoking and previous oral contraceptive use modify the probability that a conceptus will
abort. It is unlikely, although possible, that either factor
modifies the probability of aneuploidy. In our model, when
the observed distributions are attributed to a change in the
proportion of anomalous conceptions, absurd values result.
The data suggest further that interaction occurs between oral
contraceptive use and smoking. Smoking seems to ablate a
protective effect of oral contraception in sustaining pregnancy. In fact, our interest in this analysis was first
caught by the apparent interaction between two inverse effects.
We are still engaged in clarifying these results, and they may
be subject to revision.

For the epidemiologist, the demonstration that common
environmental exposures alter the ratios of 'normal' to
'abnormal' karyotype poses a warning against facile interpretations based solely on proportional distributions.

III.   UNCONVENTIONAL VIRUSES AMONG KINDRED

1. Connections with Down's Syndrome

Three separate lines of investigation have focused our
interest on brain disorders attributed to unconventional
viruses.[6]

i. Intriguing aspects of the epidemiology of Down's
syndrome include the phenomenon of premature aging, and the
high frequency of pre-senile dementia in the form of Alzheimer's disease. Alzheimer's disease is a disease of middle

---

[6]That is, viruses that cause no systemic or immune
reactions.

life and follows a characteristic clinical course of mental
and motor deterioration. Neurofibrillary tangles and amy-
loid plaques are found in the brain as they are with senile
dementia, although some hold that the pathology of
Alzheimer's disease can be distinguished from that of senile
dementia by the concentration and distribution of the
plaques. The clinical distinction between Alzheimer's
disease and senile dementia rests principally on the early
age of onset of Alzheimer's disease. In Down's syndrome,
brain autopsies of adults over 35 years of age generally
show typical Alzheimer's disease.[7]

ii. Gajdusek and colleagues established the existence
and identity of transmissible virus dementias in humans, by
transmitting a neurological disease to experimental animals
from the brains of cases of kuru and, later, from the brains
of cases of Creutzfeldt-Jakob disease (CJD)(28). A key to
the exploration and linking of 'unconventional viruses' was
that autopsy material from kuru patients caused CJD-type
changes in the brains of experimental animals. Similar experimental transmission has thus far succeeded with at least
two of about 35 cases of Alzheimer's disease. In these two
cases also, the experimental animals evinced the pathological
features of CJD and not those of Alzheimer's disease (29).
Thus the agent may be the same as those in kuru and CJD, or
have much in common with them. From the point of view of
the discussion that follows, it is noteworthy that CJD was
successfully transmitted from cases with a familial history
as well as from sporadic cases, and that both cases of
Alzheimer's disease in which transmission to animals succeeded had a familial history of dementia with onset in
middle life or earlier.

7
    An element of circularity in this assertion cannot be
avoided on the neuropathological evidence presently available. Because Down's syndrome individuals age prematurely,
it is a moot point whether the brain syndrome reflects pathology consonant with their "equivalent" chronological age -
in which case it might properly be attributed to senility -
or whether it reflects pathology premature for their
"equivalent" chronological age - in which case it might more
properly be attributed to Alzheimer's disease.

iii. Heston (30) recently reported an excess of Down's syndrome offspring among the kin of victims of Alzheimer's disease. Heston's conjecture was that the genetic transmission of some aging factor common to Alzheimer's disease kindred induced premature aging of the ova of female kin. The excess of premature aging and of Alzheimer's disease in Down's syndrome, however, is certainly not confined to those rare cases of Down's syndrome who have kin connections with Alzheimer's disease. Heston's theory cannot account for the excess.

To return to the agents transmitted to animals from cases of CJD, Alzheimer's disease and kuru, all three produced pathology that resembled that of CJD. As far as we know, no attempts to transmit viral agents from Down's syndrome, or from Alzheimer's disease occurring with Down's syndrome, have been made. In view of the suspected excess of Down's syndrome cases among the kindred of Alzheimer's victims and the frequent occurrence of Alzheimer's disease in Down's syndrome individuals, we think it not inconceivable that unconventional viruses, which have such variable manifestations, contribute either to the occurrence or to the manifestations of trisomy 21.

The finding of a transmissible agent in familial cases both of Alzheimer's disease and of CJD sharply poses a further question. Are familial distributions owed solely to a common source of exposure to an agent within families, or to genetic susceptibility of families to the agent? The link Heston reported between Down's syndrome and familial cases of Alzheimer's disease encourages closer investigation. In this regard, it seems useful to search for links between Down's syndrome and familial cases of CJD. We have identified a series of familial cases of CJD in a population subject to an unusually high frequency of the disease – to be discussed below. An imminent step is to determine the frequency of Down's syndrome in the same population.

2. The Origin of the Family Distribution of CJD

While the majority of reported cases of CJD are sporadic, in about 10% familial occurrence has been recognized (29). We shall here pursue the question of the source of this familial occurrence. Reporting bias may account for some part, but surely not for all.

The annual incidence reported has been on average about one per million. Libyan-born Israelis have an excess well above this average (31), which we estimate to be about forty-fold. (We note in passing that greater understanding of the etiology of CJD may accrue from comparative studies of incidence.) Before their mass migration to Israel in the years 1949 through 1951, Libyan Jews had survived for centuries as a small marriage isolate. In the light of this history, it occurred to one of our graduate students[8] that the high frequency of the disease among them might be the result of genetic susceptibility to the agent in the marriage isolate. We thereupon explored the familial occurrence of the disease among Libyan Jews to determine whether there was clustering within genealogies and if so, whether the pattern of clustering would support the hypothesis of genetic susceptibility (32).

Twenty-three cases of CJD had been diagnosed among Libyan-born Israelis between January, 1963 and June, 1977. The Neuguts obtained genealogies of 20 of the 23 identified cases of CJD through personal interviews of the surviving relatives. Among the 20 cases, six contributed three related pairs. A fourth related pair was constituted by a seventh case among the 20, paired with a case deceased some 20 years previous and not included in the diagnosed series. The pairs were as follows:

   i)   Mother (NM) and daughter (IM). NM died at an age
        of more than 75, and before IM who died aged 40.
        NM and her husband were first cousins.

   ii. First cousins, said never to have dwelt together in
        the same household or compound.

   iii. First cousins once removed, also said never to have
        dwelt together.

   iv. In a seventh genealogy a male case (YD) was found to
        have had an affected mother (ED) who had died 19
        years before.

In the remaining thirteen genealogies, definite cases of affected relatives of the index cases were not discovered,

---

[8]
   Rita Neugut. She and Alfred Neugut carried out the field study of CJD in Israel in the summer of 1977, with the permission and cooperation of Esther Kahana, Milton Alter, and others. Howard Levine advised on the statistical test.

although in some the disease could not be excluded. The familial clustering of CJD is obviously beyond chance. A statistical test of the chance of finding three pairs among the 20 index cases indicates a probability of < .0001. The additional pair renders the probability even less.

We first consider whether the origin of this excess of CJD can be explained primarily by common exposure to the agent. The sporadic cases cover a wide range in terms of age of onset. Date of onset is of course restricted by the period for which cases were collected (1963 to 1977), but there is as yet nothing to suggest an epidemic confined to the period of data collection. The wide age-span of onset might signify that exposure to the agent continued over decades to produce new cases among Libyan Jews. On the other hand, a point epidemic, with a long and variable latent period on the model of kuru, cannot be excluded. Whether endemic or epidemic, the agent could not have been localized. The immigrants while in Libya had lived in three separate areas, one of which was 300 miles distant from the other two, and victims came from all three areas. Within Israel also we can exclude any local environmental factor. Libyan Jews live interspersed with other Israeli ethnic groups who do not show the excess, and cases were dispersed across the country.

Further, we can safely conclude that the excess was not produced by an excess of sporadic cases alone. No previous reports of familial cases describe relationships in cousins. Leaving aside for comparison the two cousin pairs found in the Libyan Israeli series, therefore, it can be said at the least that this epidemic has no less than the proportion of familial cases expected from the literature, (2/20 or 4/20, depending on the comparison), and may have more. The solution to our question, we think, revolves around the familial cases.

Transmission in familial cases is not well understood. A common exposure to a single source, irrespective of age at exposure, is unlikely because of the rarity of occurrence in spouses. No spouse pairs were found among the Libyan Jews, and only one has been reported in a literature that now comprises some 500 to 600 cases. Both transplacental transmission and transmission through lactation can be ruled out as mechanisms; in the literature, affected paternal forebears are as frequent as maternal. If both single source exposure and vertical transmission through the mother only are ruled out on these grounds, person-to-person transmission and transmission through the genome remain to be considered.

A number of observations from this study and from the literature need to be reconciled with person-to-person transmission:

i) Susceptibility to infection upon exposure to relatives must be virtually confined to the prenubile phase because spouses are so rarely affected.

ii) Since overt CJD is a disease of middle life, with onset in parents usually after the infancy and childhood of their offspring, person-to-person transmission of an agent requires that a parent with the disease must have been infective during an asymptomatic period of at least 15 years, and perhaps more, before the onset of recognized disease. For instance, in our mother-daughter pair, a minimum of 23 years (if transmission to the daughter occurred when she was 15 years old) and a maximum of 38 years (if transmission to the daughter occurred in infancy) must have elapsed between the prenubile phase of the daughter's life and the onset of symptoms in the mother.

iii) The secondary attack rate is not constant. We can test this inference against the frequencies to be expected if it were constant. From the literature it is reasonable to assume familial infection in one of each ten index cases. Then if the source of family infection is confined to the first infected member, the probability of the occurrence of a group of three familial cases would be one in a 100, of a group of four familial cases, one in a 1,000, and so on. When more than one case exists in a family, the probability of contact is raised accordingly. Even so, the chances of a second secondary case would be very low.

Gajdusek and Gibbs (28) assembled eleven genealogies, from the literature and from their own series, with more than one case. In nine of these at least one familial case was classed as "definite". Among the nine, only three had one secondary case, and six had more than one. One had three secondary cases, three had four, and two had fourteen. (This count of familial cases includes "probable" and "possible" cases.)

FAMILIAL CJD, FROM GAJDUSEK & GIBBS (28)
Number of cases per genealogy; number of
generations affected in parentheses.

Definite cases	Probable cases added	Possible cases added
N of cases	N of cases	N of cases
(N of generations)	(N of generations)	(N of generations)
6 (3)	14 (4)	15 (4)
4 (2)	5 (3)	5 (3)
3 (3)	5 (3)	5 (3)
2 (1)	2 (1)	2 (1)
1 (1)	1 (1)	2 (2)
1 (1)	1 (1)	4 (1)
1 (1)	1 (1)	2 (2)
1 (1)	5 (3)	5 (3)
1 (1)	15 (4)	15 (4)
–	–	4 (2)
–	–	2 (2)
$\overline{20}$	$\overline{49}$	$\overline{61}$

The cases assembled in the chart above include the
index cases. Although family size and the denominators
at risk cannot be derived from the reports, these
secondary attack rates are higher than expected. If
they are not the result of reporting bias, they require
that other factors like unusual infectivity or susceptibility must interact with person-to-person transmission.

iv) Neither of the two pairs of cousins discovered among
the Libyan Jews had ever lived in the same household.
The probability that two such pairs occurred by chance,
given the incidence in this population, is less than
one in a thousand.

Thus to meet these conditions for person-to-person transmission, an agent with a long and variable latent period
must have been sufficiently widespread to infect sporadic
cases through random, extra-familial exposure, and to spread
within families only to the young and not to spouses, and yet
with a raised secondary attack rate over several generations.
In such circumstances, one might expect that non-Jewish Liby-
ans had a good chance of contracting the disease. A search
for cases of CJD in Libya, where the incidence is not known,
would provide supporting evidence. An excess of cases would

be compatible with the sequence of events postulated on this model, and would tend to exclude the alternative hypotheses discussed below.

The hypothesis that transmission of the virus in the genome of either parent could have taken place among the Libyan Jews invokes their genetic commonality. This form of transmission, after the model of murine leukemia, has not been demonstrated in humans. In order to distinguish between genome transmission and genetically controlled susceptibility, Fine (33) emphasizes that an intergenerational pattern as opposed to an intra-generational pattern would favor genome transmission.

In other respects, where genome transmission occurs the data would conform with the patterns resulting from inherited susceptibility. They would conform also if the CJD agent required a "helper" virus in the genome for its activation. The essential element in both these explanations is that the disease must be in excess among those with shared inheritance, rather than among those coming into close physical contact with affected persons. For the present we must treat them as epidemiologically indistinguishable from inherited susceptibility.

On the hypothesis of inherited susceptibility, we would expect that in each generation a proportion of susceptibles, determined by the size and the persistence of the marriage isolate, would manifest the disease in the event of sufficient exposure. On this model, there need be restrictions neither on the geographic distribution of the agent in Libya and in Israel, nor on the age of exposure, nor on the duration of the latent period. Because of the inbreeding in this population, unrelated individuals as well as distant kin (cousins, second cousins) could share high degrees of susceptibility. The small marriage isolate could account for the contrast with the large heterogeneous marriage pools in which enhanced susceptibility is apparent only among first degree relatives.

A balanced theory of interaction between inherited susceptibility and transmissible agent must accommodate variations in both these elements. An agent, more common and ubiquitous than the rarity of the disease suggests, would manifest itself in populations with a frequency depending on the distribution of susceptibility. The transmission of CJD with medical mishaps, as by a corneal transplant from a patient later found to have died of the disease, and by

SUMMARY CHART

CONDITIONS FOR TWO THEORIES OF A CJD EXCESS IN LIBYAN JEWS

A. Common Exposure to Infection

    1. Enhanced susceptibility limited almost entirely to prenubile persons.

    2. Victims infective during symptomless latent period at some stage up to 40 years before onset.

    3. Infected cousin pairs are chance events (p < .001).

    4. Either the latent period has a wide range, or the chance of exposure persisted over a long period.

    5. Chance of exposure is not localized to any area.

    6. Variable and high secondary attack rate.

B. Inherited Susceptibility or Genome Transmission of Infection.

    1. Excess of sporadic cases no greater than of familial cases.

    2. More familial cases than expected by chance.

    3. Small homogeneous marriage isolate and high co-efficient of inbreeding produce cousin pairs.

    4. No excess of cases in other population subgroups exposed to similar environment, same location, or possible common vehicles of infection e.g. indigenous Libyans, other North African immigrants to Israel.

    5. Excess of cases in subsequent generations located in Israel.

intra-cerebral electrodes previously used on a CJD patient, supports the idea that the agent may be present and harmless, only to induce the disorder when invasion of the brain is facilitated. In large heterogeneous marriage pools a powerful barrier to ordinary exposures to the agent may be postulated, a barrier under genetic control that can be penetrated when immune defenses are weak or when the attack by the agent is intense. In the small marriage isolate of Libyan Jews, the proportion susceptible because the genetic barrier is weak may be supposed to be unusually high.

If the epidemic in Libyan Jews is indeed a manifestation of inherited susceptibility or transmission in the genome, no excess of cases is to be expected in Libya. On the other hand, an excess should continue to appear among the Israeli-born offspring of Libyan-born Jews if the agent is distributed in Israel as it is in Libya. The observation of such an excess entails a wait that will probably last to the end of the century and possibly beyond. Our arguments are summarized in the accompanying chart. The excess of cases among lineages of Libyan Jews, the reported occurrence in other populations of cases in several family members, and the conditions that must be satisfied for a tenable theory limited to increased exposure to an agent, makes the theories of inherited susceptibility or of a virus in the genome the more plausible explanations of the observed epidemic.

IV. FAMILIAL AND ECOLOGICAL FACTORS INFLUENCING INTELLIGENCE AMONG WARSAW SCHOOLCHILDREN.[9]

1. Background to the Study

The city of Warsaw was seen to provide an unusual opportunity for examining the effects of an egalitarian social policy on the intellectual performance of children. The city was razed at the end of World War II, and rebuilt under

―――――――――

[9] Polish principals in the study are Magdalena Sokolowska, Anna Firkowska and Antonina Ostrowska from the Institute of Philosophy and Sociology, Polish Academy of Sciences, and Ignacy Wald from the Neuropsychiatric Institute, Warsaw. The research was assisted by Contract 19-P-58334-F, U.S., HEW, SRC, to Professor Sokolowska, and by Contract HD 42808 NIH to M. Susser.

a socialist government whose policy was to allocate dwellings
without regard to social class. Hence children of families
of heterogeneous cultural background lived side by side in
the same housing and used the same health and educational
facilities. These assumptions held good in the data later
collected to test them.

In the first phase of the study, all 11 year old children
living in Warsaw, numbering about 14,000 in all, were given
three psychometric tests. Test performance was found to be
unrelated either to school or to neighborhood factors. Performance was, however, related to occupation and education
of mothers and fathers in a strong and regular gradient.
These two parental factors account for 10.6 percent of the
total variance in test scores. From these results we concluded that an egalitarian social policy executed over a
generation had failed to override the strong association of
family factors with cognitive development that is characteristic of capitalist industrial societies (34).

2.   Study of Familial Resemblance

A main objective of the study was to evaluate the influence of specific intrafamilial processes on the chance of
rearing mildly mentally retarded or exceptionally bright
children. To this end a detailed social and clinical investigation was undertaken of a subsample of about 1,000
children and their families.

Although our central concern was the postulated influence
of intrafamilial processes on cognitive development, we believed it important to try and take genetic factors into
account. From the standpoint of our central concern, the
genetic contribution to mental performance was 'noise' that
needed to be controlled. We did not aspire to measure the
genetic component, nor gene-environment interaction. The
"family set" approach of W. J. Schull and E. Harburg (35, 36)
seemed promising for our purpose of 'noise control', and we
invited Jack Schull to advise. We decided to create family
sets, each consisting of an index child, sib, cousin, and
unrelated child, and to obtain I.Q. scores for each member.
About two hundred sets were selected from among the 14,000
index children. The unrelated child was to be selected,
according to the attributes desired for any particular analysis, from the total pool of 11-year-old children.

We begin with a look at the rationale and assumptions of this aspect of the study. For several reasons, the data seemed to be of special interest:

i)   The index and the unrelated control children can be described in the context of the total age-group.

ii)   All members of the set are similar in age, and inter-generational change will not confound the associations among them.

iii)   The first phase of the study showed that in Warsaw, school and neighborhood factors are effectively neutralized. Consequently, remaining environmental sources of variation in mental performance must be sought in the family environment.

iv)   One might expect that the levelling of Warsaw living conditions would reduce overall variation in I.Q. Hence one might expect also that the proportions of the variance explained by genetic factors on the one hand and environment on the other would be somewhat different in Warsaw from the proportions found in capitalist industrial societies.

In the United States and Western Europe the shared environment of sibs, within categories of families defined by parental occupation or education, is differentiated from other categories not only by the micro-culture within the home, but by the complex of culture, physical environment, and educational experience characteristic of neighborhoods and social classes. In Warsaw, the shared environment of sibs among the given categories of parental occupation and education is differentiated essentially and almost solely by the micro-culture found within the home or stemming from it. As a result, in Warsaw there are fewer environmental forces generating a likeness among sibs, and we anticipated that the correlation for test scores among sib-pairs would be lower than elsewhere. The data lend some support to this view. Thus in the eight heterogeneous series of sibs collected by Jencks, the correlations on I.Q. scores range from $r=.45$ to $.67$ ($n = 1935$, $\underline{r} = .5435$). In Warsaw the correlation between sibs on the Raven test was $r = .4479$.

Age of child, type of test and other factors influence such correlations, and we do not attach great significance to this finding. Yet it is of a piece with the proportion

of variance in test performance contributed by all the social
factors we could measure in the age cohort as a whole. The
total of 10.6%, all virtually accounted for by parental occupation and education, is distinctly in the lower range of
other series reported for children of comparable age.

We asked next whether we could make a statement about
the proportions of the variance in I.Q. among school children
explained by genetic and environmental factors in Warsaw as
compared with studies conducted elsewhere. We considered
two models described in the literature to estimate the
heritable proportion of variance in I.Q.: the family set
model mentioned above, and the path model of Morton and Rao
(37,38). Here we shall discuss our experience with the family
set model.[10]

Epidemiological features of the family sets bear on the
results. The index children were not a representative sample
of the total cohort. They qualified for selection only when
they had both a sib and a cousin, each within two years of
their own age and living in Warsaw. This select population
was bound to exclude one-child families (30% of the total
cohort) and to over-represent large families and those long
settled in Warsaw. The cousins over-represent maternal
relatives (54% of the total) as compared with paternal relatives. The mean and standard deviation of the scores on the
Raven intelligence test differ appreciably among index children, sibs,and cousins. We attribute these I.Q. differences
to age differences. The index children, like the total cohort, were all eleven years old, and the Raven test was
standardized on that age group. Sibs and cousins ranged in
age from 9 to 13 years.

To carry out the analysis of heritability, we used five
estimators[11] (h_i^2, i = 2, 4, 6, 8, 10), taken from Rodriguez (39). (We note that these estimators do not make use
of the unrelated individuals).

10
    Eric Dulberg, Martin Weinstock and Peeter Teedla
worked with us on the analysis.
    11
    We used Rodriguez' "unstabilized" estimators, in each
case.

$\hat{h}^2_2$ index-sib correlation

$\hat{h}^2_4$ index-cousin correlation

$\hat{h}^2_6$ multiple regression of index on sib and cousin

$\hat{h}^2_8$ the beta coefficient for the cousin taken from the multiple regression of index on sib and cousin.[12]

$\hat{h}^2_{10}$ the difference between the variances of the differences of index and cousin, and index and sib, i.e. $V(I-C) - V(I-S)$.

In Table 7 we set out the values of h^2_i we obtained for the 5 estimators applied to the I.Q. of the 200 family sets from Warsaw. The results range from .42 to 1.28. Estimators based on h^2_2 and h^2_8, to which we refer again below, are .90 and .72 respectively.

In our interpretation of this table, we greatly benefit from the work of Rodriguez in Schull's Department. Rodriguez undertook the extensive task of estimating the distribution of these several heritability estimators (h^2_2 and h^2_4 are based on the conventional correlations between relatives, and h^2_6, h^2_8 and h^2_{10} on the family set).

Using Monte Carlo simulation, he tested the accuracy and the precision of each estimator, including numerous trials for each of several sample sizes of family sets. For family sets of sample size 300, for instance (our sample was 200), he generated 460 trials without replacement. Rodriguez used several pre-set levels of heritability, and four models. His Model 4 is the most realistic for our purposes. In this model, 10 genetic loci are postulated to contribute to the characteristic under study, dominance is allowed for at each, an allowance is made for an environmental effect on the phenotype, and this environment is shared

---

12
    Rodriguez calls this "the partial regression coefficient of index on cousin holding sib constant", but we believe our term to be a less ambiguous description of the statistic he has used.

by family members. This model, however, assumes no interaction between genes at different loci. More important for
our purposes perhaps, the model also assumes random mating
and independence of genotype and environment.

Rodriguez used his results to compare the estimators for
their performance in terms of accuracy and of precision.
Accuracy was defined as the approximation, to the true level
of heritability, of the mean of many trials of the heritability estimators for given sample sizes. Precision was defined
by the confidence limits around the estimate for the estimators, again for given sample sizes. On the whole, $\hat{h}^2_2$ (based
on index sib correlation) and $\hat{h}^2_8$ (based on the family set)
were the most accurate and the most precise estimators for
Model 4. However, both these estimators overestimate heritability almost invariably, and often substantially. Overestimation was marked, especially for $\hat{h}^2_2$, with increasing
levels of environmental co-variance as defined in the model
i.e., environment shared by family members. The estimators
were also not precise. Thus although $\hat{h}^2_8$ was the most accurate
estimator, the confidence limits were wide, even for sample
sizes of 600 family sets. Other estimators generally performed less well than $\hat{h}^2_2$ or $\hat{h}^2_8$ in terms of accuracy and
precision.

The five estimators tested systematically by Rodriguez
did not include the unrelated individual. This member of the
set was included in our original design in order better to
differentiate environmental effects among individuals specified by genetic relationships. In our design, we intended
that the unrelated member would be matched at will to each
family set by selected social characteristics. When
Rodriguez included random unrelated individuals, whose environments were assumed uncorrelated with family members, the
standard deviation of the estimators was much increased. He
therefore argued that the inclusion of unrelated individuals
would increase variability of the estimators without contributing new information about heritability. This may not be the
case when the main objective is the comparison of environmental variation between and within population groups, as it is
from our vantage point. We believe the unrelated individual
might indeed contribute new information about environmental
variation. For the present, however, the necessary trials
are not available to us.

It has been our hope that a family set estimator of heritability, even one which subsumed gene-environment interaction
and covariance without specifying them, could be used in comparative studies of I.Q. variation. The purpose was not the
estimation of h^2 as such. We sought rather to employ an

estimator of heritability in the narrow sense which would meet the requirements of precision, that is reliability across populations. Whether or not it was accurate, and over-estimated or under-estimated, was of less concern to us. With a reliable estimator, we could pursue our aim of comparing the proportion of the variance remaining, under different conditions, for otherwise comparable populations.

At the present stage of development of published work on family sets, it seems one must conclude that the estimators will overestimate heritability. More important, they do not satisfy the requirements of precision. Yet the effort that has been made to test the properties of the family set model is unusual and commendable indeed, and it may be that continuing effort will overcome some of the difficulties. Meanwhile, we are experimenting with the use of the unrelated individual.

V. CONCLUSION

A presentation to an interdisciplinary audience like this one forces the authors to face their identity as epidemiologists. In pondering their differences from geneticists, they are made aware of shortcomings: less in touch with growing points in biology than are cytogeneticists; less sophisticated in mathematical skills (at least among earlier cohorts) than are population geneticists; less well-informed about a myriad of rare eponymous syndromes than are clinical geneticists. What then might their special strengths be?

In the four epidemiological problems discussed here, problems of prevalence in mental retardation, of reproductive wastage, of links between rare diseases, and of social causation in mild mental retardation, it seems to us that epidemiologists have legitimate business. This legitimacy does not depend on epidemiologic methods; we do not subscribe to the view that epidemiology is defined by its methods. Indeed we must draw on colleagues in other disciplines for measures, tools and concepts. Essentially the legitimation of epidemiologists rests on the questions they ask, questions about the distributions and determinants of health states and the control of health disorders in populations. To seek preventable causes of Down's syndrome or of mild mental retardation is to pose the purposive questions of an applied field. Because the range of outcomes is so varied and the range of determinants so broad, epidemiologists must be prepared to invade many new areas. Their armamentarium of methods has been developed in pursuit of epidemiological questions. These questions increasingly impinge on genetic issues. Geneticists, we must hope, will help us through the thickets of our ignorance.

TABLE   7

ESTIMATES OF HERITABILITY (h^2) IN RAVEN SCORES
OF 200 FAMILY SETS AMONG WARSAW SCHOOLCHILDREN
BASED ON FIVE SEPARATE ESTIMATORS ($\hat{h}_i^2$)*

Basis of estimator, $\hat{h}_i^2$	Formulas for estimators	Values derived from study	Estimated heritability
Index-sib correlation, $\hat{h}_2^2$	$[2\ \hat{\rho}_{I,S}]$	$\rho_{I,S}$ = .4479	.8958
Index-cousin correlation, $\hat{h}_4^2$	$[8\ \hat{\rho}_{I,C}]$	$\rho_{I,C}$ = .1525	1.2200
Multiple regression of index on cousin and sib, $\hat{h}_6^2$	$\dfrac{[8\ \hat{\beta}_c]}{1 - \hat{\beta}_S}$	β_C = .0905 β_S = .4350	1.2814
Beta coefficient of index on cousin (from multiple regression above) $\hat{h}_8^2$	$[8\ \hat{\beta}_c]$	β_C = .0905	.7240
Differences between variances of (I-C) and (I-S), $\hat{h}_{10}^2$	$\dfrac{[4\ \hat{d}_1]}{3\hat{v}_I}$ †	v_I= 145.054 V_S= 133.555** V_C= 88.657**	.4154

*The five estimators correspond to Rodriguez (39) h_2^2, h_4^2, h_6^2, h_8^2, h_{10}^2, respectively. I = index, S = sib, C = cousin.

†Where: $\hat{d}_1 = \hat{v}_C - \hat{v}_S + 2\ (\hat{Cov}\ (I,S) - \hat{Cov}\ (I,C)$ and

$\hat{Cov}(x,y) \equiv \hat{\rho}_{xy}\ \sqrt{\overline{\hat{v}_x \hat{v}_y}}$.

**V(I-C) = 199.125

**V(I-S) = 153.921

REFERENCES

1. Turner, G. Med. J. Austral. 2, 927, (1975).
2. Penrose, L.S. "A Clinical and Genetic Study of 1,280 Cases of Mental Defect," Medical Research Council, Special Report Series 229, H.M.S.O. London, (1938).
3. Dewey, W. J., Barrai, I., Morton, N. E. and Mi, M. P. Amer. J. Hum. Genet. 17, 237, (1965).
4. Morton, N. E., Rao, D. C., Lang-Brown, H., MacLean, C., Bart, R. D. and Lew, R. J. of Med. Genet. 14, 1, (1977).
5. Saenger, G. "Factors Influencing the Institutionalization of Mentally Retarded Individuals in New York City." Albany, (1960).
6. Stein, Z. A. and Susser, M. W. Brit. J. Prev. Soc. Med. 14, 83, (1960).
7. Lewis, E. O. "Report on an Investigation into the Incidence of Mental Deficiency in Six Areas, 1925-1927," H.M.S.O., London, (1929).
8. Kushlick, A. Proc. Roy. Soc. Med. 58, 374, (1965).
9. Tizard, J. "Community Services for the Mentally Handicapped," Oxford University Press, London, (1964).
10. Stein, Z., Susser, M. and Saenger, G. Amer. J. of Epid., 103, 477, (1976).
11. Stein, Z. and Susser, M. in "Social Psychiatry," A.R.N.M.D. (F. Redlich, ed.), Vol. 47, 62, (1969).
12. Birch, H. G., Richardson, S. A., Baird, D., Horobin, G. and Illsley, R. "Mental Subnormality: A Clinical and Epidemiologic Study in the Community," Williams and Wilkins, New Y ork, (1970).
13. Clarke, A.D.B. and Clarke, A. M. "Mental Deficiency: The Changing Outlook," Third Ed., London: Methuen, (1975).
14. Roberts, J. A. F. Eugenics Review 44, 71, (1952).
15. Clarke, A. D. B., Clarke, A. M. and Reiman, S. Brit. J. Psychol. 49, 144, (1958).
16. Conway, J. Brit. J. Statist. Psychol. 11, 171, (1958).
17. Kline, J., Stein, Z. A., Strobino, B., Susser, M. and Warburton, D. Am. J. Epidem. 106, 345 (1977).
18. Harlap, S. and Davies, A. M. Bull. World Health Organ. 52, 149, (1975).
19. Stark, C. R. and White, N. B., in Population Cytogenetics, Studies in Humans," (E. B. Hook and I. H. Porter, eds.), p. 275. Academic Press, New York, (1977).
20. Stein, Z. A. and Susser, M. W, in "Research to Practice in Mental Retardation of the Fourth Congress of the International Association for the Scientific Study of Mental Deficiency," (P. Mittler, ed.), Vol. 3, (1977).

21. Stoller, A. and Collman, R. D., Lancet 2, 1221, (1965).
22. Harlap, S., Am. J. Epidemiol. 99, 210, (1974).
23. Leck, I., Lancet 1, 1057, (1977).
24. Stein, Z. A., Susser, M., Warburton, D., Wittes, J. and Kline, J. Amer. J. Epidemiol. 102, 275, (1975).
25. Susser, M. "Causal Thinking in the Health Sciences: Concepts and Strategies of Epidemiology," Oxford University Press,(1973).
26. Infante, P. F., Wagoner, J. K., McMichael, A. J., Waxweiler, R. J. and Falk, H., Lancet 1, 1289, (1976).
27. Strobino, B., Kline, J. and Stein, Z. A. Early Human Development (1978, in press).
28. Gajdusek, C. and Gibbs, C. J., Jr., in "Advances in Neurology," (B. S. Meldrum and C. D. Marsden, eds.) Vol. 10, p. 291. Raven Press, New York, (1975).
29. Traub, R., Gajdusek, D. C. and Gibbs, C. J., Jr., in "Aging and Dementia," (W. L. Smith and M. Kinsbourne, eds.) p. 91, Spectrum Pub., New York, (1977).
30. Heston, L. L., Science, 196, 322, (1977).
31. Kahana, E., Alter, M., Brahan, J., and Sofer, D. Science, 183, 90, (1974).
32. Neugut, R. H., Neugut, A., Kahana, E., Stein, Z. and Alter, M. Neurology (in press).

33. Fine, P. E. J. of Med. Genet. 14, 399. (1977).

34. Czarkowski, M., Firkowska-Mankiewicz, A., Ostrowska, A., Sokolowska, M., Stein, Z., Susser, M. and Wald, I. in "Research to Practice in Mental Retardation of the Fourth Congress of the International Association for the Scientific Study of Mental Deficiency," (P. Mittler, ed.), Vol. 1, 89, (1977).
35. Harburg, E. and Schull, W. J. J. Chron. Dis. 23, 69, (1970).
36. Schull, W. J. and Harburg, E. J. Chron. Dis., 23, 83, (1970).
37. Morton, N. E., Amer. J. Human Genet. 26, 318, (1974).
38. Rao, D. C. and Morton, N. E. Amer. J. Hum. Genet., 26, 331, (1974).
39. Rodriguez, A. "A Monte Carlo Simulation of the "Family Set" Approach to Estimate Heritability," (unpublished dissertation), University of Texas, (1976).

454   Common Diseases

DISCUSSION

MORTON: The effect of inbreeding on incidence of mental
retardation gives risks for genetic counseling and basic
information about human genetics. Three studies yield
similar estimates of the inbred load from normal parents
(Table 1), from which we can infer that incidence of mental
retardation increases from .0124 to .0624 in the first cousin
matings (1). This clearly contradicts the conclusion of
Fraser and Biddle (2) that "the risk of first-cousin parents
with a recessively inherited disease appears to be low (< 1%)."
To be counted as a "recessive disorder" in their study a
disease present in a family coming to genetic counseling for
some other reason had to be recognized by unspecified diagnostic criteria, and in fact no recessive disorders as defined
were seen in either their first cousin group or controls.
Only a minority of recessive diseases can be easily and unambiguously diagnosed. It would be a serious error of judgment to use their measure of diagnostic precision as a morbid
risk for genetic counseling. This is part of the evidence
suggesting that licensure of medical geneticists will not
suffice to insure reasonable accuracy in the purveyance of
genetic risks.

TABLE 1

Estimates of the Inbred Load B for Mental Retardation

Population	Year	Sample	B
England	1938	case	.893
Sweden	1957	random	.716
Israel	1972	case	.790
Hawaii	1977	case	.740

Risk for MR specific to
    first cousin matings = $B/16 \doteq .05$

TABLE 2

Two Estimates of Numbers of Loci for Recessive MR

---

inbred load $\equiv B \doteq .792$

panmictic incidence $\equiv A \doteq .002$

number of loci $\equiv k > B^2/A = 314$

---

mean gene frequency $\equiv q \leq A/B = .0025$

mean IQ deficit of homozygote $\equiv t = 52.5$

regression of IQ on F (Schull and Neel) $\equiv b = -44$

number of loci $\equiv k = b/qt = 335$

contribution to genetic variance $= At^2/\sigma^2 \doteq .024$

A more fundamental question is whether the decline of IQ with inbreeding is due to polygenes or rare recessive genes. We may approach this by calculating in two ways the number of loci that can produce mental retardation: first, from the loads for mental retardation, and secondly from the observed decline of IQ reported by Schull and Neel (3) and others in the general population. These two estimates are in close agreement, with no suggestion of a discrepancy that might be due to polygenes. Rare recessive genes made an extremely small contribution to dominance deviations, which are therefore a negligible source of family resemblance for IQ.

REFERENCES

1. Morton, N.E., Matsuura, J., Bart, R., and Lew, R., Clin. Genet. (1978, in press).
2. Fraser, F.C., and Biddle, C.J., Am. J. Hum. Genet. 28, 522-526 (1976).
3. Schull, W.J., and Neel, J.V., "The Effects of Inbreeding on Japanese Children," Harper & Row, New York, 1965.

STEIN:

With regard to the risk of mental retardation in first cousin matings, given as .05 in Table 1, we cannot interpret this figure without knowledge of the grade of mental deficit. Thus in community surveys a rate of .05 which includes mild and moderate retardation is not unusual for children of 'normal' parents, particularly in unfavorable social conditions. A similar difficulty applies to the incidence figures for mental retardation of .0124 and .0624. (Cited from Morton et al., 1978.) With regard to genetic counseling, from these rates Morton suggests that there is a five-fold increase in the risk of mental retardation for the offspring of cousin matings. We think it essential to discuss the risk of severe and of mild mental retardation separately.

First, to take severe mental retardation: Schull and Neel (1965, Table 7.1) found 14 children with severe mental retardation (imbecile and idiot) out of 3,570 among the offspring of unrelated parents (.0039, entirely consistent with other prevalence data cited in our paper) and 11 severely retarded children among 1817 offspring of cousin matings (.0055). Removing the cases of Down's syndrome from each group gives .0028 among offspring of unrelated parents, and .0055 among offspring of cousins. This suggests doubling of the risk of severe mental retardation for cousin matings.

Second, to take mild mental retardation: Schull and Neel, in comparing cousin marriage offspring with the general population (excluding from the testing the severely retarded children described above) did not find evidence of 'tailing' or of 'major' modifiers in the distribution of intelligence in the offspring of cousin marriages. The modest decline in IQ that was found cannot therefore be readily stated as a relative risk for mild mental retardation that would hold true for cousin mating across all social groups.

If rare recessives contribute to mild mental retardation, we would expect them to do so evenly across the classes, as with severe mental retardation. However, children from low socio-economic status are at very much higher risk of mild mental retardation than are those from high socio-economic status. Genetic counseling on the attributable risk for cousin marriages must take these differences into account. Thus the excess attributable risk in the lowest social classes (with total prevalence of mild mental retardation up to .05) may be so slight as to be hardly evident. On the other hand, the same addition of excess risk to the much smaller frequency in the higher classes (with a total prevalence of mild mental retardation of say .0005 to .001) may make an appreciable difference.

MORTON: The family set of Schull et al. (1) is a sampling design, not a model. It will be interesting to see what models will be applied to it. For us the answer is clear: we see no competitor to our linear model of path analysis.
    The most striking finding of the Warsaw Study is that an environmental index accounts for 10.6 per cent of the variance of test scores, corresponding to a correlation of $\sqrt{.106}$ = .326. We may note in passing that such indices are not part of family sets as defined by Schull and colleagues but are incorporated in path analysis, where the expected correlation for x = m = 0 is $\underline{ic}$, according to Rao et al. (2). At this conference Rao and Morton estimated for a large American sample i = .792, c = .396, and so ic = .314. The observed correlation between child's phenotype and index is .304. Both are in close agreement with the .326 reported from Warsaw, where the index is based on more information and is therefore presumably a better estimate of the environment. While only a rough comparison is possible, we might guess that the determination of child's environment is less in Warsaw: At the upper limit of i = 1, the bound is c = .326. A reliable estimate requires path analysis of an appropriate data set. When we consider that Raven's matrices are less biased culturally than conventional IQ tests, there appears to be fair agreement with the study of Halperin et al. (3) in which "there is no evidence that the importance of cultural inheritance is diminished in a purportedly more egalitarian society" (Rao and Morton, this conference).

REFERENCE

1.   Schull, W.J., Harburg, E., Erfort, J.C., Schork, M.A., and Rice, R., J. Chron. Dis. 23, 83-92 (1970).
2.   Rao, D.C., Morton, N.E., and Yee, S., Am. J. Hum. Genet. 28, 228-242 (1976).
3.   Halperin, S.L., Rao, D.C., and Morton, N.E., Behav. Genet. 5, 83-86 (1975).

STEIN: We agree that the family set is a sampling design, not a model. We are in fact at present applying path analysis to the data.
    We also recognize the correspondence between our findings and those of Halperin et al. However, as Rao and Morton

state, the inference in that study is drawn from a "purportedly"
more egalitarian society. We aimed, in our study, to try and
provide measures of equalization to describe its degree,
rather than to rely on the assumption that it had occurred.
Thus we have demonstrated elsewhere that in Warsaw, social
policy has achieved a substantial degree of equalization of
living conditions and schooling (Firkowska et al., 1978).
Thus in our study the fact that in Warsaw egalitarian policies
did not override those forces within the family that
apparently determine mental performance among children cannot
be attributed to the ineffective implementation of policy.

Reference

Firkowska, A., Ostrowska, A., Sokalowska, M., Stein, Z.,
Susser, M. and Wald, I. Science (1978, in press).

MORTON: Geneticists tend to convert population
frequencies into "incidence among live births of persons who
will become affected if they survive according to the normal
life table". We might call this lifetime incidence (LI).

    This definition is more closely related than any other to
basic parameters like gene frequencies and mutation rates.
Usually geneticists regard lifetime prevalence (LP), defined
as the frequency of affected persons in the general population
of all ages, as an initial observation to be converted into
incidence.

    Conventional epidemiological usage is less transparent,
and I have difficulty in interpreting such concepts as
"prevalence of MR in childhood". Given that many cases are
not diagnosed until school entrance, are infants and pre-
school children included? When does childhood end? How does
this apply to institutionalized retardates of all ages? Is
specific prevalence as useful as lifetime prevalence? When
there is ambiguity in terms like incidence and prevalence, the
genetic convention should be considered because of its clear
motivation.

    Morbid risk p_x is the probability that an individual who
survives to age x is affected, and so

$$LP = \sum_{x} f_x\, p_x$$

where f_x is the frequency of age x in the general population.

STEIN: The lack of transparency in
epidemiological usage complained of by Dr. Morton is a matter
of complexity and not of ambiguity. The complexities of these
measures are elaborated in various texts (1, 2).

The term incidence is used by epidemiologists to measure the frequency of onset (or episode) of a disorder over a given time period in a defined population. Incidence can refer to inceptions (initial episodes), or to repeat episodes. An individual can contribute to incidence more than once in a lifetime. The unit of interest in an incidence rate is thus the frequency of occurrence of disease in a population through time, which is not necessarily the same as the count of individuals with the disease. Prevalence (most usefully point prevalence) refers to the number of diseased persons in a given population at a "point" in time: prevalence rates take as their denominators a census of the numbers at risk. Prevalence is a function of incidence and duration. Thus if a prevalence survey is repeated annually, the same individual may appear again in each prevalence rate. Also, one individual may contribute to the prevalence of more than one condition.

Incidence and prevalence, so defined, have many uses in epidemiology. They have required interpretations and adaptations for the study of certain chronic diseases (where the onset is often uncertain), for the study of relapsing conditions (where the 'well' state is difficult to define) and for the study of congenital anomalies (where the inception becomes visible at birth, but the initiating event took place at least 280 days earlier).

Age-specific prevalence, or as we used it, prevalence based on that captive group, the school-age child, gives a rate for severe mental retardation that can be derived accurately and economically from a reliable numerator and denominator. Those of appropriate age living in institutions can be readily included. The age group can be exactly specified, as was done for instance by Lewis, cited above (see also Stein & Susser, (3)). Age-specific prevalence at school age, as Morton rightly indicates, can not yield incidence at birth, nor prevalence in the pre-school period, nor survival between birth and six years, but it furnishes data relevant to these. It has the great advantage of being a measure retrievable from the literature and repeatable at different times and places. It has significance for medical care because it relates to survivors, who are the greatest burden in terms of families and services. A main defect of the measure is that it is too far removed from the events relating to etiology to serve the community as an early warning system. As discussed by Ernest Hook at this conference, we have as yet no entirely useful measure for this purpose.

'Lifetime prevalence' was used by earlier investigators in an attempt to assess the total impact on a community of anyone ever becoming ill with a particular disorder. This measure can have heuristic meaning if one confines one's interest to disorders 1) which will manifest themselves at different ages, and 2) which will persist in an individual, once he has manifested it. If the disorder is manifest at birth, the term is unnecessary. If there is recovery, then age-specific incidence is preferable, because it enables repeat episodes to be considered, as well as inception episodes.

The human geneticist has usually been concerned with individuals who are distinctive in that at some time they manifest a particular disorder. These individuals are of interest to the geneticist before, during, and after the disease has actually become apparent. The epidemiological measures, however, seek to measure disease frequencies in populations as well as risk in individuals. Both seem to us legitimate endeavors but discourse is not helped by using the same terms with different meanings.

REFERENCES

1. MacMahon, B., and Pugh, Thomas F., "Epidemiology: Principles and Methods," Little Brown & Co., Boston, 1970.
2. Susser, M., "Causal Thinking in the Health Sciences," Oxford University Press, New York, 1972.
3. Stein, Z.A., Susser, M., Saenger, G., and Marolla, F.A., Am. J. Epid. 103:5, 477-485 (1976).

JACOBS: During the "epidemic" was the distribution of types of trisomy different from that usually seen? Was the distribution of maternal age different from the usual? Might the excess of trisomies in the "epidemic" months not be explained by a higher success rate in culturing?

STEIN: The distribution of trisomy type did not change. For example, Trisomy 16, the commonest trisomy found in most series including ours, was present in the expected frequency, i.e. about half of all trisomies.

Mean maternal age for trisomies was slightly but not significantly higher during the epidemic. The success rate in culturing karyotypes did not explain the higher numbers of trisomies during the epidemic months. During the epidemic period (November through January) the success rate was 40 out of 81 attempts, the same as for the whole series. In two of the four months, the success rate was unusually high (68%), and the proportion of trisomies was 55%. In the ten other months with a success rate of 66.6% or more, the proportion of trisomies was 15%. In the 13 non-epidemic months with a success rate of less than 66.6%, the proportion of trisomies was also 15%.

HOOK: What action did you take once you recognized the epidemic?

STEIN: We looked for possible environmental exposures. Suspicion fell on acrylo-nitrile, a plastic briefly used in plastic sof-drink bottles. This substance had been shown to be mutagenic, and withdrawn. It was used for bottles sold in our area over the relevant period. Investigation is under way; we have as yet no results to report.

GENETIC EPIDEMIOLOGY

POPULATION SURVEILLANCE: A CYTOGENETIC APPROACH

Patricia A. Jacobs*

University of Hawaii
Honolulu, Hawaii

I.   INTRODUCTION

At a first glance the surveillance of populations for individuals with chromosome aberrations may seem a somewhat crude method for detecting the presence of an environmental agent capable of producing genetic damage. However further consideration shows that chromosomes are not quite the blunt instrument they first appear.

In an article on "Monitoring Human Populations," Vogel (1) summarized the attributes necessary of any system used to monitor mutation rates. These were: i) virtually every new mutant must be recognizable as such; ii) the penetrance must be complete; iii) the defect must be diagnosable without ambiguity; iv) the defect must be at a selective disadvantage so that there is a high proportion of mutants; v) there must be no phenocopies; vi) all cases of the defect should come to medical attention; and vii) the defect must not be rare. A well designed survey of constitutional chromosome

*University of Hawaii, John A. Burns School of Medicine, Department of Anatomy and Reproductive Biology, 1960 East-West Road, Honolulu, Hawaii 96822.

abnormalities can come very near to fulfilling all these
requirements and may well be the best mechanism available at
the present time for monitoring human mutation rates.

II.   TYPES OF ABERRATION AND THEIR SIGNIFICANCE

There are two main classes of constitutional chromosome
abnormalities, those where the structure of one or more chromosomes is clearly abnormal and those where the abnormality
is one of number.   Numerical aberrations can be subdivided
into three types, namely monosomies in which a chromosome is
lacking, trisomies in which there is an additional chromosome
and polyploids in which there are one or two additional
haploid complements.   In mutagen testing it is important to
distinguish among these different classes because they may
well be caused by different etiological factors, or alternatively by the same agent exerting its effect at a different
stage in the life cycle or on a different cell type.   The
four main types of abnormality, the mechanisms by which they
are caused and some known or suspected etiological agents are
outlined in Table 1.

A.   Structural Abnormalities

From the viewpoint of population surveillance for mutagens, the most important types of chromosome aberration in
human populations are structural abnormalities.   Virtually
every agent known to cause mutations at specific loci is also
known to produce chromosome damage that is expressed as
structural aberrations (2, 3).   As this is the only class of
chromosome abnormality in which structural damage is implicated, it is the only one we can assume to be sensitive to
many conventional mutagens.   Thus it is reasonable to postulate that any detectable increase in the number of individuals with de novo structural aberrations will be accompanied
by an increase in the number of individuals with conventional
point mutations.   Structural abnormalities can occur at any
stage in the development of the germ cell and a mutation
detectable in the Fl could be the result of an event that
occurred at any time in the life cycle of the parental
gamete.
Structural aberrations can be either balanced, that is
there is the correct amount of euchromatic material but it is
deployed in an abnormal way as the result of a translocation
or inversion, or unbalanced, that is there is the loss or

TABLE 1

Summary of Types of Cytogenetic Abnormality, Mechanism and Etiology

Type of Cytogenetic Abnormality	Structural Rearrangement	Monosomy	Trisomy	Polyploidy
Cytogenetic Mechanism	Chromosome breakage and exchange.	Non-disjunction. Anaphase lag.	Non-disjunction.	Failure of a meiotic division. Polyspermy. Failure of cleavage in zygotic division.
Known or Suspected Etiologic Factor	Ionizing radiations. Drugs. Chemicals.	?	Ionizing radiations. Advanced maternal age (only for certain chromosomes).	Pre- and/or post-ovulatory aging of oocyte. ?Ionizing radiations. ?Drugs affecting female reproduction.

gain of euchromatic material. These two types of structural
abnormality are subject to very different selective pressures
at the level of the organism and presumably also the cell,
and in any study of structural rearrangements it is desirable
to consider them separately.

Virtually nothing is known about the epidemiology of de
novo structural rearrangements in man. Jacobs and her colleagues (4) could find no effect of parental age in a study
of de novo autosomal rearrangements. However the recent
advances in detection of both cytological and biochemical
polymorphisms should enable the parental origin of many de
novo structural aberrations to be determined. Such data will
be invaluable in unravelling the etiology of this important
class of chromosome aberrations.

B. Monosomies

With the exception of the sex chromosomes, conceptuses
lacking a chromosome are extremely rare among detectable
chromosome abnormalities. Theoretically monosomies can arise
at any stage in the germ cell cycle or at an early cleavage
division of the zygote either by non-disjunction or by loss
of a chromosome at anaphase. The former mechanism would also
produce trisomies while the latter would not be expected to
produce any other type of aberration. Thus any etiological
agent whose chief mode of action was to cause anaphase lag
would only be detected by the monitoring of monosomies.

There is very little information on the epidemiology of
monosomy and the data available are based solely on the 45,X
condition. Its occurrence is independent of either paternal
or maternal age and a study of the Xg^a blood group antigens
in the tiny proportion of 45,X conceptuses who are born
alive, has shown that the single X chromosome is maternally
derived in 77% of the cases and paternally derived in the
remaining 23% (5).

C. Trisomies

Trisomy is the most frequently detected chromosome
abnormality in our species and while it can arise as a result
of non-disjunction at a mitotic or meiotic division of the
germ cell, meiotic non-disjunction is considered the most
likely mechanism of origin of the majority of trisomies. In
spite of the frequency of its occurrence very little is known
about factors which cause non-disjunction. Evidence from
four surveys of human populations (6, 7, 8, 9) suggests that
maternal but not paternal irradiation is associated with the

production of at least one type of trisomy, namely trisomy for chromosome 21. The effect of irradiation was found to be particularly marked in mothers in the older age group and seemed to accumulate over many years prior to the conception of the trisomic.

The most striking feature in the epidemiology of trisomy is the association of certain trisomies with increasing maternal age. The trisomies where maternal age is a factor are those involving the acrocentric chromosomes and also chromosome 18 (10, 11). Maternal age appears to play no part in the genesis of the other trisomies including trisomy 16, the most frequently occurring of all the human trisomies (10, 12). There has been a recent suggestion that extremely advanced paternal age plays a role in the genesis of trisomy 21 (13). However this observation awaits confirmation.

Recent advances in the technology for the detection of human chromosome heteromorphisms have made it possible to determine the parent and the meiotic division in which the non-disjunction giving rise to trisomy occurred. The great majority of observations are based on a study of liveborn children with trisomy 21 and it has been shown that the error can occur in the father or the mother and in either the first or second meiotic division in either parent (14). However, the error in the majority of cases occurs during the first maternal meiotic division. More surprising is the recently reported data on other trisomies not associated with an increased maternal age (15, 16). In these also it appears that the non-disjunctional event most often occurs at the maternal first meiotic division. It may well be that different etiological mechanisms are implicated in the two types. Thus in any monitoring program it is important to distinguish between these two major categories of trisomies.

D. Polyploids

Polyploids are a comparatively frequent type of conceptus in our species, about three-quarters being triploid and the remaining quarter tetraploid. Triploids can arise either by fertilization involving a diploid gamete or by errors of fertilization. Tetraploids are probably most frequently due to a failure of the first cleavage division of a normal diploid zygote. Increased maternal age is not an etiological factor in the production of polyploids (10) but recent evidence from Alberman and her colleagues (17) suggests that previous maternal X irradiation may be an important etiological factor associated with polyploidy. In 1970, Carr (18) suggested that oral contraceptives taken in the six months prior to conception increased the proportion of

polyploid abortuses. A number of recent surveys have failed
to confirm Carr's observations (10, 19), but this may be the
result of the changing composition of oral contraceptives.
Boue and colleagues (10) obtained some data which suggest
that overripeness in the egg, resulting either from an unusually long follicular phase of the cycle or from a long delay
between ovulation and fertilization, results in an increased
number of polyploids.

Recently a number of studies have used chromosome heteromorphisms or biochemical polymorphisms to determine the
origin of the extra haploid set in human triploids. Three of
the reports (20, 21, 22) agree that the great majority of
triploids are the result of dispermy and only that of
Lauritsen (23) found the additional set to be the result of
failure of the first maternal meiotic division in five out of
six informative cases. The mechanism which leads to poly-
spermy is not understood, but is presumably the result of an
error occurring at or immediately prior to fertilization.
Tetraploidy is most probably the result of an error occurring
immediately after fertilization (20, 24). Thus human polyploids are the only type of chromosome aberration that is
mainly caused by errors occurring around the time of fertilization. Their etiology is, therefore, rather different from
other types of aberration and their study may provide information about a class of potential mutagens that is not associated with an increase in the other types of chromosome
abnormalities.

III. TYPES OF POPULATION

The human population usually considered to be the most
suitable for the monitoring of mutation rates by cytogenetic
examination is the newborn (1, 25). Undoubtedly such a population has a number of advantages: i) it is very easy to
define non-ambiguously; ii) it is one from which blood, in
the form of cord blood, is easily obtained; iii) it is one on
which leucocyte cultures can be done to give excellent chromosome preparations easily and cheaply; iv) it is one in
which an effect can be detected relatively early in the life
cycle; and v) it is one for which excellent base line data
are already available from a number of different centers in
the world. However there are two major disadvantages to the
study of the newborn and these are: firstly, the complete
absence of certain classes of abnormality which are selected
against prior to birth and, secondly and more importantly,

the comparative rarity of chromosome aberrations in this population, only 0.5% having a detectable abnormality.

There is a population, namely spontaneous abortions, which has many advantages over any other available population for mutation rate surveillance and yet the use of this material for monitoring for mutagens and teratogens has, to my knowledge, been seriously advocated only by Dr. Zena Stein and her colleagues (26). In all the many documents on the desirability of monitoring human populations for mutagens and teratogens, spontaneous abortions receive not a single mention (1, 25). The advantages of using such a population are numerous and include availability of material, frequency of abnormalities, availability of base line data, early detection, possibility of utilizing the chromosomally normal to monitor teratogens not associated with cytogenetic abnormality, and cost effectiveness. I would like to consider some of these advantages in detail.

A.   Frequency of Chromosome Aberrations

The frequencies of the major classes of chromosome abnormality in spontaneous abortions and newborn babies are compared in Table 2. As can be seen, the total frequency of chromosome abnormalities is almost 100 times greater in spontaneous abortions than livebirths. Furthermore two major types of aberration, namely monosomies and polyploids, that account for 20% of the abnormalities in the abortions are virtually unrepresented in the liveborn.

The frequency of the different types of structural rearrangement is shown in Table 3. As can be seen, structural rearrangements are some eight times more frequent among the spontaneous abortions than the livebirths. When the different types are considered separately, the balanced rearrangements are seen to occur somewhat more frequently among the livebirths--indeed this is the only class of chromosome aberration which is not increased among abortions--but the unbalanced are ninety times more common in the abortions. However for the purposes of mutation surveillance, it is only the de novo structural rearrangements that are of interest as it is only this category that would be expected to increase after exposure to a mutagen. Table 4 shows the proportion of de novo to familial rearrangements among both abortions and livebirths where both parents were examined and the percentage in each class that are the result of a de novo mutation. Unfortunately studies of parental chromosomes are often not reported and therefore the data in several categories are rather sparse. Nevertheless it can be seen that the proportion of mutants among the abortions is twice as great

TABLE 2

Chromosome Abnormalities in Spontaneous Abortions and Livebirths

Population		Total Examined	Total Abnormal	Type of Abnormality				
				Structural	Monosomy	Trisomy	Polyploid	Other
Spontaneous Abortions	No	3,080°	1,539	61	291	810	352	25
	%	100	50	2.0	9.4	26.3	11.4	0.8
Livebirths	No	59,452*	364	124	2	177	1	60
	%	100	0.61	0.21	-	0.30	-	0.10

° Data from Kajii et al. (1973); Boue et al. (1975); Lauritsen (1976); Creasy et al. (1976); Hassold et al. (1977).

* Data from Jacobs et al. (1974); Nielsen and Sillesen (1975); Sergovich et al. (1969); Hamerton et al. (1975); Lubs and Ruddle (1970); Waltzer and Gerald (1977); Bochkov et al. (1974).

TABLE 3

Autosome Structural Abnormalities in Spontaneous Abortions and Livebirths

Population		Total Examined	Total* With Structural Ab.	Type of Abnormality						
				Balanced				Unbalanced		
				Total	Rob. Trans.	Rec. Trans.	Inv.	Total	Rob. Trans.	Other
Spontaneous Abortions	No	3,080°	52	3	1	2	0	49	28	21
	‰	1,000	16.88	0.97	0.32	0.65	-	15.91	9.09	6.82
Livebirths	No	59,452°	124	113	52	52	9	11	4	7
	‰	1,000	2.09	1.90	0.87	0.87	0.15	0.18	0.07	0.12

* Includes those with structural abnormality of autosome only.

° Data sources as in Table 2.

471

TABLE 4

Proportion of De Novo Mutants Among Autosome

Structural Abnormalities in Spontaneous Abortions and Livebirths

Population		Total	Type of Abnormality								
			Balanced					Unbalanced			
			Total	Rob. Trans.	Rec. Trans.	Inv.		Total	Rob. Trans.	Other
Spontaneous*	De novo:Total where both parents examined	25:46	2:2	-	2:2	-		23:44	11:25	12:19
Abortions	% De novo mutants	54	100	-	100	-		52	44	63
Livebirths*	De novo:Total where both parents examined	22:86	17:78	4:34	12:36	1:8		5:8	2:3	3:5
	% De novo mutants	26	22	12	33	12		62	67	60

* Data sources as in Table 2 and Reference 37.

472

as among the liveborn. This is mainly the result of there being many more unbalanced rearrangements in the abortions than in the livebirths and there being a much higher proportion of mutants among the unbalanced than the balanced rearrangements.

The frequency of the different types of trisomy is shown in Table 5. With the exception of the sex chromosomes, all trisomies are found with a much greater frequency among the spontaneous abortions than the liveborn. In the maternal age-dependent class trisomies are 50 times more frequent in the abortions and, with the exception of the XYY male and the very rare individual with trisomy 8, the class of abnormality which is independent of maternal age is not represented at all among the liveborn.

B. The Availability of Base Line Data on the Frequency of Chromosome Aberrations in Spontaneous Abortions

When the results of chromosome surveys of spontaneous abortions first became available, there were wide discrepancies in the frequency and proportion of the different types of abnormalities among different surveys, the proportion of abnormalities ranging from a low of 8% to a high of 64% (38). The variability of the results was almost, if not entirely, due to technical factors, most of which are now understood and therefore can be allowed for in the interpretation of results. For example selection for abortuses of a young gestational age, selection for an obvious phenotypic abnormality of the fetus or the placenta and a high percentage of successful cultures all tend to favor chromosomally abnormal conceptuses. Conversely a high proportion of fetuses of a relatively advanced gestational age, a low rate of successful cultures, the inclusion of the products of induced abortion and maternal contamination will all tend to increase the proportion of chromosomally normal fetuses. Among more recent surveys carried out in centers with liberal abortion laws, thus minimizing contamination by undetected induced abortions, or where a special effort was made to exclude induced abortions, the results are reasonably consistent. Table 6 shows the results of five major surveys from different parts of the world. The agreement among them is good considering that they have not been corrected for the somewhat different criteria used for including specimens in the study. For example the survey of Boué et al. (28), with the highest proportion of abnormalities, selected very heavily for early abortions while that of Creasy et al. (29), with the lowest proportion, contained a comparatively large number of late abortions. This selection bias can easily be corrected by

TABLE 5

Frequency of Different Trisomies in Spontaneous Abortions and Livebirths[+]

	Maternal Age Dependent			Maternal Age Independent		
		‰			‰	
Chromosome	Abortions	Livebirths	Chromosome	Abortions	Livebirths	
13	7	0.05	1-3	14	–	
14	14	–	4-5	7	–	
15	25	–	6-12	33	–	
18	17	0.12	16	92	–	
21	27	1.3	17,19-20	5	–	
22	23	–	Y°	–	0.45	
X*	1	0.9				
Total	114	2.37	Total	151	0.45	

* = XXX and XXY   ° = XYY

[+] Data sources as in Table 2.

TABLE 6

Chromosome Abnormalities in Five Surveys of Spontaneous Abortions

Reference	Total Examined	Total Abnormal (%)	Type of Abnormality (%)					
			Structural	Monosomy	Trisomy	Polyploid	Other
Kajii et al. (1973)	152	54	2	9	33	10	0
Boué et al. (1975)	1,498	61	2	9	33	16	1
Lauritsen (1976)	255	55	3	16	26	10	0
Creasy et al. (1976)	941	30	1	7	16	5	1
Hassold et al. (1977)	234	47	2	12	23	9	1
Total	3,080	50	2	10	26	11	1

recording the date of the last menstrual period and the date
of delivery of each pregnancy. The remaining three surveys,
those of Kajii et al. (2), Lauritsen (19) and Hassold et al.
(12) are remarkably similar. All employed essentially identical criteria for inclusion of abortions in their study and
all three had a relatively high success rate. Samples containing fetal tissue from all spontaneous abortions or from
curettage associated with incomplete, inevitable or missed
abortion presenting at a hospital were cultured with no
attempt at selection. These data suggest that it is possible
to collect and indeed that there is already available, quite
adequate base line data on the frequency of chromosome aberrations in spontaneous abortions. Furthermore if such a population were to be used for surveillance purposes, the center
or centers undertaking the project would rather quickly be
able to generate their own base line data.

C. The Use of Spontaneous Abortions to Monitor Populations
for Teratogens which are not Associated with Chromosome
Abnormalities

Spontaneous abortion is the outcome of as many as 25% of
all recognizable human pregnancies although only some half to
three-quarters of the affected women seek medical advice
(39). If we accept that approximately half of all abortions
coming to the attention of the medical profession are the
result of chromosome aberrations, other causes, including
infections, maternal-fetal incompatibility, abnormalities of
the female reproductive tract or endocrine system, environmental insults such as smoking and inadequate nutrition and
many other unknown factors must contribute to the 50% that
are chromosomally normal. In any epidemiological study of
abortions, the chromosomally normal abortions provide excellent control material for the chromosomally abnormal and vice
versa. Perhaps the best examples of the use of the chromosomally normal group as the "experimental" one were those of
Lauritsen and his colleagues (40, 41). They studied the ABO
and HLA antigens of a large series of abortions and their
parents and demonstrated a significantly higher frequency of
ABO incompatible, but not of HLA incompatible, matings in the
chromosomally normal conceptuses by comparison with the chromosomally abnormal or the population at large. They concluded that ABO incompatibility was a very important cause of
early abortion and might account for almost 40% of the chromosomally normal abortions. If these results are confirmed,
it would mean that some 70% of all abortions are the result
of either chromosome aberrations or ABO incompatibility. The
remaining unexplained 30% might well be a very sensitive

indicator of teratogens or abortifacients not associated with cytogenetic abnormalities. A significant rise in this proportion would be a cause for concern and yet might go undetected if this fraction could not be separately identified.

D.   The Time of Detection

The use of spontaneous abortions for the monitoring of mutagens and teratogens gives the advantage of the earliest possible detection of any suspicious event. The average gestational age of spontaneous abortions is 10 to 14 weeks. If we allow three weeks for the cytogenetic evaluation it is possible to detect an untoward event before the non-aborted but possibly affected fetuses are four months of age. If an alert can be given that early in pregnancy, studies can be designed to confirm or refute the suggestion by amniocentesis or investigation of the newborn on the same cohort of conceptuses. An example of this approach was given recently by Warburton and her colleagues (42) who detected an apparent increase in trisomies among spontaneous abortions in New York over a two-month period and were able to confirm that a similar increase was seen in amniocentesis specimens from the same cohort.

E.   Cost Effectiveness

It can be assumed, based on experience, that a unit of three people, an experienced scientist and two skilled technicians together with appropriate secretarial help, can analyze 250 spontaneous abortions or 1,000 livebirths with the same degree of exactitude in one year. Such an effort would be expected to detect 125 chromosome abnormalities among the abortuses but only six chromosome abnormalities among the livebirths. By this simple criterion, spontaneous abortions are 20 times as cost effective as livebirths for the monitoring of chromosome aberrations.

Sequential analysis gives another measure of cost effectiveness. Retaining the same assumptions about the number of specimens of abortions and livebirths that can be processed in a year, in sequential analysis the relative cost effectiveness of an aborted sample is

$$RCE = \left(\frac{250}{1000}\right)\left(\frac{ZA}{ZL}\right)$$

where ZA is the expected lod score per abortion and ZL is the expected lod score per livebirth. These expectations can be calculated under two conditions: i) that there is a

TABLE 7

Number of Years Effort and Relative
Cost Effectiveness in Sequential Analysis*

Hypothesis	Condition	Years of Effort		R.C.E.
		Abortions	Livebirths	
50% increase in age-dependent trisomics	Detect	0.65	6.57	10.1
	Refute	0.72	7.54	10.4
100% increase in de novo structural abnormalities	Detect	2.19	8.40	3.8
	Refute	2.74	10.62	3.9

* Type 1 Error = Type 2 Error = 0.1

specified increase in one or more types of abnormality at conception or ii) that the specified increase does not occur. Table 7 gives these measures for two hypotheses, namely a 50% increase in maternal age-dependent trisomies and a 100% increase in de novo structural rearrangements. The greater the probability that a particular abnormality will cause abortion, the greater the cost effectiveness of an abortion sample. Abortions are 10 times more cost effective than livebirths in detecting or refuting a 50% increase in age-related trisomies. Such a change would be detected in six to seven months on abortions but would take the same personnel seven years using livebirths. Similarly abortions are four times more cost effective in detecting a 100% increase in de novo structural rearrangements and such a change would be detected by a team of three people in two to three years with abortion material but eight to ten years with livebirths.

IV.   SUMMARY AND CONCLUSIONS

Chromosome aberrations fulfill most of the criteria nec-essary for a mutagen monitoring system. Furthermore the judicious study of cytological and biochemical polymorphisms in the mutant and his parents will, in many cases, enable the parental origin of the mutant to be rather precisely defined. This information would be extremely helpful in tracing the cause of any increase in mutation rate. Mutation rates should ideally be measured in gametes but as this is not pos-sible in human populations, spontaneous abortions form a very attractive alternative. Their study offers numerous advan-tages over one based on newborn babies, the most pertinent of which is a considerably increased cost effectiveness. In addition chromosomally normal spontaneous abortions provide the possibility for monitoring teratogens which are not asso-ciated with chromosome aberrations.

V.   REFERENCES

1.   Vogel, F., in "Chemical Mutagenesis in Mammals and Man" (F. Vogel and G. Röhrborn, Eds.), p. 445-452. Springer-Verlag, 1970.
2.   Evans, H.J., in "Chemical Mutagens" (A. Hollaender, Ed.), Vol. 4, p. 1-29. Plenum Publishing Corporation, 1976.

3. Perry, P. and Evans, H.J., Nature 258, 121-125 (1975).
4. Jacobs, P.A., Frackiewicz, A., and Law, P., Ann. Hum. Genet. 35, 301-319 (1972).
5. Sanger, R., Tippett, P., Gavin, J., Teesdale, P., and Daniels, G.L., J. Med. Genet. 14, 210-211 (1977).
6. Uchida, I. and Curtis, E., Lancet 2, 848-850 (1961).
7. Sigler, A.T., Lilienfeld, A.M., Cohen, B.H., and Westlake, J.E., Bull. Johns Hopk. Hosp. 117, 374-399 (1965).
8. Alberman, E., Polani, P.E., Fraser Roberts, J.A., Spicer, C.C., Elliot, M., and Armstrong, E., Ann. Hum. Genet. (Lond.) 36, 195-208 (1972).
9. Uchida, I.A., Holunga, R., and Lawler, C., Lancet 2, 1045-1049 (1968).
10. Boué, J., Boué, A., and Lazar, P., in "Aging Gametes" (Blandau, Ed.), p. 330-348. S. Kargar, 1975.
11. Taylor, A.I., J. Med. Genet. 5, 227-252 (1968).
12. Hassold, T.J., Matsuyama, A., Newlands, I.M., Matsuura, J.S., Jacobs, P.A., Manuel, B., and Tsuei, J., Ann. Hum. Genet. (Lond.), in press (1977).
13. Stene, J., Fischer, G., Stene, E., Mikkelsen, M., and Petersen, E., Ann. Hum. Genet. (Lond.) 40, 299-306 (1977).
14. Langenbeck, U., Hansmann, I., Hinney, B., and Honig, V., Hum. Genet. 33, 89-102 (1976).
15. Lauritsen, J.G. and Friedrich, U., Clin. Genet. 10, 156-160 (1976).
16. Hassold, T.J. and Jacobs, P.A., Am. J. Hum. Genet. 29, 52A (1977).
17. Alberman, E., Polani, P.E., Fraser Roberts J.A., Spicer, C.C., Elliot, M., Armstrong, E., and Dhadial, R.K., Ann. Hum. Genet. (Lond.) 36, 185-194 (1972).
18. Carr, D.H., Can. Med. Assoc. J. 103, 343-348 (1970).
19. Lauritsen, J.G., Acta Obstet. Gynecol. Scand. Supplement 52, 1-29 (1976).
20. Kajii, T. and Niikawa, N., Cytogenet. Cell Genet. 18, 109-125 (1977).
21. Coullin, P., Hors, J., Boué, J., and Boué, A., Personal communication.
22. Jacobs, P.A., Unpublished observations.
23. Lauritsen, J.G., quoted in Jacobs, P.A. and Morton, N.E., Hum. Hered. 27, 59-72 (1977).
24. Carr, D.H., J. Med. Genet. 8, 164-174 (1971).
25. Sutton, H.E., Teratology 4, 103-108 (1971).
26. Stein, Z., Susser, M., Warburton, D., Wittes, J., and Kline, J., Am. J. Epidemiol. 102, 275-290 (1975).
27. Kajii, T., Ohama, K., Niikawa, N., Ferrier, A., and Avirachan, S., Am. J. Hum. Genet. 25, 539-547 (1973).

28. Boué, J., Boué, A., and Lazar, P., Teratology 12, 11-26 (1975).

29. Creasy, M.R., Crolla, J.A., and Alberman, E.D., Hum. Genet. 31, 177 (1976).

30. Jacobs, P.A., Melville, M., and Ratcliffe, S., Ann. Hum. Genet. (Lond.) 37, 359-367 (1974).

31. Nielsen, J. and Sillesen, I., Humangenetik 30, 1-12 (1975).

32. Sergovich, F., Valentine, G.H., Chen, A.T.L., Kinch, R.A.H., and Smout, M.S., New Engl. J. Med. 280, 851 (1969).

33. Hamerton, J.L., Canning, N., Ray, M., and Smith, S., Clin. Genet. 8, 223-243 (1975).

34. Lubs, H.A. and Ruddle, F.H., in "Human Population Cytogenetics" (P.A. Jacobs, W.H. Price, and P. Law, Eds.), Pfizer Medical Monographs No. 5, p. 119-142. University of Edinburgh Press, 1970.

35. Walzer, S. and Gerald, P.S., in "Population Cytogenetics" (E.B. Hook and I.H. Porter, Eds.), p. 45-61. Academic Press, Inc., 1977.

36. Bochkov, N.P., Kuleshov, N.P., Chebotarev, A.N., Alekhin, V.I., and Midian, S.A., Humangenetik 22, 139-152 (1974).

37. Boué, J. and Boué, A., in "Les Accidents Chromosomiques de La Reproduction" (A. Boué and C. Thibault, Eds.), p. 29-55. Inserm, Paris, France (1973).

38. Carr, D.H. and Gedeon, M., in "Population Cytogenetics" (E.B. Hook and I.H. Porter, Eds.), p. 1-9. Academic Press, Inc., 1977.

39. French, F.E. and Bierman, J.M., Public Health Service Rep. 77, 835-847 (1962).

40. Lauritsen, J.G., Jorgensen, J., and Kissmeyer-Nielsen, F., Clin. Genet. 9, 575-583 (1976).

41. Lauritsen, J.G., Grunnet, N., and Jensen, O.M., Clin. Genet. 7, 308-316 (1975).

42. Warburton, D., Kline, J., Stein, Z., and Susser, M., Lancet 2, 201 (1977).

DISCUSSION

MORTON: Surveillance for a mutagenic hazard requires a
sentinel phenotype of low fitness and a correspondingly high
proportion of new mutants. This condition is satisfied by all
aneuploids and by certain autosomal dominants and sex-linked
genes. Polymorphisms are unsuitable, since only a negligible
fraction are new mutants. For example, suppose that the
mutation rate is 10^{-6}/locus/generation, the doubling dose is
40 rad, the rate of false paternity is 0.01, and the efficiency
of parentage exclusion by genetic evidence is 0.99. Then in a
population in which one parent was exposed to 200 rad the
probability that a sporadic case not excluded on genetic
evidence be due to mutation would be

$$\frac{(7 \times 10^{-6})}{7 \times 10^{-6} + 0.01\ (0.01)} = 0.07.$$

This is probably an overestimate, since mutagenic hazards are
likely to be smaller than 200 rad, parentage errors greater,
and the efficiency of parentage exclusion less. Parentage
errors are *a priori* unknown and likely to vary among groups
within a population, and therefore between exposed and control
parents. A surveillance program based on polymorphisms is
necessarily prospective, and therefore costly. On the contrary,
surveillance for aneuploidy and deleterious mutations can be
either retrospective or prospective and in favorable cases can
exploit induced and spontaneous abortions in which the yield
of mutants may be higher than for live births.
        Given these considerations, it is tragic that genetic
studies of atomic bomb survivors are directed to isozyme
mutations, when even a small study could determine dose
response for radiation induction of trisomy in a population
where the acute dose has been estimated for each survivor.
Apparently ERDA will defer consideration of spontaneous
abortions until all women at risk have passed menopause.

GENETIC EPIDEMIOLOGY

MONITORING HUMAN MUTATIONS AND CONSIDERATION

OF A DILEMMA POSED BY AN APPARENT INCREASE

IN ONE TYPE OF MUTATION RATE

Ernest B. Hook

Birth Defects Institute
Division of Laboratories and Research
New York State Department of Health
Albany, New York   12237

and

Department of Pediatrics
Albany Medical College
Albany, New York 12208

GOALS

The major purpose of surveillance of the rate of human mutations is to detect the introduction or unsuspected increase of mutagens into the human environment. The ultimate goal is to diminish, if not eliminate, the adverse public health consequences of these factors. A similar rationale applies to monitoring of rates of birth defects or cancer.
These appear such attractive goals that few have challenged the underlying assumptions that mutagens, teratogens, and carcinogens should be suppressed. No one to my knowledge has argued that diminishment of birth defects or malignancies is an unworthy social activity. But the burden of mutation is less obvious than that of embryotoxicity or carcinogenity.

Indeed, a very small proportion of mutations may be beneficial
to their carriers. Murphy has expanded upon the implications
of this to inquire: "If we could abolish mutations should we
do so?" For, he argued: "Granted that evolution has progressed by the operation of selection on mutations, it seems
evident that by abolishing mutation we will arrest evolution.
It is certainly true...that chaos is easier to create than
order and that a new mutation is much more likely to be harmful than otherwise. But it might well be argued that averages
have very little to do with progress and that avoidance of
evil is a poor excuse for sacrificing the good. Who is to
say how many deaths are a fair price to produce one Shake-
speare?" [1].

The best answer to this is that a human mutation is,
practically speaking, an irreversible process. If humanity
ever decides that there is a need, for some yet-to-be discovered reason, to increase the mutation rate, there are
ready methods to do so. But humanity cannot readily reverse
the consequences of a decision that a certain mutation rate
is tolerable and should not be lowered, even if the means and
methods to do so are at hand. Nor, even if one accepts
Murphy's perspective, does an increased mutation rate assure
us that there will be more Shakespeares in the world or more
(if any) members of society that can appreciate their sonnets?

While Murphy and perhaps others may find this argument
unpersuasive, the premise of the discussion to follow is that
in the light of our present knowledge, the optimal (germinal,
forward) mutation rate is zero.* Should it be discovered
that a small positive mutation rate is preferable, society can
quickly make the adjustment with agents readily available.

In considering monitoring mutations, an obvious distinction may be made between germinal cell mutations, which result
(usually) in changes in the entire organism, and somatic cell
mutations. Germinal cell mutations are of concern because of
(a) their direct contribution to morbidity and mortality and
(b) their contribution to the human genetic load whose effects
may not be evident for generations. Somatic mutations are of
concern becuase of (a) their plausible association with malignancy, best documented by the consistent change in the number
22 chromosome that occurs in chronic myelogenous leukemia,
(b) their plausible association with human aging, and (c) the
likelihood that agents that induce somatic mutations also induce germinal mutations, and conversely.

----

*The qualification as to germinal mutation rate here
pertains to the fact that a certain proportion of somatic
mutations in immunologic cells or their precursors may be
necessary for acquisition of host defense mechanisms.

If one defines a mutation as any heritable change in the structure of the genetic material, a number of different outcomes can be associated with mutation per se. I will deal with mutations in the relatively broad sense, considering changes in chromosome structure (at macro or micro scale, the latter including specific locus mutations) as well as chromosome number.* Data from experimental organisms indicate that nonchromosomal genetic structures such as mitochondria and other extranuclear particles are also subject to variation that may result in changes in a subsequent generation, but knowledge of the effects of mutations in these structures in humans is so sparse that it would be premature to consider them at the present time.

HISTORICAL ASPECTS

There is a large literature concerned with monitoring human mutations. Yet while human mutation rates have been under study since Haldane's and Penrose's investigations in the 1930s [3,4], it was not until the late 1960s that interest in surveillance of mutations became widespread.

The chemical mutagens first investigated experimentally in Drosophila and then in microorganisms in the 1940s were noxious toxic agents, such as nitrogen mustard and other alkylating agents, and it was initially assumed that the scale of mutagenic hazards of chemicals to the population was not likely to be large [5]. In the late 1940s and 1950s the main concern with human mutation was with the hazards of irradiation (see e.g., reference 6). A frequent implicit assumption was that human mutation rates are stable, except for modifications associated with radiation exposure from fallout and other types of ionizing irradiation. By the mid 1950s, however, this view came under challenge as evidence from studies in lower organisms accumulated. For example, in a series of comments on the effect of radiation upon human mutation, Lederberg noted in 1955 that the effects of such apparently benign substances as formaldehyde, caffeine, and hydrogen peroxide in experimental organisms appeared to contradict that assumption [7]. By the early 1960s there was extensive interest in the possible hazards of environmental chemical mutagens and in developing mechanisms for investigating their effects in humans or for proving the safety of suspicious substances such as caffeine.

---

*In the past, changes in gross chromosome structure or number were often not regarded as "true" mutations. (For examples of this, see discussion in reference 2.)

The proceedings of two extensive symposia held in 1960-61 and concerned in whole or in part with human mutation indicate that while human geneticists were then deeply concerned with the possible effects of environmental mutagens, they were not yet considering monitoring of human mutation rates as an approach to this problem [8,9]. In 1966, however, under the stimulus of recommendations from Meselson, [5]* the Genetics Study Section of the National Institutes of Health (NIH) held a small conference on the "chemical risk to future generations" [10]. While the conference was not convened to address specifically mutation monitoring, one of its recommendations was "that the feasibility of genetic monitoring of the human population for chromosome breakage and increased genetic disease be explored." This appears to have been the first published consideration of the needs and methods of mutation monitoring. The committee discussed various approaches to monitoring, including use of "gross chromosomal changes" in umbilical cord blood, sentinel phenotypes of dominant and sex-linked disorders, and sex ratio, although it was not enthusiastic about the last. The committee specifically considered the possibility that some substance presumed to be innocuous might be highly mutagenic and that large numbers might be exposed before the danger would be realized, a situation classified as a "genetic emergency." It was stated that "this could be detected by human observations only if the effect were very large--such as ten-fold increase in the mutation rate." The committee noted that although genetic monitoring of births would be both difficult and expensive, its expense might be justified if the monitoring were combined with a search "for increase in anomalies such as might arise from teratogens" [10].

That last suggestion may provide a clue as to why, between 1960 and 1966, interest had developed in mutation

---

*Meselson had written to the President's Science Advisor in December, 1964 because of the discovery that certain compounds can be intensely mutagenic in bacteria without causing much lethality (see also below). The compound of particular concern was N-methyl N' nitro-N-nitroso-guanidine. He suggested specifically in his letter that "safety guidelines and monitoring procedures" could be set up although it was not stated specifically whether the "monitoring" was to be of chemicals, populations, or both. He suggested specifically a review of a group of specialists on these issues. (Meselson, personal communication, September, 1977, and letter to Donald Hornig, December 8, 1964.)

monitoring. One factor, while nowhere cited specifically in any discussion of mutation monitoring to my knowledge, appears very likely to have provided a major impetus for concern. In 1961 and 1962 the epidemic of phocomelic limb defects was attributed to thalidomide. The consequences of this episode for public health activities in the area of teratogenesis as well as human genetics have been enormous, including the initiation of many programs for monitoring of birth defects for detection of effects of environmental teratogens [11-17]. Although not advanced openly as a reason for mutation monitoring, the timing of the thalidomide tradegy appears unlikely to be coincidental.

Another contributing factor, according to deSerres, was the discovery of "super mutagens" in the mid 1960s [18]. These are agents with very high mutagenic capabilities but with "low or negligible levels of toxicity to the cell." Most (acute) toxicity testing programs might not observe them, as there are no obvious deleterious effects. Agents cited as examples are ICR-170, AF-2, hycanthone and beta-propiolactone.

The committee report was not published until 1968, and then it appeared in a rather obscure journal [10]. Nevertheless, interest in mutation monitoring appears to have expanded considerably at this time and led to consideration of other methods which theoretically might have a greater power to detect effects. Neel in particular, who had done extensive work in human mutations, suggested that systematic study of protein variants of many systems in umbilical cord blood could pick up a relatively small increase in the overall mutation rate at specific loci, compared to use of "sentinel phenotypes" [19].

In 1969 a second NIH conference was held specifically addressed to the question of mutation monitoring [20]. This committee refined and extended the discussion of the earlier group. Several additional types of systems were now considered in some detail. In addition to sentinel phenotypes, changes in chromosome structure and number, and sex ratio, the committee considered new mutations in the structure of specific proteins (as recommended by Neel) and asymmetry, particularly in dermatoglyphics (as proposed by Lederberg).

These proposed systems will be treated in detail below. In addition, brief consideration will be devoted to two possible approaches not discussed by the committee: (a) "dominant lethals," i.e., fetal deaths, and (b) outcomes that may result from nonmutagenic toxicity of mutagens or, at least, indirect consequences of their mutagenic effects.

LOGISTICS OF MONITORING

By the early 1970s a number of criteria had been elaborated by which proposed systems might be judged. Crow suggested six specific criteria about which there appeared to have been a consensus by those at the NIH committee meetings [21].

1. Relevance of the system to human problems.
2. Speed in detection of an effect.
3. Sensitivity of the system to a small increase in incidence rate.
4. Sensitivity of the system to different kinds of mutational events.
5. Likelihood of identifying the cause of an increase in the mutation rate.
6. Availability of methodology.

These criteria of course apply to any system of monitoring, whatever the outcome, including birth defects or tumors. Additional criteria have been added by others. One author noted that cost is a key factor, particularly in choosing between systems [22]. Others have suggested that a "tie-in with experimental approaches" is useful so as to strengthen the basis for extrapolation from laboratory animals to man. [23] (The rationale for the latter criterion for the choice of a monitoring system, as opposed to an experimental system, is not clear.)

The practical difficulties in monitoring populations set major limitations on what can be achieved and have a major impact upon the costs of programs. In general, the better and the more pertinent the data collected, the more extensive and elaborate the scheme required and the greater the expense.

One may distinguish two different approaches to the logistics, depending upon the precision with which denominators are determined for calculation of rates.

The first involves systematic examination of all individuals in a particular population, e.g., biochemical or cytogenetic tests of all cord bloods, or phenotypic evaluation of all newborns by trained observers. One may define this approach as "defined population monitoring."

The other approach involves an attempt to collect only reports of cases of interest--e.g., only data on births described as abnormal in various sources, such as hospital records, birth certificate reports, and special notifications. This approach may be termed "case monitoring." While reports of cases are sought out in this way, the denominator, i.e., the numerical population base, is often not precisely known. It is frequently difficult to do more than estimate a "rate" using this approach. One reason is that the actual geographic population at risk may be only vaguely defined, depending upon the "catchment" area from which the cases are collected. Secondly, even if the population monitored is precisely defined (e.g., all livebirths recorded in a particular state), ascertainment is likely to be of uncertain completeness. Thirdly, accuracy in identification of cases may be variable, depending upon the reporting source. While this approach lacks precision, it should not be dismissed out of hand, for it is cheap and may provide leads to be followed up with other methods. Monitoring of infectious diseases is almost entirely of this type. While no one suggests that reported "frequencies" or "rates" of infectious disease reflect the actual rates of infectious disease in a defined population, study of fluctuations in these variables are extremely useful for purposes of public health policy.

The decision as to which approach should be used in mutation monitoring depends upon which goal is primary. If the main goal is precise determination of human mutation rates and elaboration of the basic mechanisms of human mutagenesis, only defined population monitoring is acceptable. If, however, the primary goal is improving public health by diminishing environmental mutagens, then the approach to methodology should be a pluralistic one, with careful attention to the cost-benefit implications of each method. I believe the latter policy is preferable, and the viewpoints expressed here will, therefore, differ from those of some other commentators whose primary interest appears to be the study of mutagenesis per se.

The discussion below will deal with the relative advantages and disadvantages of each method from a public health perspective.

SEX RATIO

Both NIH committee reports criticized the use of "special" surveillance of mutagenesis by following changes in the sex ratio. The main rationale for this decision was the view that a change would be "neither so sensitive nor so unambiguous in interpretation as an increase in known dominant conditions." [10] While this is true, it is easy to monitor the sex ratio through vital records and one might suggest that an abrupt change in the sex ratio in the absence of some plausible cause warrants investigation. Even if such a change is not necessarily attributable to mutation, it may clearly have broad public health consequences with regards to causes, consequences, and perhaps, other associated changes. However, so many different factors are potentially associated with

changes in the sex ratio that investigation and detection of
the explanation for a change may be difficult.

SENTINEL PHENOTYPES--DOMINANT DISORDERS

The second NIH committee report suggested that only
three dominant disorders--aniridia, achondroplasia, and
Apert's syndrome--warranted consideration as markers for
monitoring. These are not lethal in utero, are "recognizable
in relatives," are associated with low fertility, and are
observable at birth. The committee was not enthusiastic,
however, about use of these markers. Detection of an increase in the background mutation rates of $10^{-5} - 10^{-6}$ per
locus per generation would require screening several hundred
thousand births per year, "with the observations made more
difficult by the existence of cases transmitted from the
previous generation." The committee added: "Even with these
disorders the problems of changes of procedures for ascertainment and diagnosis and changes in illegitimacy rates are so
large as to compromise the reliability of conclusions which
might emerge from a survey" [20].
        These objections may be pertinent if the main concern is
very accurate determination of changes in mutation rates with
time. They do not seem realistic if the main concern is
monitoring for effects of environmental agents. Sources of
ascertainment can be treated as an analytical variable in the
review of data. If abrupt changes are noted in the rates,
attempts to determine the likelihood that they resulted from
changes in ascertainment may be introduced. Moreover, parental interviews concerning possible pertinent environmental
factors may be readily undertaken.
        Changes in illegitimacy rates appear even less plausible
as a source of confounding in monitoring mutation rates for
these dominant conditions. It is not clear what scenario the
committee had in mind in their objection on this point, but
the possibility of fertile achondroplastic dwarfs or individuals with Apert's syndrome suddenly spawning large numbers of
illegitimate children in various geographic areas throughout
the jurisdiction monitored appears very remote. Indeed,
these conditions were selected because of associated low
fertility. There is of course always the possibility of a
carrier individual in whom the disorder is nonpenetrant being
the biological father of an apparent sporadic case or cases.
But illegitimacy is a source of problems with any study of
mutagenesis. This is the "noise" in the system; but it seems
less likely to occur for dominant sentinel phenotypes than,
say, for biochemical mutations, as explained below.

A program for monitoring sentinel phenotypes, particularly for achondroplasia, could be readily coordinated with clinical services for short-limbed dwarfism, which often requires specialized diagnostic evaluation [24]. Such a program covering a large jurisdiction--one, say, with half a million to a million births per year--could be expected to detect 10 to 20 cases a year that were consequences of new mutations, in view of the calculated mutation rate for this condition (about 10^{-5} per gamete per generation [25]).

Such a program is of course a limited one in that only one marker is being monitored for. It has the advantage, however, that it is integrated with provision of clinical services that should be provided to these individuals in any event, so additional costs for monitoring should be relatively small.

ASYMMETRY

The second NIH committee considered the possibility that asymmetrical alterations of body forms, e.g., in dermatoglyphics (which have genetic determinants and are known to vary with chromosome constitution), might result from somatic mutations affecting only one part of the body. The "possibility arises therefore of assessing mutation through measures of asymmetry." It was recommended, however, that implementation of this approach await the determination as to whether known mosaics are in fact significantly asymmetric [20].

There is some evidence that occasional cytogenetics mosaics may develop marked asymmetry [26]. In most cytogenetic mosaics with 47,trisomy 21 however, while there may be a statistical increase in the extent of dermatoglyphic asymmetry [27], this does not seem marked enough to be useful for monitoring purposes [28]. Moreover, there are serious logistic and technical problems in examining newborns for anything other than rather gross dermatoglyphic patterns [28]. In addition, it seems likely that nonmutagenic factors, including variations in fetal environment and perhaps teratogens, may also influence dermatoglyphic asymmetry, providing a high amount of "noise" in this system [29].

PROTEIN MARKERS

Extensive consideration has been given to the use of these gene products for monitoring, particularly by Neel and colleagues [19,23,30-33], and by others [34-36].

There is general agreement that logistically, umbilical cord bloods are the best source of material. The main problems concern the very large numbers whose blood must be screened. The greater the number of gene products that may be checked, the greater the efficiency. Neel et al. estimated in 1973 that there were between about 20 and 50 useful protein systems for which the technology was developed. The outstanding question is whether adequate technology is available for automated and accurate examination of gene loci in many individuals sufficient for the purposes of monitoring, although recent progress in this area has been reported [23].

Neel and co-workers in a pilot study of the feasibility of use of umbilical cord bloods at University Hospital in Ann Arbor have obtained "trios" of blood specimens (i.e., from infant and both parents) for 65% of livebirths. Informed consent is obtained from both parents for participation [33]. They express the belief that because of a high proportion of young unmarried mothers and the "academic" nature of the town of Ann Arbor, this 35% rate of failure of completion of trios is not likely to be as high--perhaps only 20%--in obstetric services in hospitals in other, more representative communities. At some community hospitals I am aware of, however, a success rate of 65% would be astonishingly high, considering that specimens from both parents must be obtained. This success rate may depend heavily upon purely local factors within a particular hospital, such as the organization of nursing services and other administrative factors. Moreover, the logistic effort required to seek out and explain these studies to participating parents (and thus the cost) may also vary considerably between institutions.

Some Additional Problems

Neel, in a discussion of the possible utility of genetic polymorphisms, has observed that it will not be feasible to do family studies on each child exhibiting a polymorphic variant. He pointed out that this is likely to lead also to loss of undetected rare mutant variants with electrophoretic mobility similar to that of a well-established variant [30]. In this regard, as Morton has suggested to me, the calculations of Chakraborty, Shaw, and Schull are of interest [37]. Their analysis of possibilities of exclusion of paternity using various genetic markers indicates that at least in American white and black populations, using the 57 systems they discuss, in about 4-5% of instances an apparent exclusion will be detected in only one system.

If paternity discrepancy occurs with a frequency of 5×10^{-2}, the frequency of apparent exclusions may be estimated at 2.5×10^{-3} births. These occurrences, of course, will mimic a sporadic mutation, which would be far rarer than such an apparent exception because of nonpaternity. Yet this frequency will be higher than the number of individuals with a "true" mutation in at least one of these systems (estimated as about 0.5×10^{-3} if the average mutation rate is 0.5×10^{-6}) providing a very low signal-to-noise ratio in the system. (As Morton [38] and Morton and Lindsten [39] point out, this problem does not arise as frequently with chromosomal anomalies associated with diminished fitness for their carriers, although occasional fertile cytogenetic mosaics may provoke some of these types of problems.) With regard to protein variants, it would appear that only the use of mutations to rare alleles will avoid this extent of noise in the system.* This in turn will limit the number of mutations detected.

Even for rare variants a problem arises, as pointed out by Neel and collaborators, because of the possible difficulty of "parentage discrepancies" [30,33].

If (a) the average proportion of "parentage discrepancies" in the group studied is 0.05, (b) the average mutation rate is 0.5×10^{-5} per gamete per generation, (c) at each locus 90% of percentage discrepancies can be detected with precise tests, and (d) "for any system the frequency of the electrophoretic class of which the putative mutant is a member is 10^{-3}, then the probability that the presence of a variant in a child of normal parents may be attributed to undetected 'parentage discrepancy' is . . . 0.5×10^{-5} [or 0.25×10^{-5} if 95% instead of 90% of discrepancies are detectable]. If this is also the frequency of spontaneous mutation, then half of all the apparent mutations would be the result of these discrepancies." [33] If mutation rates are 10^{-6} locus per generation or lower, true mutations may be swamped by instances of parentage discrepancies, which may be very hard to detect.

In view of these considerations it may ultimately be practical to use for investigation only protein systems in which the mutation rate is known to be high, at least 10^{-5} per locus per generation. Unfortunately, just determining which systems meet that criteria may take a great deal of effort.

From a theoretical perspective, protein variants are nevertheless the most pertinent outcomes for study of specific locus mutations. The main concern with their use for monitoring is the cost involved, which is very closely related to the unresolved questions already discussed. There is hope that technological developments will make this approach more efficient. Until an estimate is available, it

---

*As noted above, this point was made by Neel earlier [30].

is not possible to say whether the resources spent on this
approach might be better put to alternative public health
goals, in particular, spent on other forms of monitoring that
are considerably cheaper and, from a public health perspective, may provide the same type of information.

NUMERICAL CHROMOSOME ABNORMALITIES

Any program for environmental mutagens must consider
numerical aneuploidy resulting from nondisjunction specifically. An agent which doubled the rate of aneuploid mutations
in liveborn individuals would have a major effect upon the
population in the first generation. The frequency of clinically significant numerical chromosome abnormalities may be
estimated as about 2.5×10^{-3} livebirths, [40] almost all of
which are due to trisomies. It is not likely that agents
which induce specific locus mutations or even chromosome
breakage and rearrangements would necessarily have the same
magnitude of effect upon nondisjunction resulting in trisomies, or conversely. Nondisjunction results from an
abnormality of chromosome segregation, whereas specific locus
mutations and translocations result from changes in gross or
fine chromosomal structure. There is evidence from experimental animals that agents inducing nondisjunction under some
experimental conditions have less effect upon gross structural
chromosomal damage [41]. Conversely, under some experimental
conditions, ionizing irradiation appears to induce chromosome
breakage more readily than nondisjunction [42].
The likely differential sensitivity of these outcomes to
environmental agents means that programs concerned with detecting all environmental mutagens must be concerned with
both types of outcomes, i.e., changes in chromosome number
as well as in chromosome structure, gross or fine.
Fortunately, the results of at least one type of nondisjunction, that for the 21st chromosome, can be monitored
fairly directly because of the ready detection of the associated phenotype. Existing programs monitoring birth defects
already are accumulating data on Down's syndrome. About 97%
of instances of the phenotype are associated with 47,trisomy
21 resulting from primary nondisjunction. Observations of
the phenotype provide an efficient mechanism for monitoring.
There is one problem latent in this approach to monitoring in livebirths, however. It has been estimated that only
about 35% of instances of Down's syndrome survive fetal life
[43]. A change in fetal survival rate of Down's syndrome
could therefore be confused with a change in the rate of
primary nondisjunction of the 21st chromosome. There would
be no specific way of separating the contribution of these

factors unless spontaneous fetal deaths were also analyzed.
This approach to monitoring, however, would be a major undertaking involving considerable cost, since it requires cytogenetic examination of the products of fetal loss and
necessitates more expensive laboratory approaches than that
required using peripheral blood in study of livebirths.

In addition, because the bulk of the fetal wastage
associated with trisomy 21 and other chromosomal anomalies
appears to occur in the first half of pregnancy [44], close
attention must be devoted to analysis of the gestational age
of fetuses examined. For example, a shift in the median age
of fetuses examined from, say, the 12th week of pregnancy to
the 10th week would be expected to be associated with an increase in the rate of chromosomal abnormalities detected,
even in the absence of any change in the rate of primary
nondisjunction.

The logistics of specimen collection in studies of fetal
wastage may also be quite variable. Women already at high
risk to conceive fetuses with cytogenetic abnormalities might
participate preferentially in such programs. Thus there will
be "noise" in the system. Theoretically it should be possible
to take account of these possible confounding factors in
statistical analyses of accumulated data. Practically, however, this may be difficult to do. Cytogenetic monitoring
of abortuses cannot be recommended on any large scale until
these problems are resolved. It is of interest, however,
that one cytogenetic study of spontaneous fetal loss has
picked up a cluster which was confirmed in another data
source (see below).

A more attractive and readily available approach to
monitoring for consequences of nondisjunction is the use of
data from prenatal diagnosis programs. This was, to my
knowledge, first suggested by Hirschhorn [45]. The advantages
of this approach are that for clinical reasons, large numbers
of fetuses are already being studied cytogenetically at a
consistent gestational age, usually between the 16th and 18th
week in a defined population, and clinical information is
available on the indications for the study. Data on both
germinal nondisjunction (e.g., trisomies) and chromosome
breakage and rearrangement (translocations, deletions, etc.)
are readily available for follow-up studies.

There are, however, two intrinsic difficulties with this
approach. First, a change in survival of affected fetuses
before the 16th week of fetal life may result in an increase
(or decrease) in the proportion surviving to the time of

amniocentesis, independent of any changes in "mutation rate."*
There is no way around this possible theoretical difficulty,
although it seems implausible. Secondly, a very strict stratification upon the indications for the cytogenetic study must
be done on the analysis. Optimally, only those studied because of elevated maternal age or because of concern with some
noncytogenetic disorder should be included in such an analysis, and the results should be stratified by single-year
maternal-age interval, for reasons discussed in detail elsewhere. [46]

The main advantage of this approach is that huge amounts
of data are or will be readily available from many jurisdic-
tions around the country. If eventually 30-40% of all pregnant women over 35 undergo amniocentesis nationwide, there
will be data on at least 45,000 pregnancies per year studied
because of maternal age, and perhaps cytogenetic data on
another 20,000 studied for other reasons (e.g., alpha-
fetoprotein determination). Thus raw data on 60,000 to 70,000
individuals per year may be generated at no additional cost.
The analysis and use of these data for monitoring purposes
would require very small additional funds. This is probably
the most cost-effective method of monitoring.

CHROMOSOME BREAKAGE AND REARRANGEMENT

As noted above, specimens from amniocentesis provide
data on the frequency of chromosome breakage and rearrangement e.g., deletions and translocations. These, resulting
from some gross change in chromosomal structure, appear likely
to be similar to specific locus mutations as indicators of
genetic sensitivity to environmental agents. To my knowledge
there are no known agents which will induce specific locus

---

*Actually this point bears on the definition of mutation
rates. Such rates, at least with regard to specific locus
mutations, usually pertain to the frequency of events in livebirths. The possibility that differential fetal survival--
or, possibly of greater significance, variations in fetal
survival of those with these mutants--may affect measured
human mutation rates at specific loci is usually not considered. If one defines mutation rates as a function of
events detected at a particular age, e.g., livebirth or some
specific gestational age, the possibility of variation in
differential survival to this age of conceptuses affected
should be considered as a nonmutational factor that may
alter the measured mutation rate.

mutations in mammals but have no effect on gross chromosomal structure, i.e., will not induce rearrangements or deletions.* If this is the case, programs which use cytogenetic data may suffice for detection of environmental mutagenic hazards having effects upon chromosome structure, gross or fine. Nevertheless, specific data on this point should be sought in experimental systems. (It is of interest that in Drosophila, according to one report, chemical mutagens can vary in their relative effects of chromosome breakage and point mutations. In particular, some agents may induce recessive lethals in the absence of chromosome breakage detectable in the system employed. [47])

An additional use of chromosome breakage and rearrangement data is monitoring rates in <u>somatic</u> cells [49,50,51,52]. The associated outcomes of consequence (e.g., malignancy) are different from those associated with germinal cell mutation. At the present time, if a point source of pollution is suspected as having potential mutagenic hazards, the most practical logistic method of <u>monitoring</u> a specific population is to follow the rates of chromosome breakage and rearrangement in the peripheral blood. This provides information much more quickly than waiting for evidence of germinal cell damage. The problems with this approach are (a) the rather tedious effort involved in evaluating breakage, (b) the fact some agents which are somatic cell mutagens may express their effects not in peripheral blood cells but in other tissues, and (c) the fact that agents other than mutagens, e.g., viral infections, may cause somatic cell breakage and rearrangement. Limiting outcomes scored to, say, chromosome dicentrics and rings (or chromosome as opposed to chromatid aberrations) would probably avoid confounding by the latter factor. However, the background frequency of dicentrics and rings under most conditions is so low (<1/1000 white blood cells) that a large number of cells from each individual would have to be studied to detect a moderate increase in the rate of these more objective events.

Nevertheless, evaluation of somatic chromosome breakage and rearrangement probably remains the most rapid method of investigating a population in an episode in which there is suspicion of exposure to mutagens. It is, in fact, used routinely in some radiobiology laboratories where undue exposure of personnel is suspected [53,54]. (Of course, there

---

*Regarding the converse it has been stated no agent has been found which breaks chromosomes without producing point mutations [48]. See below for further discussion of this.

is already knowledge that irradiation will induce somatic
chromosome breakage, i.e., the test is known to be sensitive
to the hazard in this situation.)

There is a question whether this method would be sensitive to all known human mutagens. Schinzel and Schmid [55]
found strong evidence for chromosome-type aberrations in
patients receiving mutagens as therapy for malignancies,
specifically those receiving alkylating agents (e.g.,
busulfan), cytostatic antibiotics (e.g., actinomycin D),
procarbizine, or irradiation. However, such evidence was
found in only 1 of the 20 patients who received only anti-
metabolites (e.g., methotrexate, azathioprine (6- mercapto-
purine, 5-flourouracil), or spindle inhibitors (e.g., Velban).
(Other workers have, however, reported effects of methotrexate [56,57]). It seems likely that the latter two classes
of agents have less readily detectable effects as chromosome
breakage agents. Conceivably the magnitude of their effects
as mutagenic hazards in humans may be lower than those of the
other classes of agents.

Until this method is automated, it is not practical for
routine large-scale population monitoring. The cost of careful evaluation of about 100 cells from a single individual
was recently estimated at about $200 to $300 [58], although
there are some economies of scale. Monitoring four times a
year the blood of 100 individuals living near a nuclear
reactor or working there would thus cost about $80,000 to
$120,000 per year (1977 dollars).

OTHER TYPES OF SOMATIC CELL MUTATIONS

A quick, accurate method of monitoring specific locus
mutations in somatic cells might be the most efficient for
mutation monitoring, at least for events other than those
associated with a change in chromosome number. An early
method for study of changes in blood groups was suggested by
Atwood in the late 1950s. (See discussion in reference 59.)
Unfortunately the method, depending upon immunologic detection of single-cell red blood cell variants, was not sufficiently specific. A subsequent method proposed by Sutton
[60] for detecting glucose-6-phosphate dehydrogenase variants
which metabolize 2-deoxyglucose-6-phosphate similarly foun-
dered upon technical difficulties [36,58]. A promising
immunologic method is under investigation by Stammatoyannopoulos et al. [61]. This may detect cells with hemoglobin
Constant Spring, a variant with a terminating mutation by
which additional amino acids are added onto the hemoglobin
chain. This adds immunologic specificity to the molecule
and makes the method appear especially promising.

"DOMINANT LETHALS"--FETAL WASTAGE

In experimental animals, early fetal death, particularly embryonic resorption has been used as a measure of the effect of genetic "dominant lethals" [62,63]. The rationale is usually that in experimental systems an agent known to be a mutagen on other evidence has been found associated with increased embryonic lethality. This effect is assumed to result from a genetic event which is "dominant" in the sense that it is presumably, the result of a one-hit process (i.e., it does not involve changes in two alleles).

It is difficult to test this supposition directly even in experimental animals because of the lethal outcome. There are, moreover, some theoretical objections to attributing the effect to mutation in lower organisms because the agents involved may have other effects upon litter-size, over and above their mutagenic actions [64,65]. Certainly, however, the test is one of experimental embryotoxicity, whatever the mechanism.

The concept has been extended beyond experimental animals. Suggestions have been made, at least informally, that "dominant lethals" be monitored in human populations as a way of monitoring mutations. These are in essence suggestions that early fetal wastage per se be monitored. But how much of fetal loss in humans is directly attributable to genetic factors is unknown. Recent estimates are that the overall frequency of at least chromosome anomalies among human spontaneous abortions (fetuses lost before the 28th week) may be as high as 50% [44]. This varies with fetal age. Among fetuses less than 12 weeks old the proportion associated with chromosome abnormalities may be even higher--60% in one study (see discussion in reference [44]. In addition, while there is at present no ready method for determining what proportion of human fetal wastage is attributable to de novo specific locus mutations, it may be in fact greater than 10^{-2}.

Despite the high proportion of early human fetal loss associated with genetic aberrations, there are major difficulties in simply monitoring the _rate_ of fetal wastage as a marker of _mutation_. Those marked fluctuations in the rate of spontaneous fetal wastage which have been documented are usually due to infectious disease, and there is good evidence that malnutrition during pregnancy and other environmental (presumably nonmutagenic) factors may have very strong effects upon rate of fetal wastage.

From a public health perspective, which is concerned about _all_ embryotoxins, monitoring the rate of fetal loss is still worthwhile, but the logistic problems are likely to be extraordinary because of difficulty in obtaining representative or complete sampling. These problems have been discussed in detail elsewhere [66,67].

There are ad hoc studies of fetal wastage, the results of which indirectly may show changes in the rates of embryo-toxins [66,68,69]. Shepard's program in Seattle was able to detect the rubella epidemic of embryopathy in 1964-1965 about 6 months prior to its observation in newborns [68]. But these and similar studies of fetal wastage were set up primarily for other purposes and are difficult to justify <u>exclusively</u> for monitoring, because of their cost.

Direct cytogenetic investigation of spontaneous fetal wastage has been carried out in several studies, and these may also serve a monitoring function while they continue. In one such study Warburton and colleagues found an increase ("cluster") of trisomies in spontaneous abortions to women whose last menstrual period was in December 1976 or January 1977 [70]. The increase was approximately twofold. There was also a doubling of trisomies in amniotic fluid cell cultures from women whose last menstrual period had been at the same time. The amniotic fluid finding had been "predicted" from the earlier observation of the aborted fetuses.

The most significant point about this event from a public health perspective is that it has <u>not</u> persisted [71]. As with any such cluster there is always the possibility, as the authors note, of a "random," i.e., chance, event. Still it may be important to verify this trend in other data sources if possible, and attempt to identify a possible cause.

AN EFFICIENT, INDIRECT METHOD FOR MONITORING GERMINAL CHROMOSOME BREAKAGE AND REARRANGEMENT

About 2-3% of instances of Down's syndrome [72] and about 20-25% of Patau's syndrome [58] are associated with de novo translocations.* There is to date no known physical phenotypic difference between instances associated with this cytogenetic abnormality, which results from chromosome breakage

---

*Cases of these syndromes with (Robertsonian) translocations may be referred to as "interchange trisomies." The mutation rates for livebirths resulting in interchange trisomies with Down's syndrome may be estimated at $1-2 \times 10^{-5}$ per gamete per generation [74,75,76,77]. For 47,trisomy 21 the rate in live-borns is about 10^{-3} equivalent to a mutation rate of 0.5×10^{-3} per gamete per generation. For Patau's syndrome, the mutation rates per gamete per generation resulting in affected livebirths with interchange trisomy and with 47,trisomy 13 may be estimated from available data as 0.5×10^{-5} and $2-3 \times 10^{-5}$ respectively.

and rearrangement, and those resulting from 47, trisomy produced by primary nondisjunction. The average maternal age, however, tends to be considerably older for the latter category of cases [72]. It has been proposed for these syndromes that the ratio of de novo translocation instances to those associated with 47 trisomy (stratified for maternal age) provides a sentinel index of mutagenic events likely to specifically influence chromosome structural changes [73]. The main advantage of this approach is that a defined population base is not necessary to follow trends as long as both types of outcomes are ascertained without selective bias. The most likely distorting factor (for Down's syndrome) is maternal age because of the possibility that instances born to older mothers are selectively not studied. By confining attention to cases of Down's syndrome born to mothers under 30, one diminishes the likelihood that this will be a significant confounding factor. Monitoring for G/21, D/21 interchange trisomic Down's syndrome and D/13 interchange Patau's syndrome provides three different outcomes which may be followed, all of which may be expected to be indicators sensitive to the same mutagenic factors.

Obviously, if a mutagen affects both nondisjunction and chromosome structural elements to an equal extent, this would not be reflected as a change in the genotypic ratio. For various reasons, however, changes in primary nondisjunction are likely to be readily detectable through existing methods of surveillance of rates of Down's syndrome by programs currently monitoring birth defects.

There are, of course, other theoretical difficulties with the ratio approach, including biological false paternity, and the question of possible changes in differential fetal survival of those with 47 trisomy vs. interchange trisomy. Because of diminished fertility and preferential segregation in translocation carriers, the problem with paternity is less important an issue for this method than, say, for protein variants. For example, 95% of G/21 interchange instances of Down's syndrome are de novo [72]. About 50% of D/21 interchange trisomic Down's syndrome instances are de novo; but in most cases, when they are inherited, the translocation is transmitted through the mother [72]. Practically speaking, one could analyze all interchange instances not known to be inherited (assuming that the mother had been investigated, as is almost always the case) without introducing a great deal of additional noise into the system because of the paternity issue.

This approach is discussed further below in considering a specific application of the method.

MONITORING FOR MUTATIONS BY MONITORING RATES OF
MALIGNANCIES OR BIRTH DEFECTS

As a mutagenic agent may have consequences other than
the mutagenic event itself, the possibility arises as to
monitoring effects indirectly. The correlation of mutagenity
and carcinogenity in substances tested experimentally is well
known [78].

Monitoring of malignancies is ongoing in many programs
throughout the country. Increases in rates of certain disorders (e.g., cancer of the pancreas) have been noted in
recent years, whereas some other malignancies (e.g., cancer
of the stomach) appear to be decreasing, probably because of
changes in exposure to as-yet-unidentified environmental
factors.

I suspect that if there is an increase in an environmental mutagen, this will eventually be reflected in an
increase in rates of at least some types of malignancies.
Thus monitoring of tumors probably indirectly monitors for
effects of mutagens as well.

The problem with this approach is twofold. The correlation of mutagenity with carcinogenity is not absolute [78].
There is the possibility that changes in rates of tumors may
be affected by substances with little (or no significant)
mutagenic activity but high carcinogenity. Some viruses and
hormonal agents, e.g., diethylstilbestrol, may be in this
category.

Of greater significance, changes in rates of malignancies are likely to occur many years after exposure to the
inducing agent. To my knowledge, the shortest median "incubation" periods in humans associated with exposure to carcinogens appear to be about 3-5 years, for the association of
prenatal ionizing irradiation with Wilms' tumor or leukemia
[79]. The fact that exposure to ionizing radiation occurred
prenatally may explain the relatively short incubation compared to that for some other agents.

In contrast, studies of mutations may pick up effects
very rapidly. Changes in germinal mutations might be detected
as soon as 9 months after introduction of an agent, using data
for livebirths, and even earlier if data from amniotic fluid
studies and other fetal investigations are available. If a
feasible method of continuously monitoring somatic mutations
in a population is available, the effects of introduction of
a new mutagen may be detected almost immediately. Thus,
monitoring for mutations in human populations may be an
effective method of monitoring for introduction of at least
some carcinogens.

Programs monitoring birth defects may also give pertinent data for mutation monitoring, particularly insofar as

ascertainment in livebirths of Down's syndrome, Patau's
syndrome (trisomy 13), and Edwards' syndrome (trisomy 18) is
concerned (although the latter two are rare, about 0.5 x
10^{-4} and 1 x 10^{-4} respectively).

Such programs, then, may be adequate for monitoring for
environmental causes of nondisjunction. Aside from such outcomes, however, most birth defects that may be presumed to be
the result of a new mutation are either sufficiently rare
and/or detected too long after birth to be useful for mutation monitoring. Therefore special ad hoc studies are
necessary to get adequate data. The reasons for this have
been indicated above and elaborated upon in detail elsewhere [67]. Most monitoring programs for birth defects still
lack the resources and extent of data sources available for
monitoring of malignancies [80].

OBSERVATION OF AN INCREASE IN ONE TYPE OF MUTATION RATE

There has been attention in the literature to methods of
monitoring but, to my knowledge, no discussion of what should
be done once an increase in mutation rate is suspected or
detected. The following example illustrates the nature of
some of the difficulties that arise and describes a further
investigation that may be undertaken when an apparent increase in mutation rate is observed.

In 1976 the proportional analysis of genotypes (de novo
translocation/47 trisomy) described above [73] was first
applied to data on Down's syndrome collected by the New York
State Chromosome Registry. The analysis revealed that an
apparent change, an approximate doubling, had occurred in
1973 (i.e., for cases born in that calendar year) compared
to previous years and that the rise had apparently continued
into 1974 and 1975. An increase in ratio was observed for
both D/21 and G/21 interchange trisomies. It occurred for
cases reported to be known mutants (i.e., both parents had
been investigated); it was also noted if analysis was
limited to those born to mothers whose age at conception was
less than 30. A similar trend, although many fewer cases
were involved, occurred for Patau's syndrome. (See tables
1-3 for the data on trends in the interchange trisomies reported to January 1, 1977.)

This observation was provocative, but it was not clear
how to proceed. It was decided therefore to make two quite
different working assumptions regarding the observation. The
first was one of scientific caution--that the observed increase was purely artifact and that further investigation of
the data would reveal its source. (No other readily available sources of data were known that could quickly and

TABLE 1

Trends in Ratios of Sporadic Unbalanced Translocations to 47 Trisomies Associated with Down and Patau Syndromes Reported to New York State Chromosome Registry by all Centers by January 1, 1977*

Syndrome and defect	Before 1968	1968	1969	1970	1971	1972	1973	1974	1975	1976	Not Stated	Total
Down syndrome												
G/31 translocation												
Number	3(4)	1	3	1(1)	3	2	5(1)	6	7(1)	4(1)	0	35(8)
Ratio to 47,+21	$\frac{7}{815}=.009$	$\frac{1}{92}=.011$	$\frac{3}{151}=.020$	$\frac{2}{169}=.012$	$\frac{3}{192}=.016$	$\frac{2}{165}=.012$	$\frac{6}{174}=.034$	$\frac{6}{197}=.030$	$\frac{8}{250}=.032$	$\frac{5}{148}=.034$	$\frac{0}{288}=0$	$\frac{43}{2641}=.016$
D/21 translocation												
Number	4(6)	2(1)	3	3	2	2	5(1)	6(1)	3(1)	1(0)	1(0)	32(11)
Ratio to 47,+21	$\frac{10}{815}=.012$	$\frac{3}{92}=.033$	$\frac{3}{151}=.020$	$\frac{3}{169}=.018$	$\frac{2}{192}=.010$	$\frac{2}{165}=.012$	$\frac{6}{174}=.034$	$\frac{7}{197}=.036$	$\frac{4}{250}=.016$	$\frac{2}{148}=.014$	$\frac{1}{288}=.003$	$\frac{43}{2641}=.016$
All translocations												
Number	7(10)	3(1)	6	4(1)	5	4	10(2)	12(1)	10(2)	5(2)	1(0)	67(19)
Ratio to 47,+21	$\frac{17}{815}=.021$	$\frac{4}{92}=.043$	$\frac{6}{151}=.040$	$\frac{5}{169}=.030$	$\frac{5}{192}=.026$	$\frac{4}{165}=.024$	$\frac{12}{174}=.069$	$\frac{13}{197}=.066$	$\frac{12}{250}=.048$	$\frac{7}{148}=.047$	$\frac{1}{288}=.003$	$\frac{86}{2641}=.033$
Patau syndrome												
D/13 translocation												
Number	(1)	0	0	1	1	1(1)	2(1)	3	2	1	0	11(3)
Ratio to 47,+13	$\frac{1}{4}=.250$	$\frac{0}{1}=0$	$\frac{0}{2}=0$	$\frac{1}{4}=.250$	$\frac{1}{10}=.100$	$\frac{2}{6}=.333$	$\frac{3}{6}=.500$	$\frac{3}{10}=.300$	$\frac{2}{17}=.118$	$\frac{1}{9}=.111$	$\frac{0}{4}=0$	$\frac{14}{73}=.192$

*Numbers in parentheses indicate cases of unknown origin, i.e., those in which parental carrier state has not been excluded. Other numbers are presumed mutant cases. Ratios are calculated including both categories.

504

TABLE 2

Trends in Rates of Mutant Unbalanced Translocation to 47 Trisomies Associated with Down and Patau Syndromes Reported by Founding Centers Only. Instances are Restricted to Those Born to Mothers Under Age 30*

Syndrome and defect	Year of birth											Total
	Before 1968	1968	1969	1970	1971	1972	1973	1974	1975	1976	Not Stated	
Down syndrome												
G/21 translocation												
Number	3(1)	1	2	1(1)	2	1	2(1)	5	4(1)	2(1)	0	23(5)
Ratio to 47,+21	$\frac{3}{195}=.015$	$\frac{1}{34}=.029$	$\frac{2}{55}=.036$	$\frac{1}{56}=.018$	$\frac{2}{71}=.028$	$\frac{1}{68}=.015$	$\frac{2}{55}=.036$	$\frac{5}{59}=.085$	$\frac{4}{56}=.071$	$\frac{2}{27}=.074$	$\frac{0}{37}=0$	$\frac{23}{713}=.032$
D/21 translocation												
Number	3(1)	2	2	1	2	0	4(1)	3(1)	3(1)	0(1)	0	20(5)
Ratio to 47,+21	$\frac{3}{195}=.015$	$\frac{2}{34}=.059$	$\frac{2}{55}=.036$	$\frac{1}{56}=.018$	$\frac{2}{71}=.028$	$\frac{0}{68}=0$	$\frac{4}{55}=.073$	$\frac{3}{59}=.051$	$\frac{3}{56}=.054$	$\frac{0}{27}=0$	$\frac{0}{37}=0$	$\frac{20}{713}=.023$
All translocations												
Number	6(2)	3	4	2(1)	4	1	6(2)	8(1)	7(2)	2(2)	0	43(10)
Ratio to 47,+21	$\frac{6}{195}=.031$	$\frac{3}{34}=.088$	$\frac{4}{55}=.073$	$\frac{2}{56}=.036$	$\frac{4}{71}=.056$	$\frac{1}{68}=.015$	$\frac{6}{55}=.109$	$\frac{8}{59}=.136$	$\frac{7}{56}=.125$	$\frac{2}{27}=.074$	$\frac{0}{37}=0$	$\frac{43}{713}=.060$
Patau syndrome												
D/13 translocation												
Number	0	0	0	0	1	0(1)	1	1	1	0	0	4(1)
Ratio to 47,+13	$\frac{0}{4}=0$	$\frac{0}{1}=0$	$\frac{0}{2}=0$	$\frac{0}{4}=0$	$\frac{1}{8}=.125$	$\frac{0}{3}=0$	$\frac{1}{4}=.250$	$\frac{1}{6}=.167$	$\frac{1}{12}=.083$	$\frac{0}{7}=0$	$\frac{0}{1}=0$	$\frac{4}{52}=.077$

*Numbers in parentheses indicate translocation cases of unknown status, i.e., for whom parental carrier state has not been excluded. Other numbers are presumed mutant translocation cases. All ratios given are for new mutants only, i.e., only the latter group.

TABLE 3

Comparison of Genotypic Ratios for 1973-1976 with Those of Previous Years

	Prior to 1973	1973	1974	1975	1976
Down syndrome					
All translocations not known to be inherited	$\frac{41}{1584}=.03$	$\frac{12}{174}=.07^a$	$\frac{13}{197}=.07$	$\frac{12}{250}=.05$	$\frac{7}{148}=.05$
Founding center reports mothers < 30, known mutant translocations only	$\frac{20}{479}=.04$	$\frac{6}{55}=.11^b$	$\frac{8}{59}=.14^b$	$\frac{7}{56}=.13$	$\frac{2}{27}=.07$
Patau syndrome					
All translocations not known to be inherited	$\frac{5}{7}=.19$	$\frac{3}{6}=.50$	$\frac{3}{10}=.30$	$\frac{2}{17}=.12$	$\frac{1}{9}=.11$
Founding center reports, known mutant translocations only, mothers < 30	$\frac{1}{22}=.05$	$\frac{1}{4}=.25$	$\frac{1}{6}=.17$	$\frac{1}{12}=.08$	$\frac{0}{7}=0$

[a] If starting with 1969, the founding year of the registry, each year's experience is compared with previous cumulative experience for translocations not known to be inherited, 1973 was the first year for which a difference significant at the .05 level emerged (chi^2 = 7.7, p < .01).

[b] If starting with 1969, each year's experience is compared with previous cumulative experience, in 1973 the difference was not significant at the .05 level (p = .06, Fisher's exact test, 2 tailed) but became so in 1974. (p = .03, Fisher's exact test, 2-tailed).

independently confirm the trend.) For this reason it was decided initially not to report the data, but to continue to investigate and analyze the nature of the data in a search for some artifact, e.g., systematic changes in ascertainment or differential reporting, that might account for the observation.

The second working assumption, made from the public health perspective, was paradoxically the exact opposite-- that the change in genotypic ratio resulted from a true increase in the frequency of interchange trisomies owing to some environmental effect. On this assumption it was obviously important to attempt to determine if some associated environmental factor could be identified. As there was a 2-3 fold excess, it was hoped a quick case-control study could reveal the source of the change. The greatest concern was (and is) the fact that the increase in the ratio in 1973 did not abate.

Initially we decided to interview all mothers of interchange-trisomy patients born in 1974 and 1975, along with a series of controls (mothers of patients with 47,trisomy 21) matched by maternal age and birth date of the child. Since the interviews were first attempted in 1976, we felt that the patients born in those years would be easier to track down and that the parents would have better recall than for patients born in 1973. As it was, we could locate for interview only about half of the mothers of interchange trisomic Down's syndrome patients born in 1974 and 1975. Similarly, we could obtain interviews with only half of the mothers of initially designated controls, and alternate controls had to be chosen. Then, despite a good deal of effort, including up to hour-long interviews concerned with many possible environmental factors, hobbies, occupations, illnesses, drugs, etc., we were unable to develop a clear lead as to an environmental agent that might have been responsible for the increase. We concluded that if the change was real, it was not due to an obvious, easily detectable factor. These investigations are, however, continuing.

The investigation of the trend itself focused on a number of possible artifacts in reporting. The increased ratio was due, not to a fall in the number of 47 trisomies reported, but to an increase in the frequency of reported interchange trisomies.

One possibility, to which strong consideration was given, was that the phenotypes of interchange and 47 trisomies are not identical and that some dramatic uniform change in ascertainment had occurred for patients born in 1973. For example, suppose that the interchange trisomies are expressed as significantly milder cases of Down's syndrome and that, for some reason, there was increased cytogenetic study of instances of mild Down's syndrome cases born in 1973 and thereafter. This would produce a slight rise in denominators and steeper rise in numerators. For several reasons, however, this appears implausible. First of all, in the group investigated, the associated morbidity and mortality rate was higher for interchange trisomic than for 47 trisomic instances. While the difference was not significant, there was no evidence for a markedly milder phenotype in the interchange instances. (For cases and initially designated controls whose parents could not be interviewed concerning phenotype, questionnaires were sent to reporting centers concerning associated morbidity and mortality.) Secondly, there is no reason why there should have been any abrupt changes in ascertainment or study of individuals with the Down's syndrome phenotype by cytogenetic laboratories in 1973 and thereafter. No director of any participating laboratory was aware of any change in procedure at this time that could be pertinent to the observed change.

If the opposite phenotypic effect occurs, i.e., de novo interchange trisomies are more severely expressed than the 47 trisomies, then to explain the changes in genotypic ratio one would have to postulate that severely affected instances were selectively not detected if born before 1973 and that a great change occurred abruptly in 1973. Again, there is no independent evidence for such a change in detection of cases and no plausible reason why it should occur.

The literature provides no evidence for any definitive difference between the physical phenotypes of the interchange and 47 trisomic instances. There is a very slight hint that the phenotypes may be milder in the interchange trisomies [81,82]; but unfortunately, these reports do not indicate whether the cases studied were inherited or sporadic, and the differences are trivial or inconsistent (see e.g., reference 83). Our own observations suggest that the de novo interchange trisomies may be more likely to have higher associated morbidity and mortality, but we can make no definite statement about this.

After reviewing all the available data we concluded that some difference in "average" phenotype between interchange trisomic and 47 trisomic instances of Down's syndrome cannot be excluded. But if so, this cannot explain the change in the genotypic ratio observed in 1973 and thereafter.

Analysis of all data collected by 1977 indicates no explanation other than that a true increase, a doubling or greater in the rate of interchange trisomies in the jurisdiction, occurred in 1973 and may still be persisting.

The obvious questions, in addition to whether an environmental cause can be identified, are: Is the increase in interchange trisomies (and perhaps other outcomes) found only in the jurisdiction covered by the registry, or does it occur elsewhere? Is the increase limited to interchange trisomies, or are other types of chromosomal damage, gross and subtle, involved? And what additional steps should be taken?

Inquiries are still outstanding at other chromosome registries, although some may not have the necessary data to analyze the genotypic ratios, and do not cover the same jurisdiction.* The latter is pertinent in that putative environmental factors associated with the observed increase may be limited in their geographic distribution. Even if available data from the U.S.A. interregional registry or others prove to be negative (and are of magnitude sufficient to exclude any substantial increase with high confidence), this could not refute a true increase in the jurisdiction in which the trend was first observed.

With regard to other outcomes, a prima facie case can be made that an increase in interchange trisomies may also be associated with an increase in other types of germinal chromosome breakage and rearrangement, as well as specific locus mutations. To my knowledge, there are no readily available data on specific locus mutations in the jurisdiction in question that can allow one to infer with any degree of confidence if a change in the mutation rate occurred in 1973. With regard to other types of chromosome breakage and rearrangement, there is no defined population base and hence no way to establish a reliable rate. (Prenatal diagnosis was not sufficiently widespread in 1973 and prior years for adequate data to be collected in a defined population base.)

If we consider deletions of the B, G, and E chromosomes, which are associated with clinically defined syndromes likely to be detected in the early years of life, there was a peak in 1973 in reported cases but the number is very small, and a strict correlation with the frequency of interchange trisomies was not observed. Most deletions of the X chromosomes are only detected in late childhood or adolescence so a trend to an increase in these outcomes in individuals born in 1973 or later may not be evident for some time.

Obviously other types of events can be associated with germinal chromosome breakage and rearrangement, e.g., somatic cell chromosome changes. The difficulty here is that back-

---

*The interregional U.S. chromosome register coordinated by the University of Oregon as of October 18, 1977 had provided data on G/21 interchange trisomic Down's syndrome from two centers which were consistent with a change in 1973 and 1974. Data on D/21 instances are still being analyzed.

ground rates vary so widely among populations that detection
of doubling in a population that has not been systematically
monitored over time is difficult if not impossible to establish. One might expect an eventual increase in the disorder
associated with, for example, the Philadelphia chromosome,
but the length of the "incubation" or "gestation" period
between somatic mutation and observed disease is unknown.
One cannot know when to expect a change, if any, that would
be correlated with evidence for increased meiotic chromosome
breakage and rearrangement in 1973. Nevertheless, as this
example implies, while the immediate significance of the
observations may be limited to interchange trisomies, there
may be other serious implications, and these are not necessarily limited to disorders associated with the Philadelphia
chromosome. Investigations of this are also under way.

It is, of course, still possible that chance or artifact
accounts for the change in genotypic ratios. Nevertheless,
the fact that the changes in interchange trisomies are consistent, and that the change was abrupt, make it more likely
than not I believe, that the observed trend results from a
true increase in rate of interchange trisomies and must be
regarded with concern, from a public health perspective, particularly because the ratio appears to be remaining above the
pre-1973 level.*

ANALYSIS OF DATA ACQUIRED IN MONITORING AND FOLLOW-UP
PROCEDURES

Some discussions of monitoring imply that with appropriate resources the decision as to which changes in mutation
rates are real and which are due to chance will be straightforward. In fact, as the example above may illustrate, such
a decision may be extremely difficult and require careful
examination of assumptions and data sources in a search for
possible artifacts. Even if none are found, there is always
the possibility of a chance cluster of events.
Several statistical procedures may be used for surveillance. The discussion below attempts to relate these to
public health goals, logistics of investigation, and cost-
benefit considerations.
First consider a surveillance scheme that examines a
single outcome, e.g., the rate of Down's syndrome only, or

---

*The data in tables 1-3 are reports received as of the
end of 1976. Additional data received in the first 6 months
of 1977 indicate ratios in 1976 and 1977 are still above pre-
1973 levels.

the <u>overall</u> frequency of mutant variants. Presumably at the start of the analysis there is a historical base of some type which allows calculation of an "expected" rate from which to seek deviations. (For rare protein variants this may take some time to accumulate.) One may expand this reference base with time and accumulation of new data or, perhaps, maintain the old reference base. Then suppose that an apparent abrupt increase in the rate of the event being monitored is noted. One may test this against the baseline data to determine its significance readily enough, and for such an episode this may be the easiest and most straightforward approach. (The further consequences are discussed below.) Suppose, however, that one is also concerned with more gradual changes over time, which may of course also result from an introduction of some hazard but which become apparent on a different time scale. Testing the data each month or each quarter against some historical base may miss this gradual change for some time, <u>particularly</u> <u>if</u> <u>the</u> <u>historical</u> <u>base</u> <u>itself</u> <u>is</u> <u>expanded</u> <u>with</u> <u>the</u> <u>acquisition</u> <u>of</u> <u>new</u> <u>data.</u>

One alternative approach would be to use Wald's method of sequential analysis, as suggested by Morton and Lindsten [39]. This is a much more powerful method of picking up a gradual trend. It has, however, the drawback that interpretation of an abrupt increase may be influenced by events in the recent past. The sequential analysis model, which had its origins in industrial quality control, is applicable if one assumes that the increase in rates of events monitored is analogous to the progressive increase in rejected items made by a machine that is gradually failing. But the rate of events monitored in the population may both wax and wane (not just because of random fluctuations, but as associated events change). Thus the analogy with industrial quality control is not exact. Conceivably an abrupt increase judged significant by the simpler tests may not be detected as significant by sequential analysis.* It would appear worthwhile to use both statistical approaches.†

---

*In such an instance, change in values of alpha, beta, background rate, and rejection criteria may considerably raise sensitivity of sequential analysis to a recent abrupt change in rates, but this would I believe, in general, result in hypersensitivity to fluctuations.

†Another sequential method, the use of "cusums" (cumulative sums), has been employed by groups monitoring defects [12,13]. The calculations are lengthier than those required by sequential analysis per se, and this method may be less likely to detect gradual trends, although it may more readily detect abrupt changes. Morton and Lindsten express the view that in practice, sequential analysis is preferable to use of cusums [39].

If one is monitoring many events simultaneously, as is usually the case for birth defects, the situation is more complicated. At least for "abrupt" increases one can be reasonably sure that each time the data are examined for changes, some chance "increase" is going to be "significant" (using reasonable criteria) in some jurisdiction. Each month, for example, in the Birth Defects Institute, examination of the most recent rates (by 1-, 3-, and 12-month intervals) of about 70 categories of birth defects in the 57 counties in upstate New York reveal several that appear significantly (p <.01) increased over the "expected" value. A proportion of these--and perhaps all--may be attributable to chance alone.

We follow up each such observation with a search for "internal consistency"--e.g., determining if an increase in the same defect has occurred in geographically adjacent counties and if a slight, albeit insignificant increase had occurred in the previous month or months in the same locality. These searches for consistency are in essence, subjective approaches using criteria not easily quantified, since they depend upon the nature of the defect involved, the reporting practices and population size of the counties, and the reported rate of defect itself. Depending upon the results, a decision is made whether to follow up with a detailed, time-consuming survey. One can never be certain that an observed increase in rate is a chance event simply because it does not meet this test of consistency; but if the increase does not persist, at least it is not a <u>continuing</u> public health problem.

In addition to issues of statistical testing and searches for consistency in analysis, a decision whether to follow up an increase depends on a host of other variables, in particular administrative ones. For example, a recent, very marked rise in "all birth defects" reported on birth certificates in one county was not followed up because we knew that the hospitals in this county had begun to report birth defects, as they should have been doing earlier. Had the increase been limited to a specific birth defect, this would have been of more concern, although we have also seen "administrative epidemics" of single defects, and such episodes have been reported in the literature [12,14]. These administrative epidemics for specific defects are usually due either to enthusiastic physicians who report (or perhaps overreport) defects (e.g., noting "phimosis" on the certificate of each child circumcised [14]) or else to greater medical awareness of specific defects. Sometimes tracking

down such causes of increased rates is quite time-consuming.
In a sense the search for consistency described above is an
attempt to limit this type of confounding.

These considerations illustrate some of the difficulties
that may arise with mutation monitoring as well, particularly
for programs that monitor various types of outcomes. For
example, even if only specific protein variants are considered, the observation of an apparent increase in mutation
rates in many different systems has the virtue of consistency
as discussed above (similar to the increase noted in G/21,
D/21, and D/13 interchange trisomies). But an apparent increase in mutation rate at only one structural protein locus,
although it could be due to a mutagen with specificity,
should be suspect as reflecting an artifact of some type.
Thus each observation of a putative increase in a mutation
rate must be treated separately with regard to judgments
about follow-up investigations.

The approach discussed above for investigating the increased ratio of interchange trisomies is one plausible
strategy to follow up suspected increases in mutation rates.
Interviews or questionnaires to determine possible associated
environmental factors can be undertaken promptly, even if the
increase is not yet certain--particularly if the absolute
number of affected individuals is not large. This has the
advantage of diminished loss of cases for investigation and
better recall concerning possible associated environmental
events. From a public health perspective this approach may
be even more important than an attempt to "confirm" the
trend in another source. Obviously the choice of approach
will depend upon available resources, the magnitude of the
effort involved, and the number of trends that may present
themselves for investigation. If eventually, for example,
20 or more different mutagenic events are monitored simultaneously, it may be practical to follow up only those
trends exhibiting the strongest change, if they are not all
correlated.

ACKNOWLEDGMENTS

I thank Dr. James Crow and Dr. Newton E. Morton for the
benefit of discussion and suggestions and Dr. James V. Neel
for a preprint of his article. Regarding the trends in the
genotypic ratios for Down's syndrome and Patau's syndrome, I
thank Geraldine Chambers, Susan Albright, and Duane Damiano
for assistance with the tabulations. Ms. Chambers did the
interviews. Laboratories currently affiliated with the New
York State (now the Northeastern Regional) Chromosome
Registry and their directors are: New York State Birth

Defects Institute* (I. H. Porter, M.D.), State University of
New York at Buffalo School of Medicine* (R. M. Bannerman,
M.D.), Columbia University College of Physicians and Sur-
geons* (D. Warburton, Ph.D.), Grasslands Hospital (P. B.
Farnsworth, M.D.), Letchworth Village* (L. R. Shapiro, M.D.),
Jewish Hospital and Medical Center of Brooklyn* (H. Dosik,
M.D.), Mt. Sinai School of Medicine* (L. Y. F. Hsu, M.D.),
New York Blood Center* (J. German, M.D.), New York State
Psychiatric Institute (J. D. Rainer, M.D.), Buffalo Chil-
dren's Hospital* (R. Neu, Ph.D.), State University of New
York at Syracuse Upstate Medical School* (L. Gardner, M.D.),
University of Rochester Clinical Genetics Center* (P. L.
Townes, M.D., Ph.D.), University of Rochester Prenatal
Diagnosis Center (R. Doherty, M.D.), Albert Einstein College
of Medicine* (H. M. Nitowsky, M.D.), Beth Israel Medical
Center (H. Kim, M.D.), State University of New York Down-
state Medical Center (G. I. Solish, M.D.), Nassau County
Medical Center (C. T. Doyle, Ph.D.), New York University
Medical Center* (S. R. Wolman, M.D.), Brooklyn-Cumberland
Medical Center (G. Frohlich, M.S.), Long Island Jewish-
Hillside Medical Center (E. Lieber, M.D.), North Shore
Hospital (J. Davis, M.D.), New York State Institute for
Basic Research in Mental Retardation (E. C. Jenkins, M.D.),
Dartmouth Medical School (D. H. Wurster-Hill, Ph.D.), Yale
University School of Medicine (W. R. Breg, M.D.), Massachu-
setts General Hospital (L. Atkins, M.D.), Rhode Island
Hospital (T. Mendoza, M.D.), and University of Connecticut
Health Center (R. M. Greenstein, M.D.). The laboratories
indicated with an asterisk are "founding" centers of the
registry. The Northeastern Regional Chromosome Registry has
been supported in part by the National Foundation--March of
Dimes.

I thank Dr. Gerald Prescott and Linda Stanbeck for data
from the U.S. Interregional Cytogenetic Registry. The
directors of the cytogenetic laboratories from the University
of Tennessee and the University of Oregon are Dr. R. L.
Summitt and Dr. R. E. Magenis, respectively. The U.S. interregional registry is supported in part by the National
Institute of Child Health and Human Development.

REFERENCES

1. Murphy, E. A. Why monitor? in Hook, E.B., Janerich,
    D. T., and Porter, I. H., eds., Monitoring, birth
    defects and environment--The problem of surveillance,
    Academic Press, New York, 1971, 7-19.

2. Auerbach, C.: Mutation Research--Problems, results and perspectives, Champion and Hall, London, 1976, pp. 504. (See especially 1-54.)

3. Haldane, J.B.S.: The rate of spontaneous mutations of a human gene. Journal of Genetics 31: 317-326, 1935.

4. Gunther, M., Penrose, L. S.: The genetics of epiloia. J. Genetics 31: 413-419, 1935.

5. Crow, J. F.: Personal communication.

6. Carter, T. C.: The genetic problem of irradiation to human populations. Bull. Atom. Scient. 11: 362-363, 1955.

7. Lederberg, J.: Letter to the editor. Bull. Atomic Scient. 11: p. 368, 1955.

8. Burdette, N. J., ed.: Methodology in Human Genetics, Holden-Day Inc., San Francisco, 1962, pp. 436.

9. Schull, W. G., ed.: Mutations, University of Michigan Press, Ann Arbor, 1962, pp. 248.

10. Crow, J. F.: Chemical risk to future generations. Scientist and Citizen 113-117 (June-July), 1968.

11. Milham, S.: Congenital malformation surveillance system based on vital records. Public Health Reports 78: 448-452, 1963.

12. Hill, G. B., Spicer, C. C., Weatherall, J.A.C.: The computer surveillance of congenital malformations. Brit. Med. Bull. 24: 215-218, 1968.

13. Weatherall, J.A.C., Haskey, J.C.: Surveillance of malformations. Brit. Med. Bull. 32: 39-44, 1976.

14. Milham, S.: Experience with malformation surveillance, in Hook, E. B., Janerich, D. T. and Porter, I. H., eds., Monitoring, birth defects and environment--The problem of surveillance, Academic Press, New York, 1971, 137-142.

15. Banister, P.: Evaluation of vital record usage for
     congenital anomaly surveillance, in Hook, E. B.,
     Janerich, D. T. and Porter, I. H., eds., Monitoring,
     birth defects and environment--The problem of sur-
     veillance, Academic Press, New York, 1971, 119-131.

16. Flynt, J. W., Ebbin, A. J., Oakley, G. P., Falek, A.,
     Heath, C. W.: Metropolitan Atlanta Congenital Defects
     Program, in Hook, E. B., Janerich, D. T., Porter, I. H.,
     eds., Monitoring, birth defects and environment--The
     problem of surveillance, Academic Press, New York,
     1971, 155-158.

17. Center for Disease Control, Congenital malformations
     surveillance, Annual Summary 1974, Issued July 1975
     (Atlanta, Georgia), 1-20.

18. deSerres, F. J.: Prospects for a revolution in the
     methods of toxicological evaluation. Mutation Research
     $\underline{38}$: 165-176, 1976.

19. Neel, J. V., Bloom, A. D.: The detection of environ-
     mental mutagens. Med. Clin. N. Amer. $\underline{53}$: 1243-1246,
     1969.

20. Anonymous: Report of the Committee for the study of
     monitoring of human mutagenesis, Teratology $\underline{4}$: 103-
     108, 1971.

21. Crow, J. F.: Human population monitoring, in Hollaender,
     A., ed., Chemical Mutagens--Principles and methods for
     their detection--Volume 2, Plenum, New York, 1971,
     591-605.

22. Hook, E. B.: Some general considerations concerning
     monitoring: Application to utility of minor defects
     as markers, in Hook, E. B., Janerich, D. T., and
     Porter, I. H., eds., Monitoring, birth defects and
     environment--The problem of surveillance, Academic
     Press, New York, 1971, 177-190.

23. Neel, J. V., Tiffany, T. U., Anderson, N. G.: Approaches
     to monitoring human populations for mutation rates and
     genetic disease, in Hollaender, A., ed., Chemical
     Mutagens--Volume 3, Plenum, New York, 1973, 105-150.

24. Smith, D. W.: Discussion in Hook, E. B., Janerich, D. T.
     and Porter, I. H., eds., Monitoring, birth defects and
     environment--The problem of surveillance, Academic
     Press, New York, 1971, 273-274.

25. Vogel, F., Rothenberg, R.: Spontaneous mutation in man, Adv. Hum. Genet. 5: 223-318, 1975.

26. Hook, E. B., Yunis, J. J.: Congenital asymmetry associated with trisomy 18 mosaicism, Amer. J. Dis. Child. 110: 551, 1965.

27. Polani, P. E., Polani, N.: Chromosome anomalies, mosaicism and dermatoglyphic asymmetry. Ann. Hum. Genet. 32: 391, 1969.

28. Hook, E. B.: The possible value of dermatoglyphic patterns and asymmetry as teratogenic markers, in Hook, E. B., Janerich, D. T. and Porter, I. H., eds., Monitoring, birth defects and environment--The problem of surveillance, Academic Press, New York, 1971, 199-203.

29. Hook, E. B., Harper, R. G., Achs, R.: An investigation of dermatoglyphic asymmetry in Rubella embryopathy. Teratology 4: 405-408, 1971.

30. Neel, J. V.: The detection of increased mutation rates in human populations. Perspectives in Biology and Medicine 14: 522-537, 1971.

31. Neel, J. V.: The detection of increased mutation rates in human populations, in Sutton, H. E. and Harris, M. I., eds., Mutagenic effects of environmental containments, Academic Press, New York, 1972, 99-119.

32. Neel, J. V.: Developments in monitoring human population for mutation rates. Mutation Research 26: 319-328, 1974.

33. Neel, J. V., Mohrenweiser, H., Satoh, C., Hamilton, H. B.: A consideration of two biochemical approaches to monitoring human populations for a change in germinal cell mutation rates, in K. Berg, ed., Proceedings of a conference on the detection of genetic damage caused by environmental factors, Oslo, 1977, in press.

34. Vogel, F.: Monitoring of human populations, in Vogel, F. and Rohrborn, G., eds. Chemical mutagenesis in mammals and man, Springer-Verlag, New York, 1970, 445-452.

35. Weitkamp, L.: Prospects for the automated typing of
     biochemical markers for the purpose of monitoring the
     human germinal mutation rate, in Hook, E. B., Janerich,
     D. T. and Porter, I. H., eds., Monitoring, birth defects
     and environment--The problem of surveillance, Academic
     Press, New York, 1971, 217-232.

36. Clark, M. C., Goodman, D., Wilson, A. C.: The bio-
     chemical approach to mutation monitoring in man, in
     LeCam, L., Neyman, J., and Scott, E. L., eds.,
     Proceedings of the Sixth Berkeley Symposium on Mathe-
     matical Statistics and Probability, Volume VI: Effects
     of Pollution on Health, University of California,
     Berkeley, 1972, 393-399.

37. Chakraborty, R., Shaw, M. and Schull, W. J.: Exclusion
     of paternity: The current state of the art, Amer. J.
     Hum. Genet. 26: 477-488, 1974.

38. Morton, N. E.: Concluding remarks, in Inouye, E. and
     Nishimura, H., eds., Gene-environment interaction in
     common diseases, University of Tokyo Press, Tokyo,
     1977, p. 226.

39. Morton, N. E. and Lindsten, J.: Surveillance of Down's
     syndrome as a paradigm of population monitoring. Hum.
     Hered. 26: 360-371, 1976.

40. Hook, E. B., Hamerton, J. L.: The frequency of chromo-
     some abnormalities detected in consecutive newborn
     studies--Differences between studies--Results by sex
     and by severity of phenotype involvement, in Hook,
     E. B. and Porter, I. H., eds., Population cytogenetics
     --Studies in Humans, Academic Press, New York, 1977,
     63-69.

41. Hansmann, I.: Chromosome aberrations in metaphase II-
     oocytes-States sensitivity in oogenesis to amethopterim
     and cyclophosphamide. Mutation Research 22: 175-191,
     1975.

42. Russell, L. B.: Numerical sex chromosome anomalies in
     mammals: Their spontaneous occurrence and use in
     mutagenesis studies, in Hollaender, A., ed., Chemical
     Mutagens--Volume 4, Plenum, New York, 1976, 55-91.
     (See particularly pp. 80-85.)

43. Creasy, M. R., Crolla, J. A.: Prenatal mortality of
     trisomy 21 (Down's syndrome) Lancet 1: 437, 1973.

44. Carr, D. H., Gedeon, M.: Population cytogenetics of human abortuses, in Hook, E. B. and Porter, I. H., eds., Population cytogenetics--Studies in Humans, Academic Press, New York, 1977, 1-9.

45. Hirschhorn, K.: The possible use of amniocentesis for monitoring, in Hook, E. B., Janerich, D. T. and Porter, I. H., eds., Monitoring, birth defects and environment --The problems of surveillance, Academic Press, New York, 1971, 25-27.

46. Hook, E. B.: Differences between rates of trisomy 21 Down's syndrome and other chromosomal abnormalities diagnosed in livebirths and in cells cultured after second trimester amniocentesis--Suggested explanations and implications for genetic counseling and program planning, in Bergsma, D. and Summitt, R. L., eds., Proceedings of the 1977 Birth Defects Conference, Birth Defects Original Article Series, Alan R. Liss, Inc., New York, 1978. (in press).

47. Vogel, E.: Mutagenicity of cyclophosphamide, tri-phosphamide, and ifosfamide in Drosophila melanogaster. Specific induction of recessive lethals in the absence of detectable chromosome breakage. Mutation Research 33: 221-228, 1975.

48. Bateman, A. J., Epstein, S. S.: Dominant lethal muta-tions in mammals, in Hollaender, A., ed., Chemical Mutagens, Volume 2, Plenum, New York, 1971, 541-568.

49. Cohen, M. M., Bloom, A. D.: Monitoring for chromosomal abnormality in man, in Hook, E. B., Janerich, D. T. and Porter, I. H., eds., Monitoring, birth defects and environment--The problem of surveillance, Academic Press, New York, 1971, 249-272.

50. Buckton, K. E., Evans, H. J., eds.: Methods for the analysis of human chromosome aberrations, World Health Organization, Geneva, 1973, pp. 1-66.

51. Evans, H. J., O'Riordan, M. L.: Human peripheral blood lymphocytes for the analysis of chromosome aberrations in mutagen tests. Mutation Research 31: 135-148, 1975.

52. Bloom, A. D.: Induced chromosomal variation in man. Adv. Hum. Genet. 3: 99-172, 1972.

53. Purrott, R. J., Lloyd, D. C.: The study of chromosome
     aberration yield in human lymphocytes as an indicator
     of radiation does 1. Techniques, National Radiological
     Protection Board (Publication NRPB-R2), Harwell, Didcot,
     United Kingdom, 1972, pp. 1-15.

54. Purrott, R. J., Lloyd, D. C., Dolphin, G. W.: The study
     of chromosome aberration yield in human lymphocytes as
     an indicator of radiation does V. A review of cases
     investigated, 1974. National Radiological Protection
     Board (Publication NRPB-R35), Harwell, Didcot, United
     Kingdom, 1975, pp. 1-15.

55. Schinzel, A., Schmid, W.: Lymphocyte chromosome studies
     in humans exposed to chemical mutagens. The validity
     of the method in 67 patients under cytostatic therapy.
     Mutation Research 40: 139-166, 1976.

56. Locher, H., Franz, J.: Chromosome--veranderungen bei
     Methotrexatebe handlungen, Med. Welt 34: 1965-1966,
     1976, cited by Schinzel, A. and Schmid, W., Mutation
     Research 40: 139-166, 1976.

57. Kaung, D. T., Swartzendruber, A. A.: Effect of chemo-
     therapeutic agents in chromosomes of patients with
     lung cancer. Dis. Chest 55: 98-100, 1969, cited by
     Schinzel, A. and Schmid, W., Mutation Research 40:
     136-166, 1976.

58. Hook, E. B., Hatcher, N. H., unpublished observations
     or unpublished review of literature.

59. Atwood, K. C.: Problems of measurement of mutation
     rates, in Schull, W. J., ed., Mutations, University
     of Michigan Press, Ann Arbor, 1962, 1-77.

60. Sutton, H. E.: Prospects of monitoring environmental
     mutagenesis through somatic mutations, in Hook, E. B.,
     Janerich, D. T. and Porter, I. H., eds., Monitoring,
     birth defects and environment--The problems of
     surveillance, Academic Press, New York, 1971, 237-248.

61. Stammatoyannopoulos, G.: Possibilities for demonstrating
     point mutations in somatic cells, as illustrated by stud-
     ies of mutant hemoglobins, in Berg, K., ed., "Proceedings
     of a conference on the detection of genetic damage caused
     by environmental factors," Oslo, 1977, in press.

62. Bateman, A. J., Epstein, S. S., Dominant lethal mutations
     in mammals, in Hollaender, A., ed., "Chemical Mutagens,
     Vol. 2," Plenum, New York, 1971, 541-568.

63. Rohrborn, G.: The dominant lethals: Methods and cyto-genetic examination of early cleavage stages, in Vogel, F. and Rohrborn, G., eds., Chemical mutagenesis in mammals and man, Springer-Verlag, New York, 1970, 148-155.

64. Rohrborn, G.: Mutagenicity tests in mice I. The dominant lethal method and the control problem. Humangenetik 6: 345-361, 1968.

65. Auerbach, C., Kilbey, B. J.: Mutation in eukaryotes, Ann. Rev. Genet. 5: 163-218, 1971.

66. Miller, J. R., Poland, B. J.: Monitoring of human embryonic and fetal wastage, in Hook, E. B., Janerich, D. T. and Porter, I. H., eds., Monitoring, birth defects and environment--The problem of surveillance. Academic Press, New York, 1971, 65-81.

67. Hook, E. B.: Monitoring human birth defects: Methods and strategies in LeCam, L., Neyman, J., Scott, E. L., eds., Proceedings of the Sixth Berkeley Symposium on Mathematical Statistics and Probability, Volume VI: Effects of Pollution on Health, University of California, Berkeley, 1972, 355-366.

68. Shepard, T. H., Nelson, T., Oakley, G. P., Lemire, R. J.: Collection of Human Embryos and Fetuses: A centralized laboratory for collection of human embryos and fetuses: Seven years experience: I. Methods, in Hook, E. B., Janerich, D. T., and Porter, I. H., eds., Monitoring, birth defects and environment--The problem of surveillance, Academic Press, New York, 1971, 29-43.

69. Nelson, T., Oakley, G. P., Shepard, T. H.: Collection of human embryos and fetuses: A centralized laboratory for collection of human embryos and fetuses: Seven years experience: II. Classification and tabulation of conceptual wastage with observations on type of malformations, sex ratio and chromosome studies, in Hook, E. B., Janerich, D. T., and Porter, I. H., eds., Monitoring, birth defects and environment--The problem of surveillance, Academic Press, New York, 1971, 45-64.

70. Warburton, D., Kline, J., Stein, Z., Susser, M.: Trisomy cluster in New York, Lancet 1: 201, 1977.

71. Warburton, D.: Personal communication.

72. Hamerton, J. L.: Human cytogenetics, Volume II,
     Clinical cytogenetics, Academic Press, New York, 1971,
     1-336.

73. Hook, E. B.: Ratios of de novo translocation to 47
     trisomy resulting in Down's syndrome (DS) or Patau
     syndrome in humans: Potential utility of chromosome
     registry data in monitoring populations for germinal
     mutations associated with chromosomal breakage and
     rearrangement (CBR). Genetics 83: s33, 1976.

74. Polani, P. E., Hamerton, J. L., Gianelli, F., Carter,
     C. O.: Cytogenetics of Down's syndrome (mongolism) III.
     Frequency of interchange trisomies and mutation rate of
     chromosome interchanges. Cytogenetics 4: 193-206,
     1965.

75. Kikuchi, Y., Oshi, H., Tonomura, A., Yamada, K.,
     Tanaka, Y., Kurita, T., Matsunaga, E.: Translocation
     Down's syndrome in Japan: Its frequency, mutation rate
     of translocation and parental age. Jap. J. Hum. Genet.
     14: 93-106, 1969.

76. Jacobs, P. A.: Structural rearrangements of chromosomes
     in man, in Hook, E. B., and Porter, I. H., eds.,
     Population cytogenetics--Studies in humans, Academic
     Press, New York, 1977, 81-97.

77. Walzer, S., Gerald, P. S.: A chromosome survey of
     13,751 male newborns, in Hook, E. B., and Porter, I. H.,
     eds., Population cytogenetics--Studies in humans,
     Academic Press, New York, 1977, 45-61.

78. Miller, E. C., Miller, J. A.: The mutagenicity of
     chemical carcinogens; Correlations, problems and
     interpretations, in Hollaender, A., ed., Chemical
     Mutagens, Volume 1, Plenum, New York, 1973, pp.
     83-119.

79. Armenian, H. K., Lilienfeld, A. M.: The distribution
     of incubation periods of neoplastic diseases. Amer.
     J. Epidemiol. 99: 92-100, 1974.

80. Miller, R. W.: Studies in childhood cancer as a guide
     for monitoring congenital malformations, in Hook, E. B.,
     Janerich, D. T., and Porter, I. H., eds., Monitoring,
     birth defects and environment--The problem of surveil-
     lance, Academic Press, New York, 1971, 97-111.

81. Gibson, D., Pozsonyi, J.: Morphological and behavioral consequences of chromosome subtype in mongolism. Amer. J. ment. defic. <u>69</u>: 801-804, 1965.

82. Rosner, F., Ong, B. H., Paine, R. S., Mahanand, D.: Blood-serotonin activity in trisomic and translocation Down's syndrome. Lancet <u>1</u>: 1191-1193, 1965.

83. Berman, J., Hultén, M., Lindsten, J.: Blood serotonin in Down's syndrome. Lancet <u>1</u>: 730-732, 1967.

DISCUSSION

CHAKRABORTY: Dr. Hook in his expository presentation points out some of the practical issues relating to monitoring human mutation rate. For the sake of completeness I want to make some brief remarks which may be of some import here.

First of all, I want to emphasize the fact that the studies of protein variants by electrophoresis does not detect all mutations at the codon level. In some circles there is a belief that electrophoresis detects only one-third of all mutations. Actually our analytic as well as empirical studies indicate that it is not always true (see 1, 2, 3). The amount of hidden variability within an electromorph shown by these studies depends on the effective population size as well as the frequency of the electromorph in the population.

Second, I am a little apprehensive about the use of our work on exclusion of non-paternity (4) to detect the existing mutations in a population. It is theoretically plausible that the analytical approach can be extended to incorporate the possibility of mutations. This would algebraically be similar to our treatment of misclassifications as is done in our previous publication. In a later publication (5) we actually worked out the distribution of the number of exclusions to be expected in paternity testing. If the mutation rate is assumed to be the same at all loci, this distribution will shift towards the right and the expected displacement may provide estimates of the incorporated mutation rate. If the mutation rate varies from locus to locus (which is probably the case as documented by Dayhoff (6), Wilson, Carlson and White (7), Nei, Chakraborty and Fuerst (8)) this analysis will still be valid provided reasonable assumptions regarding the distribution of mutation rates are made. In practice, however, any deviation from random mating as well can cause such displacement. It is usually difficult to assert, as

experienced by our case studies, that all the disputed
paternity cases are randomly drawn from the population. Any
deviation from this assertion would grossly affect the mutation rate estimate from the amount of displacement in the
distribution, since by mutations alone the expected displacement will usually be very small.

References

1.   Chakraborty, R., and Nei, M., Genetics 84, 385 (1976).
2.   Nei, M., and Chakraborty, R., J. Mol. Evol. 8, 381 (1976).
3.   Chakraborty, R. J. Mol. Evol. 9, 313 (1977).
4.   Chakraborty, R., Shaw, M., and Schull, W.J.,
     Am. J. Hum. Genet. 26, 477 (1974).
5.   Chakraborty, R., and Schull, W.J., Am. J. Hum. Genet.
     28, 615 (1976).
6.   Dayhoff, M.O., (Ed.) "Atlas of Protein Sequence and
     Structure, Vol. 5, Suppl. 2," National Biomedical
     Research Foundation, Silver Spring, MD, 1976.
7.   Wilson, A.C., Carlson, S.S., and White, T.J.,
     Ann. Rev. Biochem. 46, 573 (1977).
8.   Nei, M., Chakraborty, R., and Fuerst, P.A.,
     Proc. Natl. Acad. Sci. USA 73, 4164 (1976).

MORTON: Sex ratio has not been a popular indicator of
mutagenesis, and yet it is more efficient and specific than
most methods and has given good results in a variety of
organisms. The general impression that the secondary sex ratio
in man shows "noise" from epidemics of other factors has
little support and can in any case be controlled by stratification and covariance analysis.

Elegant techniques have shown that the mutation rate is
about 3.0×10^{-5} lethals per chromosome per acute rad in
spermatozoa of Drosophila melanogaster (1). If irradiated
males are mated to attached-X females, the sex ratio change
corresponds to $6.9 \pm 1.4 \times 10^{-5}$ lethals per rad (Morton,
unpublished). There are several possible causes for this
discrepancy, which is not due to detrimental mutations (2).
The most likely explanation is chromatid (or half-chromatid)
mutation leading to death of the F_1 mosaic but only a proportion of F_2 descendants. While these and other special features
of F_1 tests must be considered, the mutation rate estimate
from sex ratio in Drosophila is fairly satisfactory.

Comparable results have been published for three mammals,
where the radiation response of the sex ratio has been
estimated as 1.6, 1.7, and 2.3×10^{-4} sex-linked recessive
lethal mutations per gamete per rad in the rat, mouse, and

man (3, 4). The last (nonsignificant) figure is from the
data of Hiroshima and Nagasaki, using crude estimates of
radiation dose, since the refined estimates made by the
Atomic Bomb Casualty Commission at great labor and expense
have never been applied to the genetic data, nor has attention
been given to the reported decline of mutation frequency with
interval between exposure and conception in female mice (5).

These figures are in excellent agreement with other
evidence. For example, Abrahamson et al. (6) estimated the
mutation rate to lethals and near lethals as 2.6×10^{-7} per
locus per rad in man, corresponding to

$$n = \frac{2.3 \times 10^{-4}}{2.6 \times 10^{-7}} = 885$$

loci on the X chromosome at which lethal mutation may occur.
By mitotic length this is .058 of the haploid euchromatic
genome, giving n/.058 = 15,000 lethal-producing loci per
gamete. The spontaneous mutation rate has been estimated as
.1 per gamete per generation (4), and therefore 6.7×10^{-6}
per lethal-producing locus per generation. Therefore the
acute doubling dose is

$$r = \frac{6.7 \times 10^{-6}}{2.6 \times 10^{-7}} = 26 \text{ rad}$$

All of these estimates are well within accepted ranges,
and justify confidence in sex ratio as an indicator of mutagenesis. Of course other medical and social factors which
may affect sex ratio must be controlled by covariance analysis
and stratification. Sex ratio shares with chromosomal
analysis of spontaneous abortions the capability of discriminating between maternal and paternal gametes: the sex ratio
should be depressed from high-risk mothers but not fathers,
and from high-risk maternal grandfathers but not other grandparents.

Given these demonstrated advantages, the reluctance of
expert committees to advocate sex ratio as an indicator of
mutagenesis can be understood only as genetic drift in a small
isolate. The sex ratio data from Hiroshima and Nagasaki cry
out for quantitative analysis.

References

1.   Muller, H.J., Am. Sci. 38, 25, 126, 399 (1950).
2.   Abrahamson, S., Genetics 46 (part 2), 845 (1961).
3.   Havenstein, G.B., Taylor, B.A., Hansen, J.C., Morton, N.E.,
     and Chapman, A.B., Genetics 59, 255 (1968).

4.   Morton, N.E., Am. J. Hum. Genet. 12, 348 (1960).
5.   Russell, W.L., Proc. Natl. Acad. Sci. USA 54, 1552 (1965).
6.   Abrahamson, S., Bender, M.A., Conger, A.D., and Wolff, S.,
     Nature 245, 460 (1973).

HOOK: If, analogous to the characteristics of a diagnostic
test, the "sensitivity" of a monitoring method for mutagens is
the complement of "false negatives" and the "specificity" is
the complement of "false positives", then it would appear, in
view of the considerations above, that use of sex-ratio is
likely to have high sensitivity (at least for agents which
have effects upon specific locus mutations). But it is not
likely to have high "specificity" because of all the other
factors which may influence sex-ratio. Covariance analysis
and stratification may allow a control on those non-mutagenic
factors already known to affect sex-ratio and on which data
are available. But a change in sex-ratio may be caused by
introduction of unsuspected agents with non-mutagenic effects,
e.g. a virus which induces fetal mortality preferentially in
one sex. A multivariate analysis may not enable one to detect
whether or not mutagenic factors per se are responsible for
an observed change, although it could in some instances help
to exclude changes in the already identified non-mutagenic
factors such as birth order.
       Nevertheless, whatever the likely cause of a significant
change, it would be worth investigation from a public health
perspective.

WHITE: Do you think of your program as concerned with
scientific research in which hypotheses have not been formed
in advance of data collection? In certain types of surveillance such as the monitoring of air pollution, or the detection of lowered levels of immunity to common infections, or
the collection of data on the build-up of influenza virus,
the appropriate response to the findings is fairly clearly
defined. This feature, however, is not present, except in a
non-specific sense, when one monitors for cytogenetic
abnormalities. What is your view of the function of such
monitoring?

HOOK: There are four levels of investigation pertinent to
monitoring for birth defects or other events whose environmental determinants can not in general be specified prior to
monitoring.
       The first is that of what may be termed the "null

hypothesis of surveillance": that the observed proportion of
affected individuals in a particular population in some period
deviates (positively) from the "expected" proportion (defined
in some suitable way) by no more than what may be attributed
to "chance" alone. This hypothesis (and the α level) of course
is formed in advance of data collection.

If one rejects the null hypothesis--or rather a null
hypothesis about a specific defect in a specific period--one
is then at the second level of investigation. As discussed
above, what one does may be strongly influenced by a number of
factors, including the magnitude of the change and the
clinical significance of the defect. At this level one may
attempt to generate hypotheses concerning the explanation of
the observed increase. (A possible hypothesis that must
always be considered is some "artefact" in reporting or
analysis.)

Once one identifies a plausible "cause", one is at the
third level of investigation. One may evaluate the plausibility of the hypothesis on the basis of readily available
information and, if possible, attempt to confirm it by doing
further studies using other data sources. Finally, at the
fourth level, a hypothesis concerning intervention may also be
structured and investigated, although such may not always be
obvious.

A difference between surveillance for birth defects and
say, for polio, is that if one observes a polio outbreak there
is an obvious environmental intervention which may be immediately postulated as likely to curtail the increase: increased
immunization. In this instance, enough is known about polio
to enable one to go from the first level of investigation
directly to the fourth. (It does not follow however, even if
this is effective, that lack of immunization is the only
cause of the epidemic. Obviously the virus had to be introduced to the population as well. Moreover, that the intervention strategy for polio will work is a hypothesis until
confirmed. It might fail if a new virus type was responsible
for the outbreak.)

For birth defects or cancer, there is usually no analogous
intervention that is obvious in advance of investigation of a
cluster, although some outcomes may provide exceptions, e.g.
Rubella embryopathy. Such exceptions aside, about all one
may do initially is investigate affected cases in a suitable
population to generate second level hypotheses for further
investigation. Not until this is done, may one reasonably hope
to come up with an intervention strategy.

Prevention strategies need not of course, await definition
of all ultimate causal factors. The Broad street pump-cholera
episode for example, occurred prior to identification of the

responsible microbe. Similarly, if one observed a cluster of
some very rare defect in infants of women working in one
building of a chemical plant, one could readily suggest steps
that would appear likely to end the episode in this group even
if the responsible teratogen were still unidentified.

Success of a prevention strategy may in fact confirm that
a postulated factor is one element of a causal chain that has
resulted in the cluster.

The social costs of a cluster of birth defects or
mutations are usually clear, so that there may be great
pressure to undertake some prevention strategy in the absence
of careful and critical analysis at the "third level" of
investigation. The social costs of a prevention strategy
however, are often hidden, and may turn out to be much higher
than expected, so these should be carefully considered before
policy is made.

The spray adhesive ban provides an example of an episode
in which intervention concerning an alleged teratogen and
mutagen was undertaken on inadequate evidence. While the
initial findings did not come out of a formal surveillance
program, the example is still pertinent to the possible
adverse consequences of a false identification of an agent as
a teratogen or mutagen (1, 2).

Since this paper was submitted for publication, I have
had an opportunity to review data from three cytogenetic
laboratories in Philadelphia and one laboratory in
Indianapolis. These, as well as summary data from Atlanta,
provide no evidence for an abrupt change in de novo interchange-
trisomy Down syndrome births in 1973 or 1974 in the experience
of the centers in these localities. Although data from the
University of Tennessee and University of Oregon are consistent
with an increase in 1973, only few cases are involved at these
institutions. These results from centers outside New York and
New England suggest that if an environmental agent was
responsible for the increase in ratios (and inferred increase
in rates of interchange trisomies) in the jurisdiction covered
by the New York-New England chromosome registry, such an agent
may have (or have had) limited geographic distribution within
the United States.

References

1.   Oakley, G.P., in "Birth Defects--Risks and Consequences,"
      (S. Kelly, E.B. Hook, D.T. Janerich, and I.H. Porter,
      Eds.), p. 185. Academic Press, New York, 1976.
2.   Hook, E.B. and Healy, K.M., Science 191, 566 (1976).

GENETIC EPIDEMIOLOGY

IRA HISCOCK LECTURE*

CHARACTERISTICS OF THE HEPATITIS B VIRUS

Baruch S. Blumberg

The Institute for Cancer Research
The Fox Chase Cancer Center
7701 Burholme Avenue
Philadelphia, Pennsylvania 19111

*This paper was presented as the Hiscock Lecture of the School of Public Health, University of Hawaii.

This work was supported by USPHS grants CA-06551, RR-05539 and CA-06927 from the National Institutes of Health and by an appropriation from the Commonwealth of Pennsylvania.

529

An objective of population biology is to construct a
model of a natural system and from this develop mathematical
and quantitative descriptions of the system which, among
other things, can be used to make predictions of future
events. In most cases the model chosen is relatively simple.
When dealing with complex biological systems this presents
something of a paradox. On the one hand, a simple model
facilitates the mathematics without the necessity of including many variables. On the other hand, if the model is too
simple, it fails to describe the complexity and richness of
the system under study.

In the case of hepatitis B virus (HBV), we are currently
concerned with two projects which may be of significant
practical importance and which might be advanced by mathematical models: 1) We are planning a strategy for the
prevention of persistent infection with hepatitis B in order
to decrease the probability of developing chronic liver
disease and primary hepatocellular carcinoma (1, 2, 3).
This may have application in regions of the world where
hepatitis B is common and includes vast tropical areas of
the world, in Africa, Asia and Oceania. There are several
factors which contribute to the transmission of hepatitis
and to the development of the persistent carrier state. We
would like to have quantitative information on the transmission, infection, vectors, and the variation in response
of infected hosts. This will help to devise the most
efficient strategy for controlling infection and response
and at the same time do as little damage as possible to
the environment.

2) The agent of hepatitis B has many unusual characteristics. For heuristic reasons, a new name to designate
infectious agents with characteristics similar to those of
hepatitis B virus has been proposed. We have suggested the
term "Icron" which is an acronym on The Institute for Cancer
Research (ICR), the laboratory where the early work on
hepatitis B virus was done (4). At present, we know in
detail of only one agent in this class, the hepatitis B
virus. Are there other agents which have similar characteristics? Can we use the known characteristics of
hepatitis B in a qualitative and quantitative manner that
would aid in the discovery of other infectious agents of the
"Icron" class?

A question with which I would like to leave with you
is whether the construction of a mathematical model will

help in reaching these goals, and if so, what additional information about the virus would be required to construct a useful model.

A Description of the Virus

The "Dane" particle is thought to be the whole virus. It is approximately 42 nm in diameter with an electron dense core of about 27 nm. The core contains DNA and a specific DNA polymerase, an unusual combination. In addition, there are particles of about 22 nm diameter and elongated particles of the same diameter and a variable length. The latter two particles appear to contain only surface antigen and this is the same as the surface coat of the Dane particle. The DNA is also of an unusual character. It is in part double-stranded and in part single-stranded with a gap of variable length in each of the circular strands (5). Some of the biochemical characteristics of the surface antigen have been determined. In addition to protein it appears to include lipoproteins and glycoproteins.

On the basis of genetic, biochemical and immunological evidence, we have hypothesized that the surface antigen of the virus may share antigenic specificities with human antigens, including serum proteins. If this is true, then the antigenic makeup of the virus would be at least in part a consequence of the antigenic characteristics of the host from whence it came. In our discussion of the "Icron" we pointed out that the responses of the putative host to HBV may be dictated in part by the nature of the "match" between the antigens of the host and virus (that is, the virus acts as if it were a polymorphic antigen). London et al. (6) and Werner and London (7) have described this in a review of these concepts. If a person A is infected with HBV particles that contain proteins antigenically very similar to his own, then he will have little immunologic response and will tend to develop a persistent infection with the virus. On the other hand, if the proteins of HBV are antigenically different from his, he may develop an immune response to the virus (that is, anti-HBs) and will have a transient infection. During the course of infection in person A, new particles will be synthesized which contain antigenic characteristics of A. In turn, person A can infect person B and the same alternatives present themselves. If the relevant proteins of person B are antigenically similar to the antigens of person A and the antigens of the HBV produced by A, then B could develop a persistent infection. If they

are different, then antibody can form, as described above. (A
corollary of this hypothesis is that inflammatory disease
of the liver is associated with the immune response to the
infectious agent rather than solely with replication of the
agent.). A further possibility is that the virus has complex
antigens, that some may match the host and some may not and
that both persistent infection and development of antibodies
may occur. The persistent antigens and the antibody in the
same individual would have different specificities, and this
occurrence has been described.

This view of the agent as an Icron introduces an interesting element into the epidemiology of infectious agents in
which not only the host and virus are factors, but also the
previous host or hosts of the agent, since they influence the
antigenic characteristics of the virus. Hence, the dynamics
of infectious spread may depend not only on the agent and
host but on previous hosts and neighbors.

Modes of Transmission

Hepatitis B may be transferred by blood transfusion or
by purposeful or accidental transmission of blood or blood
products by other means. Presumably, transfer of bloods by
the use of shared objects (i.e. toothbrush) may also play a
role in the transmission of the agent among household members.
The virus has been identified in sputum although it is not
generally considered that respiratory spread represents an
important route of transmission. A variety of folk methods
which could inadvertently lead to the transmission of blood
from one individual to the next may also result in the spread
of hepatitis B. These include tatooing, ritual circumcision,
decorative and ritual cicatrix formation and a variety of
other folk practices (8). There is also substantial evidence
that certain insects carry the virus. These include several
species of mosquitoes and a very high percentage of bedbugs
collected in beds whose main occupants are hepatitis carriers
(9, 10, 11). It has not yet been demonstrated that these
infectious agents can transmit hepatitis to susceptible
experimental animals, but it is possible that this high frequency of hepatitis in biting and blood sucking insects could
account for a large amount of transmission in tropical areas.

At present, it is not clear if fecal-oral spread is an
important mechanism for transmission of hepatitis B. Hepatitis B is not consistently identified in the feces of
individuals infected with the virus. However, some epidemiologic observations are consistent with fecal-oral spread,

particularly the general observations that a high frequency
of infection is often associated with deficient sanitary
measures.

Hepatitis B virus appears to have evolved many methods
for its transmission and perpetuation. For example, it has
been reported to have been transmitted by computer cards
used in a clinical laboratory (12). Apparently. the cards
became contaminated with blood containing the virus in the
laboratory, and this virus was transmitted to others in the
hospital when they incurred small cuts from the edge of the
cards. It is difficult to suppress admiration for an organism which according to our definition has only the bare
characteristics of life that can adapt so readily to a
complex and rapidly changing environment.

Responses to Infection

1) The most common result of infection with hepatitis
B virus in most environments is the development of antibody
to the surface antigen, anti-HBs. Individuals who respond
in this manner will usually not have symptoms. Indeed, they
may not even be aware of infection and they are conferred
with extended and possibly life-long protection against subsequent infection with hepatitis B virus. Titers of antibody may be increased if the individuals are subjected to
subsequent infections with HBV.

2) Development of the carrier state. Carriers are
individuals who have detectable hepatitis B surface antigen
(HBsAg), often in high concentration, in their peripheral
blood. They do not have symptoms or gross findings of the
disease. However, a variable number of carriers (in some
populations, as many as 1/3) may have biochemical evidence
of mild liver disease. In some cases, it is believed, carriers may go on to the development of chronic liver disease
and/or primary hepatocellular carcinoma. Antibody against
the core antigen (anti-HBc) is nearly always present in
carriers. It has been suggested that this indicates replication of the virus, but there is not substantial evidence
to support this view.

3) Development of acute hepatitis proceeding to complete recovery. This is accompanied by the transient
appearance of HBsAg early in the disease, often before the
onset of symptoms. Anti-HBc appears transiently during the
active stage of the illness, but often decreases as the
disease progresses. During recovery anti-HBs nearly always

appears in the blood and may remain for long periods. This
appears to confer immunity against further infection.

4) About 5%-10% of acute hepatitis cases will go on
to chronic hepatitis, and the consequences of this can be
severe. Anti-HBc usually persists in these patients.

5) Chronic hepatitis may occur without any apparent
episode of acute hepatitis.

6) Persistent HBsAg is found in higher than expected
frequency in certain chronic diseases associated with immune
deficiencies. This includes Down's syndrome, lepromatous
leprosy, chronic renal disease, some forms of leukemia, and,
as has already been mentioned, hepatocellular carcinoma.
This infection is usually associated with chronic anicteric
hepatitis.

7) Under some circumstances, HBsAg/anti-HBs antigen-
antibody complexes may develop. This may be associated with
certain "immune" diseases including periarteritis nodosa,
forms of chronic renal disease and mixed cryoglobulinemia.

These striking differences in response could be a
result of infection with different strains of virus; but
in many cases, this appears to be unlikely. In several
studies, different individuals infected with what is
probably the same strain of the virus have shown very
different responses. For example, London showed that
patients with renal disease in a dialysis unit when
infected are likely to develop chronic anicteric hepatitis
while the staff are much more likely to develop acute
hepatitis if they become ill (13).

The response to infection with hepatitis B is an
inherent biological characteristic and an indication of
how individuals may deal with other biological phenomena.
For example, in some studies, it has been shown that end
stage renal patients who respond to HBV infection by the
development of anti-HBs are more likely to reject trans-
planted kidneys (particularly when the donors are males)
than renal patients who become carriers as a consequence
of infection (14). Males have a higher probability of
becoming carriers and females of developing anti-HBs when
infected with HBV (15). In areas where primary hepatocellular carcinoma is common, carriers have a very much

higher risk of developing primary hepatocellular carcinoma
than individuals who develop anti-HBs following infection
(16).

The ratio of hepatitis carriers to those who develop
anti-HBs is an interesting biological characteristic of
patient groups and of populations. For example, in patients
with Down's syndrome a large percentage will become carriers
and a smaller percentage will develop antibody or acute
hepatitis compared to hemophilia patients who are more
likely to develop high titers of antibody and less likely
to become carriers.

Non-patient populations also differ markedly from each
other in this respect. In normal U.S. populations infected
individuals are more likely to develop antibody while only
a very small number, say 1-5 per thousand will become
carriers. In New Hebrides, by contrast, exposed people are
about equally likely to become carriers or develop antibody
and carriers may be extremely common, say 10-15%. Hence
the ratio of responses can be construed as an interesting
biological characteristic of the population or disease group
and this may be a reflection of how, on a population basis,
responses to other biological situations may develop.

Age of Infection

The age of infection may also have a bearing on
response. Acute hepatitis B is uncommon in people under
about 19 years. The development of the carrier state may
be age-dependent since the frequency of hepatitis carriers
peaks in a young age group (i.e. about 10-15 years).
The frequency of carriers decreases with advancing age,
possibly due to changes in the immune status with age or
conceivably to differential mortality. The frequency of
anti-HBs increases with advancing age. This is unlikely
to be due to increased probability of exposure alone, since
the frequency of anti-HBc and the carrier state does not
increase with age. Infection at a very early age, as a
consequence of maternal or paternal infection, may have a
profound effect on the infected individual and increase the
probability for the development of chronic liver disease and/
or primary hepatocellular carcinoma. This hypothesis, if
confirmed, could have an important bearing on the control of
hepatitis and its consequences.

Family Infection

     In our first major paper on Australia antigen (Au) we described family clustering of HBsAg in a large Samaritan family from Israel (17). From it we inferred the hypothesis that the persistent presence of Au was inherited as a simple autosomal recessive trait. The genetic hypothesis has proved to be very useful not in the sense that it is necessarily "true" [exceptions to the simple hypothesis were noted by us and others very soon], but because it has generated many interesting studies on the family distribution of responses to infection with hepatitis B. We suggested that HBV may have several modes of transmission. It can be transmitted horizontally from person to person similar to the trans- mission of "conventional" infectious agents. This is seen in the transmission of HBV by transfusion. Other forms of direct and indirect horizontal transmission exist; for example, by sputum, by the fecal-oral route, and, perhaps, by hematophagous insects (see above). HBV may also be trans- mitted vertically. If a genetic hypothesis were sustained, then it would imply that the capacity to become persistently infected is controlled (at least in part) as a genetic trait. The data are also consistent with the notion that the agent could be transmitted with the genetic material; that the virus could enter the nucleus of its host and in subsequent generations act as a Mendelian trait. The data also suggest a maternal effect. A reanalysis of our family data showed that in many populations more of the offspring were persis- tent carriers when the mother was a carrier than when the father was a carrier. Many investigators have now shown that women who have acute type B hepatitis, just before or during delivery or women who are carriers can transmit HBV to their offspring, who then also become carriers. This may be a major method for the development of carriers in some regions, for example, Japan. Interestingly, this mechanism does not appear to operate in all populations. This suggests that some aspects of delivery and parent- child interaction, differing in different cultures, as well as biological characteristics may affect transmission.

     The family is an essential human social unit. It is also of major importance in the dissemination of disease. A large part of our current work is directed to an under- standing of how the social and genetic relations within a family affect the spread of hepatitis virus.

Sex of Offspring

In many areas of the world, including many tropical regions (for example, the Mediterranean, Africa, southeast Asia, and Oceania) the frequency of HBsAg carriers is very high. In these regions, most of the inhabitants will eventually become infected with HBV and respond in one of the several ways already described. Family studies and the mother-child studies show that there is a maternal effect. Hesser et al. collected information on the sex of the offspring of parents in a Greek town in southern Macedonia (18). In this community the probability of infection with HBV is very high and a majority of the parents had evidence of infection, that is, detectable HBsAg, anti-HBs, or both in their blood. It was found that if either parent was a carrier of HBsAg there were significantly more male offspring than in other matings. Using the Greek data in subsequent studies, London, et al. (in preparation) have found that there is a decreased male to female sex ratio in the offspring of parents who have anti-HBs compared to the sex ratio of the offspring of carrier parents. This had led London and his colleagues to test the hypothesis that anti-HBs has specificities in common with Hy or other histocompatibility antigens determined by genes on the Y chromosome. Subsequent studies in Kar Kar, New Guinea and Scoresbysund, Greenland, are consistent with the Greek findings. If these observations are supported by additional studies then HBV may have a significant effect on the composition of populations in places where it is common, which includes the most populous regions of the world. The ratio of males to females in a population has a profound effect on population dynamics as well as on the sociology of the population.

Discussion

This brief summary may give some indication of the fascinating complexity of hepatitis B virus and its interactions with humans. Would it be useful to use these biological characteristics to develop a hereditary environmental model for mathematical analysis in order to help us further understand the population dynamics of this infectious agent and others which may be similar to it?

REFERENCES

1. Blumberg, B.S., Larouzé, B., London, W.T., Werner, B.,
    Hesser, J.E., Millman, I., Saimot, G., and Payet, M.
    Am. J. Pathol. 81, 669 (1975).
2. Larouzé, B., London, W.T., Saimot, G., Werner, B.G.,
    Lustbader, E.D., Payet, M., and Blumberg, B.S. Lancet
    2, 534 (1976).
3. Nishioka, K., Mayumi, M., Okochi, K., Okada, K., and
    Hiraymam, T. in "Analytic and Experimental Epidemiol-
    ogy of Cancer" (W. Nakahara, T. Hirayama, K. Nishioka,
    and H. Sugano, Eds.), pp 137-146. University Park
    Press, Baltimore, 1973.
4. Blumberg, B.S. Science 197, 17 (1977).
5. Summers, J., O'Connell, A., and Millman, I. Proc. Nat.
    Acad. Sci. 72, 4597 (1975).
6. London, W.T., Sutnick, A.I., Millman, I., Coyne, V.,
    Blumberg, B.S., and Vierucci, A. Canadian Med. Assoc.
    J. 106, 480 (1972).
7. Werner, B., and London, W.T. Ann. Internal Med. 83,
    113 (1975).
8. Blumberg, B.S., and Hesser, J.E. in "Physiological
    Anthropology" (A. Damon, Ed.), pp 260-294. Oxford
    University Press, New York, 1975.
9. Prince, A.M., Metselaar, D., Kafuko, G.W., Mukwaya,
    L.G., Ling, C.M., and Overby, L.R. Lancet 2, 247
    (1972).
10. Wills, W., Saimot, G., Brochard, C., Blumberg, B.S.,
    London, W.T., Dechene, R., and Millman, I. Am. J.
    Trop. Med. Hyg. 25, 186 (1976).
11. Wills, W., Larouzé, B., London, W.T., Millman, I.,
    Werner, B.G., Ogston, W., Pourtaghva, M., Diallo, S.,
    and Blumberg, B.S. Lancet 2, 217 (1977).
12. Pattison, C.P., Boyer, K.M., Maynard, J.E., and Kelly,
    P.C. J. Am. Med. Assoc. 230, 854 (1974).
13. London, W.T., DiFiglia, M., Sutnick, A.I., and
    Blumberg, B.S. New Eng. J. Med. 281, 571 (1969).
14. London, W.T., Drew, J.S., Blumberg, B.S., Grossman,
    R.A., and Lyons, P.J. New Eng. J. Med. 296, 241 (1977).
15. London, W.T., and Drew, J.S. Proc. Nat. Acad. Sci.
    (U.S.A.) 74, 2561 (1977).
16. Larouzé, B., Blumberg, B.S., London, W.T., Lustbader,
    E.D., Sankale, M., and Payet, M. J. Nat. Cancer Inst.
    58, 1557 (1977).
17. Blumberg, B.S., Alter, H.J., and Visnich, S. J. Am.
    Med. Assoc. 191, 541 (1965).
18. Hesser, J.E., Economidou, J., and Blumberg, B.S. Human
    Biol. 47, 415 (1975).

CONCLUSION

The dialogue between epidemiologists and geneticists in the workshop had both successes and failures. Genetic epidemiology still represents the efforts of geneticists to become epidemiologists. The latter are sympathetic, although repelled by the Procrustean temper of quantitative genetics, which cannot forget that Mendel triumphed through mathematics. One might be tempted to hope that statistical complexities will wither away, except that conclusions which ignore them tend to be invalid whether the phenotype is biochemically appealing or not. On the other hand, elaborate analysis of phenotypes that are not biochemically simple can be disappointing, especially if heterogeneity is not sought for. Refinements of phenotype and analysis are complementary, not competitive.

The workshop began with epidemiology and ended with infective heredity. In the interval statistical methods which admit limited etiological heterogeneity were confronted by evidence of greater complexity. Undoubtedly this challenge will be taken up in more specialized articles and symposia. Arno Motulsky gives an appraisal.

GENETIC EPIDEMIOLOGY

THE GENETICS OF COMMON DISEASES

Arno G. Motulsky

University of Washington
Seattle, Washington

Some diseases such as the common birth defects, the common diseases of middle life, and the common psychoses occur more often in families. Various research designs have demonstrated genetic rather than environmental causes to account for familial aggregation. Multifactorial inheritance involving many undefined genes (polygenes) in conjunction with usually unknown environmental factors is generally postulated to explain these findings. Heritability calculations and various powerful statistical techniques have been used to analyze complex data in this field.

Currently studied phenotypes in these diseases are often remote from gene action and may be ultimately unsuitable for in-depth genetic analysis. Several functional approaches to the study of gene action in common diseases are described. The results of the Seattle study of hyperlipidemia in myocardial infarct survivors are referred to. It is considered likely that relatively few genes determine a large portion of the genetic contribution in most common diseases. A plea is made for more biologic-genetic approaches. More collaboration between laboratory-oriented biomedical researchers, statistical geneticists, and epidemiologists is essential for better insights.

Genetic diseases are commonly categorized as (a) chromosomal aberrations, (b) Mendelian (monogenic) diseases, and (c) multifactorial (polygenic) diseases. The advent of cytogenetic techniques has clarified some birth defects and has been useful for understanding of some neoplastic diseases. Better understanding of gene action at the biochemical level

541

has led to elucidation of the pathophysiology, management, and prevention of many Mendelian diseases. While the total impact of cytogenetic and Mendelian diseases on public health is significant, the multifactorial diseases are potentially likely to have the greatest impact of genetics on medicine. Three broad groups of conditions are included among the multifactorial diseases:

a.   Common birth defects (i.e., neural tube defects, cleft lip and cleft palate, club foot, congenital heart disease, etc.) (1)

b.   Common psychoses (schizophrenia and affective disorders) (2)

c.   Common diseases of middle life (diabetes (3), hypertension (4), coronary heart disease (5))

In all these conditions, an unspecified number of genes of usually unknown action is claimed to interact with generally unknown environmental factors to produce the disease. The involved genes are referred to as polygenes. The concept of polygenes usually assumes that a large number of genes, each of small effect, contributes additively to the observed variation. The combined genetic and environmental factors are designated as multifactorial agents. Random or stochastic factors may also play a role, particularly in the pathogenesis of birth defects, and may have neither a genetic nor environmental basis. A threshold is often postulated for birth defects assuming that when the numbers of genes exceeds a certain threshold the defect will occur. (See Carter (1, 6) and Fraser (7) for recent reviews.)

I.   FAMILIAL AGGREGATION

Evidence for the hypothesis of genetic etiology usually comes from familial aggregation of the disease which does not fit Mendelian proportions and comparison of identical twins to fraternal twins with greater disease concordance in identical twins. Familial aggregation, however, may be caused by similar family environments. Resemblance of identical twins reared in different environments, absent spouse correlations, failure of expected familial aggregation in biologic and adopted sibs living in the same household, and similar disease outcomes in biologic sibs living in different environments are findings which suggest a genetic rather than an environmental etiology. Evidence from such research strategies is extensive for the psychoses (2, 8) and accumulating for most of the other common diseases cited.

The participation of genetic factors in most diseases is not surprising since all of development, growth, and metabolism is under genetic control. Based on genetic markers

(blood groups and HLA types, serum and enzyme types, etc.)
each person on this planet (except for identical twins)
probably is unique. Genetic variation for some of these polymorphic traits is likely to contribute to etiology of many
diseases. Most diseases, therefore, will have some genetic
basis. Usually not every person with a given genotype will
develop the disease and specific environmental factors may
precipitate the disease.

II. HERITABILITY

The relative contribution of heredity to a phenotype is
often computed from family data and is known as "heritability." Many geneticists do not find the concept useful for
understanding and management of disease since it fails to deal
with the specific causal mechanism (9).

The heritability concept is derived from breeding studies
of domestic animals whose environments can be randomized or
specifically controlled. Heritability data from twins are
particularly treacherous since identical twins may search out
similar environments because of their genetic identity. The
dissection of heredity and environment therefore becomes
difficult and has been criticized by some quantitative geneticists as logically impossible (10). "Heritability" studies
usually deal with phenotypes remote from individual gene
action and cannot provide any information regarding the number
of genes nor their mechanisms. When the underlying genes are
understood, heritability measurements usually become super-
fluous. Newer and more powerful statistical methods such as
path analysis and segregation analysis have been useful for
better analysis of genetic data (11) but are also unable to
get at mechanisms of gene action.

III. DETECTION OF MENDELIAN GENES IN COMMON DISEASES

Further understanding therefore requires concern with
the pathophysiology of the disease under study. It is likely
that for many common diseases, a relatively small number of
major potentially identifiable genes may contribute to their
genetic etiology and explain most of the genetic variance.
The remaining "polygenes" can be considered as the genetic
background. The action of such major genes ideally should be
studied by appropriate laboratory techniques since demonstration of Mendelian genes by combined laboratory and family
studies is usually convincing.

Strategies to understand common disease involve:

A. Heterogeneity Analysis.

1. Distinction of the rare monogenic disease from the "waste-
basket" of the polygenic category (e.g., various Mendelian
syndromes from multifactorial cleft lip and palate, Zollinger-
Ellison syndrome from peptic ulcers, α-antitrypsin deficiency
from usual type of chronic obstructive pulmonary disease,
etc.).

2. Clinical, laboratory, and genetic study of unselected
cases of broad heterogeneous disease groupings such as mental
retardation, deafness, blindness, and coronary heart disease
using genetic, clinical, and functional techniques in attempts
to sort out genetic from nongenetic cases (clinical population
genetics) (12). Among patients with genetically determined
diseases, further categorization into different entities or
syndromes is often necessary.

3. Search for better ways using biochemical, clinical,
genetic, and other leads for subcategorization of current
diagnostic categories which are likely to be heterogeneous
("schizophrenia", "hypertension", "diabetes", etc.).

B. Study of the relationship of common genetic markers to the
disease, i.e., HLA-D as a locus involved with immune response
for association with various autoimmune diseases (13). This
approach will be most successful if markers which are patho-
physiologically related to the disease can be studied. Random genetic markers investigated in random disease are not
likely to produce meaningful data.

C. Study of the hypothesis that the frequent heterozygote
carriers for rare inborn errors of metabolism may be at
higher risk for a disease suggested by the symptomatology of
the inborn error, i.e., cancer among carriers for diseases
such as Fanconi's and Bloom's syndromes (14) where malignancy
is commonly seen and can be related to chromosomal breakage.

IV. CORONARY HEART DISEASE AS A MODEL

Family data, particularly among younger affected patients,
suggest the operation of genetic factors in coronary atherosclerosis (see 5 for references). A variety of risk factors
are recognized as increasing the probability of coronary

disease. These include hyperlipidemia, hypertension, diabetes, and heavy smoking. Other risk factors such as the hard driving personality, lack of exercise, and obesity are less certain. An approach to the multifactorial genetics of coronary heart disease therefore should study possible genetic contributions to the various risk factors. Our Seattle project (15, 16) was designed to elucidate the frequency of hyperlipidemia among unselected patients with myocardial infarction and to study the genetics of hyperlipidemia. We have interpreted our family studies to indicate that autosomal dominant familial hypercholesterolemia occurs in 4% of male survivors of myocardial infarction, aged 60 and below. Autosomal dominant hypertriglyceridemia occurred in 5% and familial combined hyperlipidemia which we believe is also a unitary autosomal dominant Mendelian trait occurred in 11% of males in that age group (16). Thus, about 20% of men with premature myocardial infarction were believed to have a monogenic defect of lipid metabolism. Patients with these disorders were over 10 years younger than patients with myocardial infarction without these defects (5). Using similar techniques of analysis, we have data to suggest that in a normal male middle aged population, 0.2% of individuals have familial hypercholesterolemia, 0.8% familial hypertriglyceridemia, and between 1-2% have familial combined hyperlipidemia (17).

In the analysis of both normal and myocardial infarct data presorting of the data was practiced using empirical rules. Statisticians who make no prior assumptions about lipid metabolism have criticized such analysis. A variety of statistical techniques are now being applied to these data. Final assessment of the putative three single gene defects will require biochemical methods for their demonstration. The lipoprotein phenotype system did not contribute additional information to make a genetic diagnosis of hyperlipidemia over that already available by fasting cholesterol and triglyceride values (18). The fundamental defect of familial hypercholesterolemia appears to be failure of a cell receptor to bind (19) and to internalize low density lipoprotein and can be demonstrated by appropriate techniques (20).

The diagnosis of the different hyperlipidemias is practically difficult (21). Hyperlipidemia may be caused by environmental, presumably dietary, factors and may occur for unknown reasons. Better laboratory tests are required.

V. PERSPECTIVES

Scientific workers studying common disorders need to realize the etiologic heterogeneity of each of these diseases.

Our current phenotypes used for genetic analysis are similar to phenotypes such as "jaundice", "anemia", or "bleeding diathesis" used in the past as diagnoses. We now realize the remarkable genetic and environmental heterogeneity of such diagnoses. Biologic techniques are required to open the "black box" of the currently recognized phenotypes. Advanced statistics methods of various sorts are required to analyze our current data. However, as our biologic understanding increases, the need for complex statistical methods is likely to decline. We should therefore avoid erecting superstructures on statistical interpretations which may lack biologic reality. Both biomedical and statistical approaches must be used and be validated against each other.

Statistical and quantitative human genetics enters a new era. From concern with evolutionary phenomena and population structure, quantitative geneticists are becoming involved with disease. Research in this new genetic epidemiology (11) must stay in touch with the biologic facts and collaboration with biomedical researchers is essential. Similarly, medical researchers need to become much better acquainted with the relevant genetic and epidemiologic concepts.

The combined use of such techniques aims at the identification of persons susceptible to common diseases. A more rational and selective preventive medicine is likely to come from such approaches.

REFERENCES

1. Carter, C.O., <u>Brit. Med. Bull.</u> 32, 21 (1976)
2. Childs, B., Finucci, J.M., Preston, M.S., and Pulver, A.E., <u>Adv. Hum. Genet.</u> 7, 57 (1976).
3. Zonana, J., and Rimoin, D.L., <u>N. Engl. J. Med.</u> 295, 605 (1976).
4. Tyroler, H.A., <u>J. Chron. Dis.</u> 30, 613 (1977).
5. Motulsky, A.G., and Boman, H., in "Atheroclerosis III" (G. Schettler, A. Weizel, Eds.), p. 438. Springer-Verlag, Berlin, 1975.
6. Carter, C.O., <u>Brit. Med. Bull.</u> 25, 52 (1969).
7. Fraser, F.C., <u>Teratology</u> 14, 267 (1976).
8. Worden, F.G., Childs, B., Matthysse, S., and Gershon, E.S., <u>Neurosciences Res. Prog. Bull.</u> 14, 1 (1976).
9. Feldman, M.W., and Lewontin, R., <u>Science</u> 190, 1163 (1975).
10. Lewontin, R.C., <u>Am. J. Hum. Genet.</u> 26, 400 (1974).
11. Morton, N.E., in "Gene-Environment Interaction in Common Diseases," (Japan Medical Research Foundation), p. 21. University of Tokyo Press, 1977.

12. Motulsky, A.G., <u>Am. J. Hum. Genet.</u> 23, 107 (1971).

13. McMichael, A., McDevitt, H., <u>Prog. Med. Genet.</u> 2, 39
     (1977).

14. Swift, M., in "Genetics of Human Cancer," (J.J. Mulvihill,
     R.W. Miller, and J.F. Fraumeni, Jr., Eds.), p. 209.
     Raven Press, New York, 1977.

15. Goldstein, J.L., Hazzard, W.R., Schrott, H.G., Bierman,
     E.L., and Motulsky, A.G., <u>J. Clin. Invest.</u> 52, 1533
     (1973).

16. Goldstein, J.L., Hazzard, W.R., Schrott, H.G., Bierman,
     E.L., and Motulsky, A.G., <u>J. Clin. Invest.</u> 52, 1544
     (1973).

17. Boman, H., Ott, J., Hazzard, W.R., Albers, J.J., Cooper,
     M.N., and Motulsky, A.G., <u>Clin. Genet.</u> 13, 108 (1978).

18. Hazzard, W.R., Goldstein, J.L., Schrott, H.G., Motulsky,
     A.G., and Bierman, E.L., <u>J. Clin. Invest.</u> 52, 1569
     (1973).

19. Brown, M.S., Goldstein, J.L., <u>N. Engl. J. Med.</u> 294, 1386
     (1976).

20. Bilheimer, D.W., Ho, Y.K., Brown, M.S., Anderson, R.G.W.,
     and Goldstein, J.L., <u>J. Clin. Invest.</u> 61, 678 (1978).

21. Motulsky, A.G., <u>N. Engl. J. Med.</u> 294, 823 (1976).

ACKNOWLEDGEMENT

Supported by NIH Grant GM 15253.

DISCUSSION

SING: The work of the Seattle group to establish the genetic
heterogeneity of the quantitative variability in serum cholesterol has provided valuable directions for research in this
area.   The question has been clearly stated and the inference
that there is more than one genetic locus for determination of
cholesterol will undoubtedly stand the test of time.   Recently
Motulsky has expressed doubt about utility of statistics in
this work.   Is he implying that the virtues of a proper
statistical analysis are overstated or is it possible that he
is suggesting that statistical analyses could lead to the
wrong conclusions?   I would like to suggest that the studies
on lipoproteins represent an under-utilization of statistics
in that stronger inferences could be drawn by proper application of statistical methodology.   For instance, rejection of
the one-locus determination of extreme lipid levels has given

no indication whether two or three loci are necessary to
explain the observations. Is it possible that although a
simple one-locus model is not appropriate, a one-locus model
with a complex penetrance function, polygenic background or
substantial environmental influence might fit the data?   I
believe present standards do not give a proper analysis of
competitive hypotheses to explain the segregation of hyper-
lipid levels in pedigrees.

MOTULSKY: Our studies on the genetics of hyperlipidemia were
an attempt to define the role of hyperlipidemia in coronary
atherosclerosis and to sort out various types of genetic
hyperlipidemia. It is likely that we have underutilized all
possible ways of analyzing our data. Several statistical
geneticists elsewhere and members of our groups are further
analyzing these data to extract more information, if possible.
        My remarks regarding statistics were made to point out
that the very best and sophisticated statistical methods alone
are unable to provide new biologic and medical insights.
Specifically, measurements of fasting cholesterol and triglyceride values in families followed by statistical analysis
of such data are unlikely to elucidate the genetic basis of
the hyperlipidemias. We will need laboratory techniques
similar to those developed in other areas of human biochemical
genetics for ultimate understanding. Analogous reasoning
applies to hypertension, diabetes, and other common diseases.
Phenotypes such as blood pressure readings and serum glucose
levels will not give the answers even if analyzed by superb
statistics.

Index